PHYSIOLOGY OF NERVOUS SYSTEM

ENCYCLOPAEDIA OF ANIMAL PHYSIOLOGY SERIES

PHYSIOLOGY OF NERVOUS SYSTEM

Edited by
M. PRAKASH
C. K. ARORA

ANMOL PUBLICATIONS PVT. LTD.
NEW DELHI-110 002 (INDIA)

ANMOL PUBLICATIONS PVT. LTD.
4374/4B, Ansari Road
Daryaganj, New Delhi-110 002

Physiology of Nervous System

First Edition, 1998

ISBN 81-7488-889-6

PRINTED IN INDIA

Published by J. L. Kumar for Anmol Publications Pvt. Ltd., New Delhi, Typeset by Chitra Computers, Delhi and Printed at Mehra Offset Press, Delhi.

Contents

Preface

The present volume has been designed for the introductory course in Physiology. It is prepared for students in biological, medical, and health oriented programs. Among the students specifically served by this volume are those aiming for a career as a nurse, medical assistant, radiologist, physical therapist, mortician, or medical record keeper.

Because the structures of the body are exquisitely designed to carry out specific functions one can best appreciate and understand anatomy and physiology when structure and function are studied together.

Accordingly the authors have integrated both anatomy and physiology as much as possible throughout the text of the book. Authors have used a system rather than a regional approach, and although anatomy has not been slighted, an emphasis has been placed on physiology.

This volume has been devoted to the central nervous system, neurons and their interaction with emphasis on transmission of impulses. Peripheral and autonomic nervous system have been dealt separately. The volume also presents the nervous disorders.

Special care has been taken to make the reading level appropriate for today's college student. New technical terms are described separately and new concepts are thoroughly explained. Students will find the writing style easy to read and enjoyable.

Though, the authors have taken special care to present a current account, yet they are fully aware about their limitation, and the readers may come across the mistakes of various types. For all types of mistakes they extend their due apology.

The authors have freely consulted other standard books and research papers while preparing the manuscript, so the authors claim no originality of the work.

It has often been said that a man never writes a book alone and this was never more true than in the present case. In the actual compilation of the book the authors could not have done without the conscientious and enthusiastic help of their friends and colleagues, too numerous to mention individually, who influenced our approach to related subject. Some of the outstanding contributors nevertheless merit special acknowledgement—Prof. K.S. Rao, Head of the Department, School of Studies in Zoology, Vikram University, Ujjain for making exceptional efforts as providing illustrative material and Prof. (Mrs.) R. Kaul, Department of Zoology for enriching intellectual ideas.

We are also thankful to Km. Neeru Nayar, for her help on diverse occasion during the work on the manuscript.

The authors are also thankful to Shri J.L Kumar, Managing Director, Anmol Publications Pvt. Ltd., New Delhi, for bringing out a handsome print of this book in a comparatively short time.

Constructive criticisms and suggestion for improvement of the books will thankfully be acknowledged.

—Authors

1

Introduction

The human brain has been characterized as "nature's master contrivance," yet it must be remembered that the great majority of organisms on the earth fill out their cycle of existence, accomplishing successfully the two major activities of self maintenance and the continuation of their kind without the aid of so elaborate a mechanism as that which in man becomes the "most complicated organ known" (Minot). Nevertheless with a human brain it becomes possible to *live a human life*, which involves something more than metabolism and reproduction. This lofty goal has been gained, as comparative anatomy reveals, only after much evolutionary travail.

The vertebrate brain is the enlarged anterior end of the medullary tube. Like the cord it is a continuous tubular structure, the walls of which are composed of neurons that are arranged in communicating tracts and adjusting centers, supported and protected by non-nervous elements.

The brain became differentiated from the cord as the result of a mobilization of nerve elements in the neighborhood of the important sense organs of smell, sight, hearing, and taste, which are on guard near the entrance of the digestive canal. Whenever these sense organs are reduced or absent, as in deep-sea or cave animals, or in sessile forms, the brain diminishes in corresponding degree. Although the sense organs of the head unquestionably take a prominent part in determining the modifications which the brain undergoes, they by no means set the limit to its differentiation, for there are many animals with inferior brains whose sense organs are superior to those of man. It is primarily the *associative centers* that form the outstanding feature of the brain. Its general mass and contour, unlike that of the cord with its brachial and lumbar enlargements, are not solely dependent upon the area of stimulus-receiving surface involved, or the amount of glandular tissue supplied.

In other words, the conspicuous enlargements that characterize the walls of the brain are not so much due to incoming and outgoing limbs of reflex arcs that relate the animal directly to its environment, as to internal associative connections which, at least in man, enable the brain which "sits in darkness" not only to reconstruct the outside world but also to preserve the accumulations of memory and even to provide for creative flights of imagination.

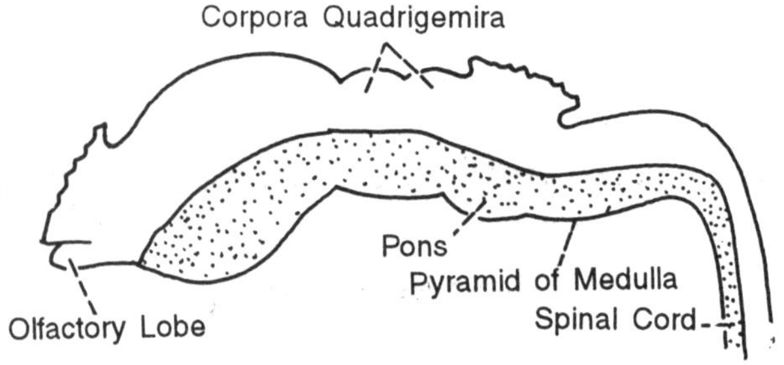

Fig. 1.1. Dorsal sensory and ventral motor regions of the brain stem.

The primary axis, or *brain stem,* is directly concerned with peripheral nerve relations, the *motor* centers and pathways, both somatic and visceral, being located along the ventral region as in the cord, while the visceral and somatic *sensory* neurons occupy the dorsal area (Fig. 1.1). Upon this primary cordlike axis of simple reflex-arc systems, is superimposed the relaying association centers of correlation and coordination, the complex *cerebrum* and *cerebellum,* which are once removed from direct sense reception and muscular response. *Correlation centers* concern the adjustment of incoming sensory stimuli, while *coordination centers* regulate the outgoing motor responses. These superimposed centers of the brain may be compared to the switchboard of a telephone exchange, where messages are received and distributed.

Meninges. Both brain and spinal cord are surrounded by membranes, or meninges (singular, *meninx*), the complexity in arrangement of which increases according to advance in the evolutionary scale. These membranes protect and give some support to the central nervous system.

Cartilage and bone are covered with a tough, vascular membrane known as the *perichondrium* or *periosteum,* as the case may be. The cavities of the cranium, and the neural canal of the vertebral column, are thus lined with perichondrium or periosteum, depending upon whether the skeleton is composed primarily of cartilage or bone. In either case the lining membrane is called the *endorachis.* It is not considered to be a true meninx.

In cyclostomes and fishes a single membrane, the *meninx primitiva,* forms a close union with brain and spinal cord, which it covers. Between the meninx primitiva and the endorachis is a space, the *perimeningeal* space, filled with mucoid and fatty tissue. Delicate strands of connective tissue cross the perimeningeal space, connecting the meninx with the endorachis.

Beginning with urodele amphibians, instead of a single meninx, two more or less distinct layers are present, an inner *pia-arachnoid* layer and an outer *dura mater*. The pia-arachnoid layer apparently has its origin, at least in part, from neuralcrest cells, whereas the dura mater is composed mostly of connective tissue. The pia-arachnoid is a very vascular membrane in intimate contact with the surface of brain and cord. Between pia-arachnoid and dura mater is the *subdural space;* the cavity between the dura mater and the endorachis is the *epidural space*. A small amount of fluid is present in the subdural space, but the epidural space is filled largely with alveolar tissue, fat, and numerous veins.

In mammals the pia-arachnoid membrane differentiates further into two layers, an inner, very vascular pia mater and an outer, nonvascular *arachnoid membrane*. A network of fine trabeculae composed of collagenic and elastic fibers joins the arachnoid membrane and pia mater. A *subarachnoid space,* filled with cerebrospinal fluid, makes its appearance between the two membranes. In the brain region the *cranial dura mater* fuses with the endorachis and the epidural space thus disappears. The *subdural space* between the dura and arachnoid membrane is shallow and contains only a minimum of fluid which is not cerebrospinal fluid. Melanocytes are usually present in the portion of the pia mater of mammals on the ventral side of the medulla oblongata.

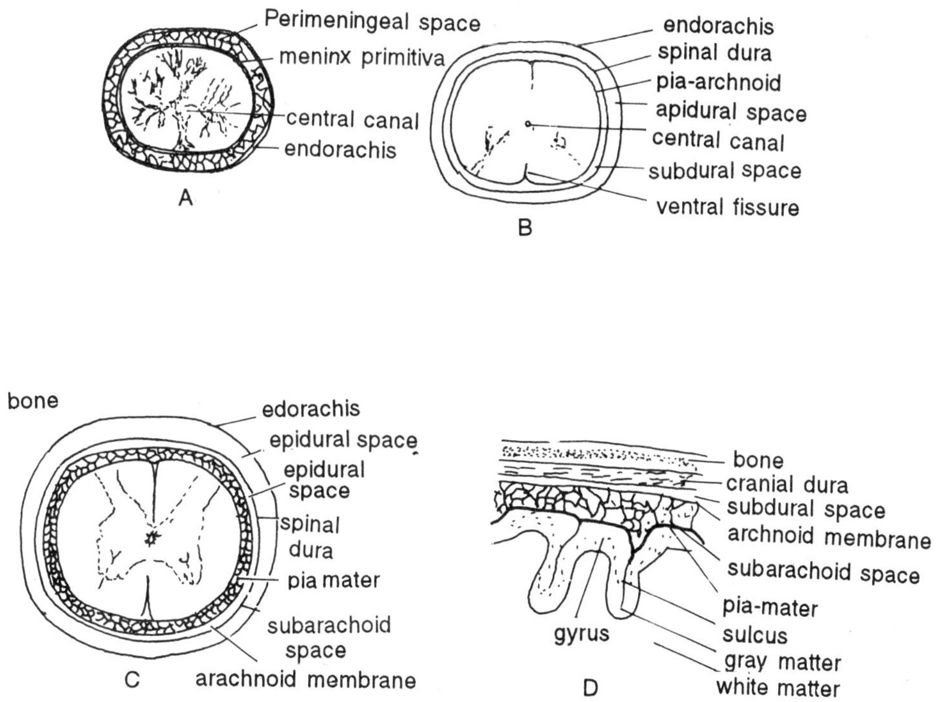

Fig. 1.2. Diagrams illustrating the relations of the meninges to the spinal cord and brain. A and B, cross sections through spinal cords of dogfish and salamander, respectively; C and D, sections of spinal cord and brain of mammal, respectively.

About the spinal cord a fusion of *spinal dura* and endorachis does not occur, and the epidural space, which thus persists in this region, contains fatty and other connective tissues as well as a number of veins. The cranial dura is continuous with the spinal dura at the foramen magnum.

The cranial dura is a tough, dense membrane loosely attached to the cranium except at the sutures and the basal portion of the skull. The pia mater and arachnoid membrane, known collectively as the *leptomeninges*, are of a loose, delicate consistency. Those of the brain and cord are of similar structure and appearance.

Near the posterior end of the spinal cord the subdural space disappears and the spinal dura forms a close-fitting sheath around the filum terminale. At the points where cranial and spinal nerves emerge, the dura forms sheaths around the nerves and their roots. The sheaths pass through the intervertebral foramina and are continuous with the periosteal covering of the bones. The dura is firmly attached to the margins of the foramen magnum.

The cerebrospinal fluid, which is present in the ventricles of the brain, the central canal of the spinal cord, and the subarachnoid space, and which is similar in composition to tissue fluid, circulates slowly through these various cavities and spaces. Elaborated, for the most part, by the anterior choroid plexus, the fluid passes into the lateral ventricles, through the interventricular foramina to the third ventricle, and thence through the cerebral aqueduct to the fourth ventricle. Three openings in the roof of the medulla oblongata—a single, median *foramen of Magendie* and two lateral *foramina of Luschka*-serve for the passage of cerebrospinal fluid into the subarachnoid space. Thus the surfaces of brain and cord are constantly bathed by cerebrospinal fluid. The fluid is formed continuously and must be absorbed continuously in order to ensure an even flow and a constant intracranial pressure. Absorption is partially through lymphatic vessels, but most of it passes through small protrusions of the arachnoid membrane, the *arachnoid*

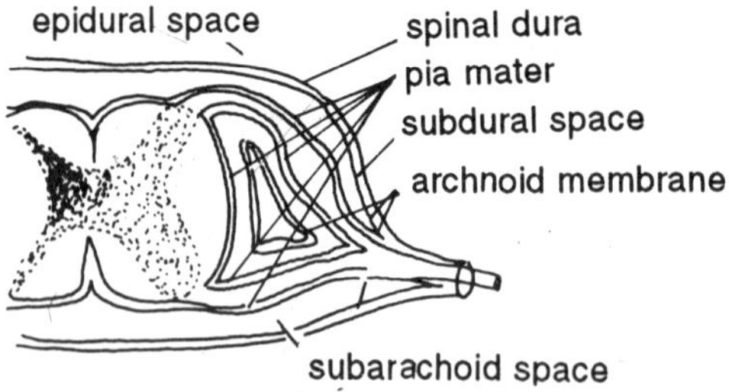

Fig. 1.3. Relations of the meninges to the roots of a spinal nerve in a mammal.

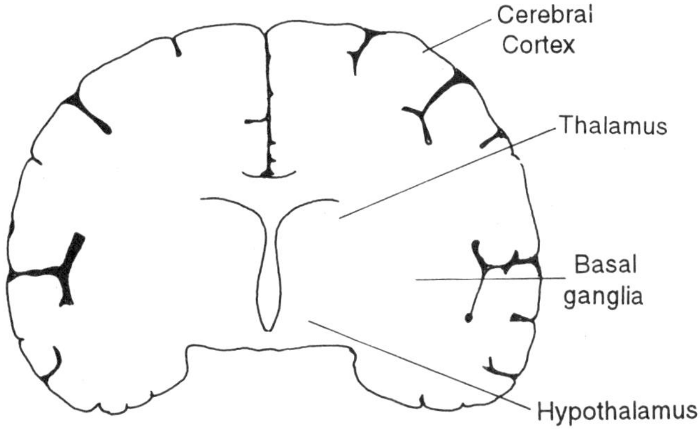

Fig. 1.4. Section of the brain showing the major features of the cerebrum.

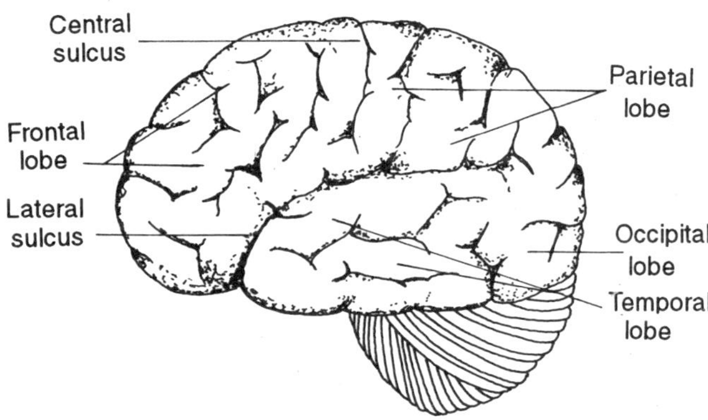

Fig. 1.5. The cerebral cortex. This superficial layer of the cerebrum is thrown into many folds. grooves (sulci) divide the cortex into four lobes.

villi, which project into the cavities of certain large venous sinuses in the dura mater. Only the thin mesothelial membranes of the arachnoid villi separate the cerebrospinal fluid in the subarachnoid space from the blood in the venous sinuses.

Certain modifications of the meninges are to be observed in mammals. The cranial dura sends a process, or fold, the *falx cerebri,* down into the fissure separating the two cerebral hemispheres. A similar process, the *tentorium,* pushes down between the cerebral hemispheres and cerebellum. In some forms, as in the cat, the tentorium becomes ossified and fused to the parietal bones. On the ventral side of the brain, the dura encapsulates the pituitary gland but also forms a fold, the *diaphragma sellae,* over the sella turcica, or depression in the dorsal face of the sphenoid bone, in which the pituitary gland lies. The stalk of the infundibulum, together with the pars tuberalis, if present penetrates the diaphragma sellae.

Fluid circulation through the brain. The brain is perfused with two fluids: blood and cerebrospinal fluid (CSF).

The brain has an extemely rich blood supply which is essential to support its high level of metabolic activity. It is easily damaged by interruption of its blood supply; this is the cause of the symptoms which may occur after a stroke. The blood circulation through the brain and spinal cord is unusual since their cells do not become stained by dyes injected into the blood. This inaccessibility of the CNS to dyes and many other materials has given rise to the term 'blood-brain barrier.' The exact nature of this 'barrier' is unknown: it appears that it consists of both actual barriers to the penetration of some materials and of active transport systems which regulate the concentration of different substances in the brain. Nerve cells are extremely sensitive to a number of substances in the blood circulation and the 'blood-brain barrier' is essential for the maintenance of the constant environment necessary for the normal working of the nervous system.

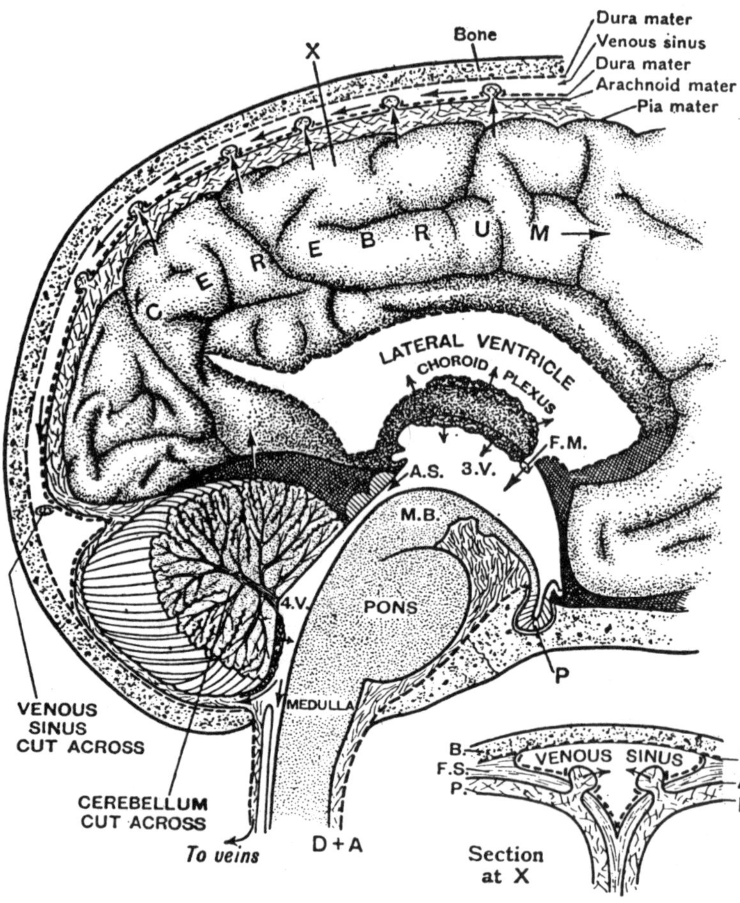

Fig. 1.6. Diagram showing by means of arrows the origin and destination of the cerebrospinal fluid. The diagram is really of a medial section of the brain except that one lateral ventricle is shown with cerebral convolutions.

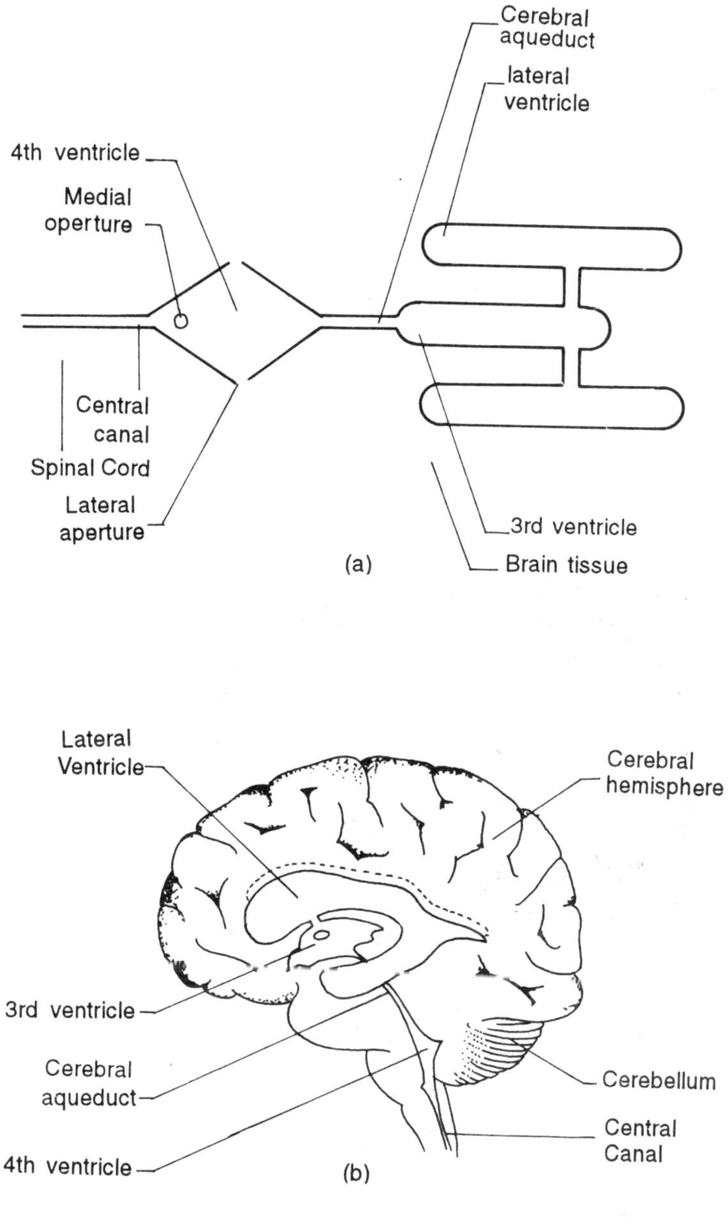

Fig. 1.7. The ventricular system of the brain. Within the brain is a series of fluid-filled spaces—the cerebral ventricles. (a) Diagrammatic representation of the ventricular system: these spaces are connected to the external surface of the brain and spinal cord by the medial and lateral apertures (after Bowsher). (b) Lateral view of the cerebral ventricles (after Netter). (c) Frontal view of the cerebral ventricles (facing page) (after Noback & Demarest). (d) Circulation of cerebrospinal fluid. The cerebral ventricles are filled with a liquid—cerebrospinal fluid—which is formed within the ventricles by the choroid plexes. Cerebrospinal fluid circulates through these spaces and then passes to the external surface of the CNS via the medial and lateral apertures; it is finally taken back into the blood through 'valves' in the arachnoid granulations on the upper surface of the brain (facing page).

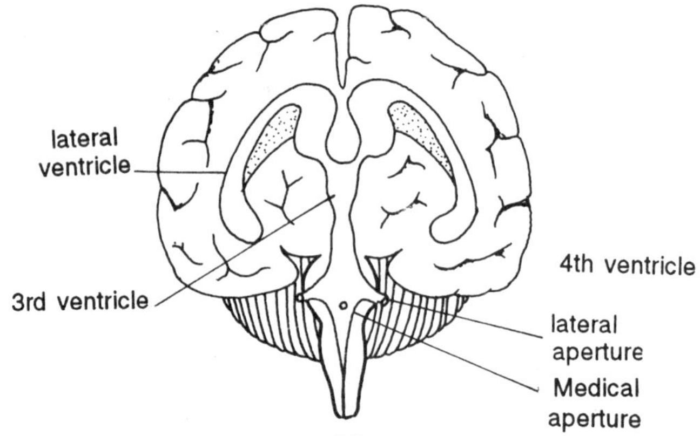
lateral
ventricle
3rd ventricle
4th ventricle
lateral
aperture
Medical
aperture

(c)

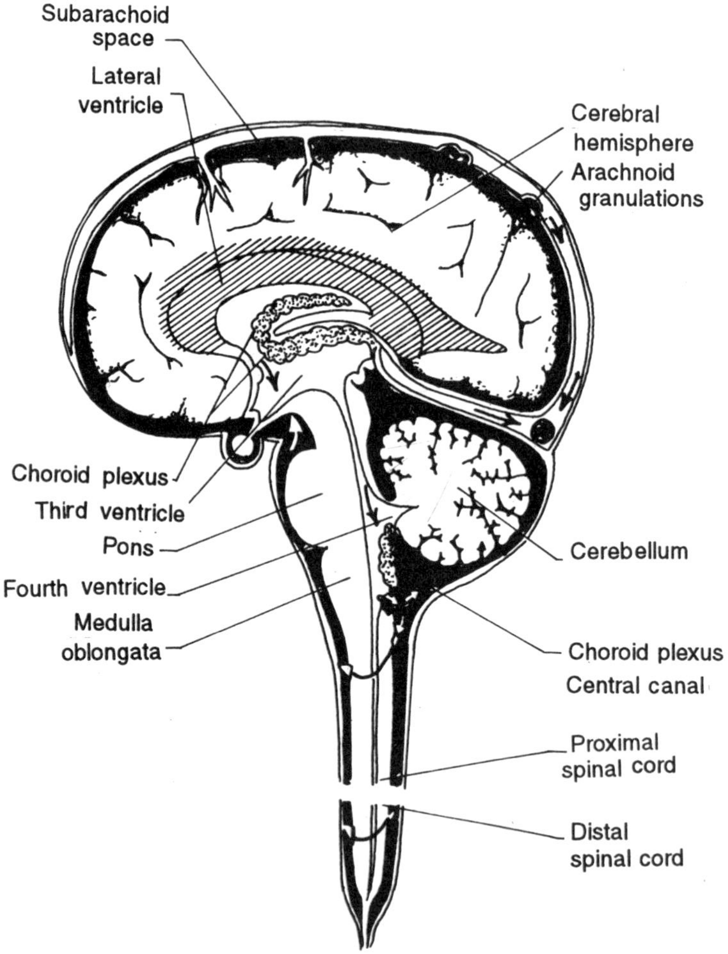
Subarachoid
space
Lateral
ventricle
Cerebral
hemisphere
Arachnoid
granulations
Choroid plexus
Third ventricle
Pons
Fourth ventricle
Medulla
oblongata
Cerebellum
Choroid plexus
Central canal
Proximal
spinal cord
Distal
spinal cord

(d)

Fig. 1.7. (d)

Within the brain there are four interconnected fluid-filled spaces, known as the cerebral ventricles. These ventricles are continuous with the central canal of the spinal cord. Within each ventricle there is a highly vascular structure known as a choroid plexus. The choroid plexes are responsible for the production of cerebrospinal fluid, which fills the ventricles. Cerebrospinal fluid is isotonic with blood plasma, but is not merely produced by a process of filtration since it differs from plasma in several ways. It contains only a small amount of protein and less potassium and calcium than plasma. The concentrations of sodium and chloride, on the other hand, are greater than those in plasma. The choroid plexes form approximately 300 ml. of cerebrospinal fluid per day. Once formed the cerebrospinal fluid flows through the ventricles and finally passes out to the external surface of the CNS via one medial and two lateral apertures. The cerebrospinal fluid then circulates over and bathes the brain and spinal cord. Cerebrospinal fluid is finally returned to the blood circulation via 'valves' within arachnoid granulations on the upper outer surface of the brain. Because cerebrospinal fluid is being formed continuously obstruction of its circulation causes a rise in hydrostatic pressure within the ventricular system. This leads to the condition known as hydrocephalus which can produce severe brain damage. Cerebrospinal fluid apparently provides the CNS with mechanical support, acts as a buffer against mechanical shock, controls the chemical environment of the brain (together with the blood circulation), and exchanges nutrients and waste materials with the brain tissue.

Table 1.1
Composition of Cerebrospinal Fluid

Constituent	*Plasma*	*CSF*
Na^{+}	150 mM	147 mM
K^{+}	4.6 mM	2.9 mM
Cl^{+}	99 mM	113 mM
Ca^{2+}	2.3 mM	1.1 mM
Protein	6000 mg/100 ml	20 mg/100ml

Primitive Nervous Systems

It took a long time to develop the complex human nervous system. In a simple animal like an Amoeba, the whole body is a single cell mass of protoplasm, possessing a generalized capacity for irritability and contractility whenever a stimulus impinges at some spot on such a body there results a direct local response at the point of stimulation, but the of it travels slowly to other parts of the cell. The fact that an Amoeba in escaping from danger extrudes a preuclopod on the side opposite to the point of stimulation is an indication that some degree of protoplasmic conduction is present even here. It is out of the question in such a case to speak of sense organs or receptors of communicating nerve fibres, adjusting center or of reacting muscles, because they have not yet developed.

It has been suggested that the coelentrates show what may have been the first steps in the evolution of the neuromuscular mechanism. In hydra, for example, the inner ends of some of the surface ectodermal cells developed muscular processes. When these cells are stimulated their inner portions contract without mediation of any sensory receptor. Parker has given the name independent effector to this type of cell which serves as both receptor and effector.

In most animals, including many coelentrates, these two functions are perforated by seperate cells. In the simplest arrangement sensory cells, exposed to the outside, are indirect contact, through these branching inner ends, with underlying contractile muscle cells (effectors). Usually, however, a second nerve cell, a motor cell, is inserted between the sensory and muscular elements. In coelentrates the motor cell, is inserted between the sensory and muscular elements. In coelentrates motor cells unite into a continuous network, nerve net, in which impulses may pass freely in any direction and consequently spread through the net to give a diffuse response to a localized stimulation. Nerve net works are found on vertebrate blood vessels.

Simple localized reflex arcs including two short neurons persist in the walls of the digestive tube of man. By means of large numbers of these arcs, located in the plexus of Auerbach and the plexus of Meissna the peestaltic response to the stimulating presence of food is brought about without the intervention of the cord or brain.

The final step is taken by the flatworms in which the synapses between sensory and motor neurons as well as the cell bodies of the latter are located in nerve cords. Also nerve impulses are transmitted in only one direction similar simple reflex arcs, involving a central nervous system, are found in most invertebrates and in the vertebrates.

Primarily the cell bodies of sensory neurons are located in the surface epithelium, as we have seen in the coelentrates and worm. But frequently they shift deeper into the body and develop dendrite, which may be of considerable length if the cell body lies at some distance from the surface of the animal's body.

The Embryonic Rise of the Nervous System

In invertebrates generally the inward migration of the central nervous system comes about through a process of disemination, that is, the splitting off of a thickened band of cells from the hypodermis along the ventral side of the body.

In the case of some vertebrates, on the contrary, the central nervous system is buried by a process of invagination. In cyclostomes and in many teleosts, however, the embryonic foundation of the central nervous system is probably laid down first as a solid rod of cells which afterwards becomes hollowed out.

The first step in the formation of the vertebrate nervous system occurs toward the end of the gastrula stage when the ectoderm in front of the blastoporic lip thickens to form the neural or medulary plate, which extends lengthense along the dorsal side of the elongated embryo. This structure is morphologically continuous and since the embryonic ectoderm is not conspiciously given to metameric expression, it is never marked off into segments, as in the underlying mesoderm in the formation of somites.

The lateral edges of the long flat medullary plate next become elevated, thus transforming it into a trough like canal, the medullary groove. Continuing their growth upward, the edges eventually meet and grow together forming the medullary tube. The cavity with in this embryonic tube is the forerunner of the ventricles of the brain and the central canal of the spinal cord. The closure of the tube begins in the middle region and extends both ways so that for a time both ends still remain open. At the posterior end there may exist, in addition to the trough like opening to the outside, a temporary inward passage way around into the primitive enteric cavity through the blastopore. This is the neurentric canal, which remains open upto the fourth week in the human fetus, although the medullar groove begins to close about the fifteenth day. The anterior end of the medullary tube remains unclosed longer than the posterior end in the form of the so-called neuropore. Aniphioxus retains the neuropore throughout life. Possibly in this forerunner of the vertebrate it may serve as some sort of a sense organ.

As the medullary tube closes there form on either side along the seam of fusion two distinct ridges of medullary tissue, the neural crests. At first continuous with the tube, these crests later again independence by the insertion of invading mesenchymal tissue between the medullary tube and the tube itself. Eventually the crests break up into chains, forming both the sensory dorsal ganglia of the spinal nerves and the ganglia of

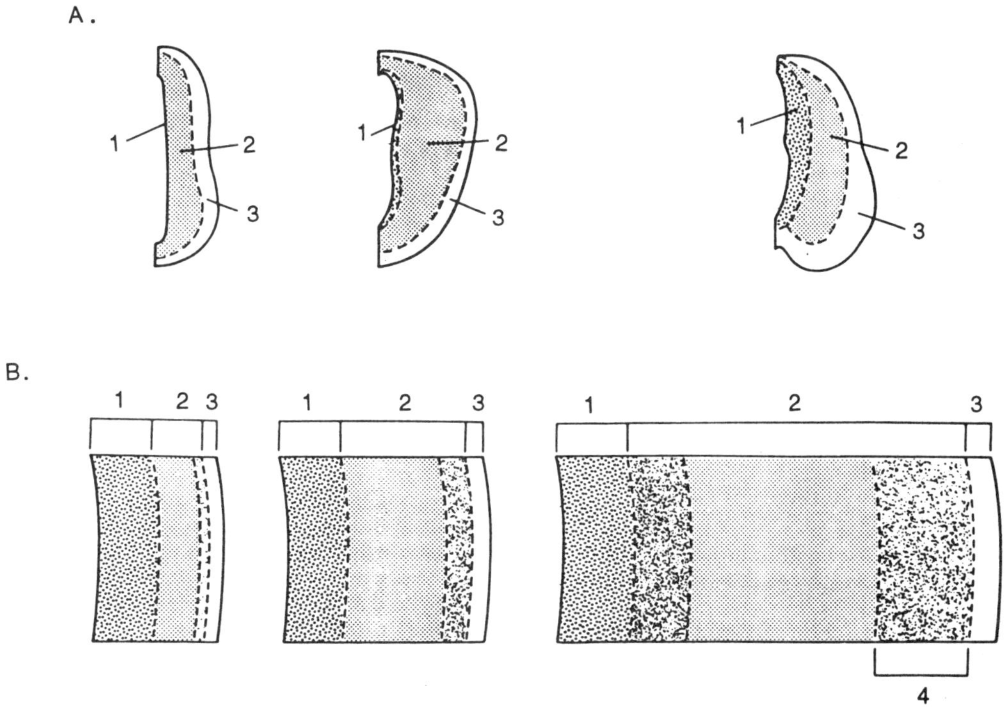

Fig. 1.8. The progressive formation of the spinal cord (A) and the cerebral cortex (B) in the human embryo. In A, the successive layer, from within outward are: 1. Ependymal layer. 2. Mantle layer. 3. Marginal layer. In B, the successive cortical layers (1, 2, 3) are the same as in the cord, however the outermost region of the mantle layer of the cortex differentiates into the pyramidal layer of the embryonic cortex (4).

the autonomic system, which are of motor function when the neurons of the dorsal ganglia sprout they send their dendrites into the various organs of the body while their neuriles establish a secondary connection into the cord.

The autonomic ganglia also becomes connected with the cord, but by neuriles, which grow out from the cells with in the cord itself. Similar relationships are established in the brain region. All of the nervous tissues of the body are derived, either directly or indirectly from the medullary tube, with the exception of cells and fibres that contribute to the olfactory epithelium.

Factors that Influence the Growth and Development of the Nervous System. Although the factors that are responsible for governing the developmental patterns within the nervous systems are, in general, unknown, certain physicochemical influences can be recognized.

Among the important physical processes that regulate patterns of nerve growth and development is the hydrostatic pressure developed within the neural tube that is caused by an accumulation of fluid secreted by the ependymal cells. As noted earlier, this pressure, combined with the differential rates of hypertrophy and hyperplasia of the cells in different regions of the brain, results in profound alterations in the anatomic relationship among the various gross structural elements present in the embryonic and adult brain. Consequently, mechanical factors are significant, at least in the development of the central nervous system.

The protoplasm of the tips of growing axons is capable of active ameboid movement; hence these neuronal processes are capable of penetrating the intercellular spaces between other cell types. In this regard, the highly organized microfibrillar and microtubular elements of the neurons play an important role in determining this movement. Furthermore, ameboid movement of entire neurons (as well as most other embryonic cell types) during embryogenesis is an important factor in determining their ultimate disposition within the nervous system.

A major problem in neuroembryology is: How do neuronal processes become associated with their ultimate target structures or organs during embryogenesis? The adult patterns of innervation throughout the entire body are highly specific; therefore the progression of entire nerve cells (as in the formation of the cerebral cortex and the peripheral ganglia) or their axonal processes (as during the innervation of particular muscles by individual nerve fibers) is a highly selective process. It is clear that chemical factors must play a very decisive role in guiding these developmental patterns. Although the specific biochemical regulatory mechanisms that underlie most of these events in the embryo are unknown, one compound has been isolated and characterized that exerts profound effects upon the generation, growth, and maintenance of specific types of neurons. This compound, known as nerve growth factor (NGF), is a protein that resembles insulin both structurally and functionally.

NGF has been demonstrated to enhance the growth of peripheral sensory neurons in general as well as to stimulate the growth and maintenance of sympathetic neurons in particular. Furthermore, NGF has been demonstrated to affect the regenerative growth of severed axons that arise from centrally located adrenergic neurons, indicating a role of this protein in central nervous functions. Like insulin, NGF appears to act upon specific receptors located on its target cells through stimulation of the biosynthetic and bioenergetic processes of those cells. Hence it has been proposed that sympathetic nerve outgrowth toward particular effector cells in the periphery is through the attractive action of NGF that is bound to the specific receptor sites for NGF upon the target cells. In this regard, it is significant that a quantitative relationship exists between the number of NGF binding sites upon particular cells and the extent of sympathetic innervation of those cells. The nonneural glial cells of the nervous system have been implicated in NGF production, but these elements also appear to elaborate other, as yet unidentified, nerve growth factors.

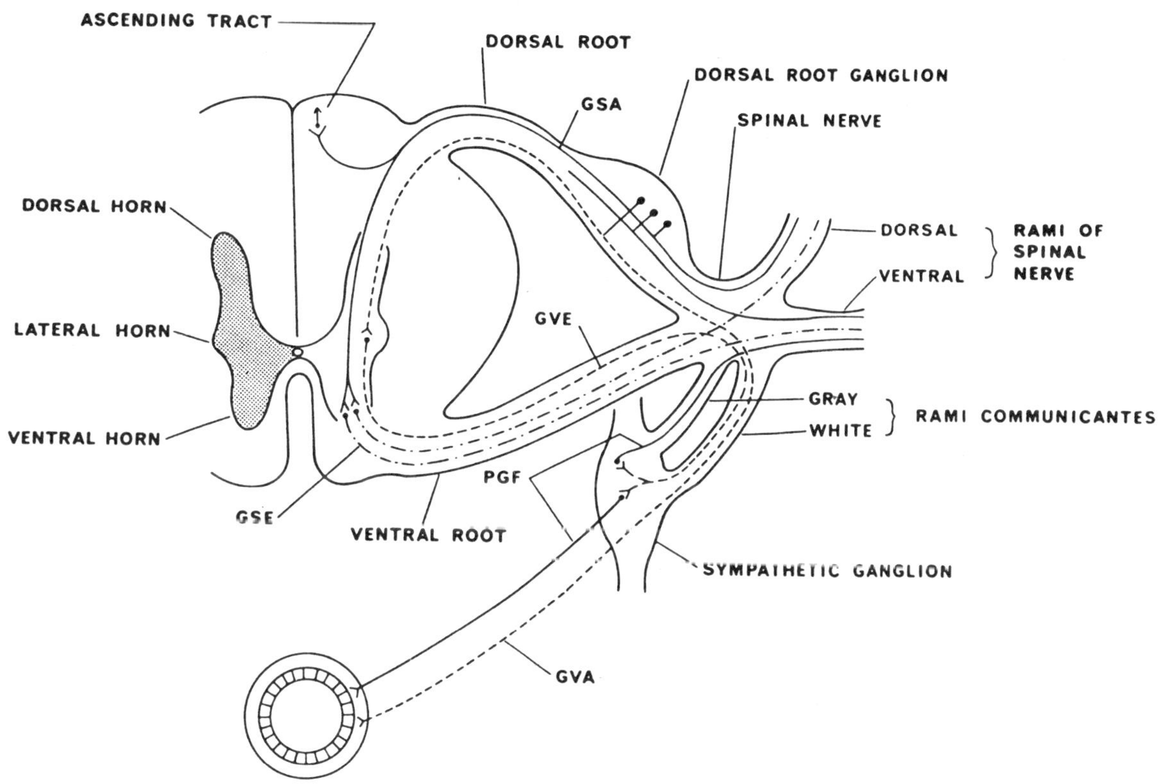

Fig. 1.9. Cross section of the adult spinal cord illustrating the components of a typical spinal nerve and its connections. Nerve cell bodies are indicated by black dots, and synapses by "V" terminations of presynaptic fibers on the nerve cell bodies. The abbreviations used for particular types of fiber are: GSA = general somatic afferent; GSE = general somatic efferent; GVA = general visceral afferent; GVE = general visceral efferent; PGF = postganglionic sympathetic fibres.

Interestingly, the functional roles of NGF in vivo do not appear to be confined to neural and related tissues. In fact, NGF has been implicated experimentally as a substance that may be involved in wound healing as well as in carcinogenesis. In this regard, the elaboration of NGF by nonneural glial cells as well as by fibroblasts is particularly significant.

At one time it was believed that neural migration, growth, and organization took place along electric gradients developed between the axons and dendrites of individual neurons. This concept, known as "neurobiotaxis," remains wholly unsupported by direct experimental evidence. Therefore, it would appear that chemotactic mechanisms involving various as yet unidentified biochemical factors are responsible for the growth and development of the nervous system.

Differentiation of the Brain

The transforming embryonic brain is a key to the adult structure. The modification of the simple tubular brain into the exceedingly complex structure found in man is brought about through the following phases of growth: (a) constriction; (b) unequal thickenings of the walls; (c) invagination and evagination; and (d) bending.

(a) *Constriction.*— The original, somewhat inflated anterior region of the medullary tube, which is formed upon the closure of the medullary groove, is called the *encephalon*.

Very early in embryonic life (the third week in man), the encephalon becomes marked off into three regions by two constrictions. These primitive regions are designated as the *prosencephalon*, *mesencephalon*, and *rhombencephalon*, the latter so called because of the kite-shaped appearance of the ventricle, or cavity, showing here.

A little later (the fourth week in man), the prosencephalon becomes further constricted into two subregions, the *telencephalon* and the *diencephalon*. The rhombencephalon likewise (about the fifth week in man) is subdivided into a *metencephalon* and a *myelencephalon*, the mesencephalon remaining unconstricted as it was before. The brain is now marked off into five definite areas, arranged in order from anterior to posterior as follows: telencephalon, diencephalon, mesencephalon, metencephalon, and myelencephalon.

Certain of these primary regions of the brain are destined to take on special importance, because of the sense organs with which they are intimately connected. The telencephalon may be regarded as the "nose brain," the mesencephalon as the "eye brain," and the myelencephalon as the "ear brain," with the additional assignment to the latter of "skin brain" and "visceral brain."

Cyclostomes throughout life remain with the brain constricted into only three regions, but from fishes onward the five fundamental parts of the brain are clearly represented.

(b) *Unequal Thickening of the Walls of the Brain.*— The walls of the primitive encephalon are at first of approximately equal thickness, but as neurons develop

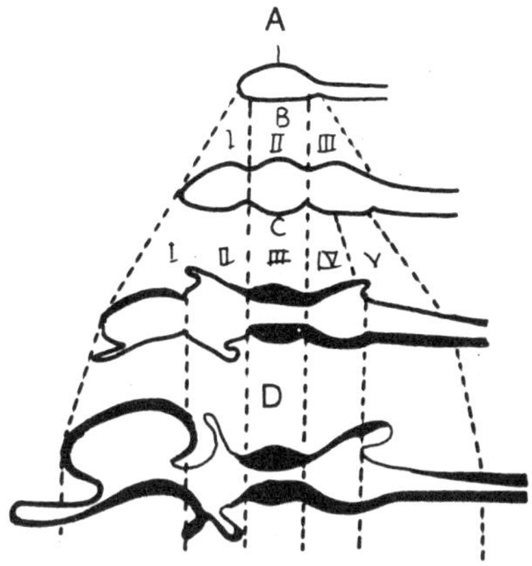

Fig. 1.10. Diagrams of the differentiation of the encephalon. A, primitive encephalon; B, division into an anterior prosencephalon, a mesencephalon, and a posterior rhombencephalon; C and D, further division into the five regions of the brain.

and collect into centers and transmission tracts, the disposition of these collections of nerve elements brings about decided contrasts in the thickness of the walls of the brain in different places.

The thinnest regions are at two points, the roofs, or *vela,* (1) of the diencephalon and small median portion of the telencephalon and (2) of the myelencephalon. Each velum includes only the thin ependymal layer.

The thickest areas, on the other hand, are the *cerebellum,* which develops from the dorsal part of the metencephalon, and the walls of the *cerebral hemispheres,* the paired antero-lateral outgrowths which make up most of the telencephalon. The cerebral hemispheres, the crowning hope of the evolving brain, become so enormously thickened and enlarged in mammals that they overshadow and entirely cover up both the diencephalon and the mesencephalon, concealing them from dorsal view.

(c) *Invaginations and Evaginations.*— There are two places where the brain wall is pushed in or invaginated, namely, in the regions of the thin vela just mentioned. Over the outside of these thinnest places in the walls of the brain extends a network of capillaries in the *pia mater,* the vascular meninx that intimately envelops the brain. These capillary nets are the *choroid plexuses,* which by invagination are pushed down into the cavities of the brain below, carrying the thin wall with them. They provide a blood supply for the inside of the brain.

From the walls of the diencephalon, there also occur various *evaginations.* In certain vertebrates these are two finger-like outpushings of the wall, one behind the other, on

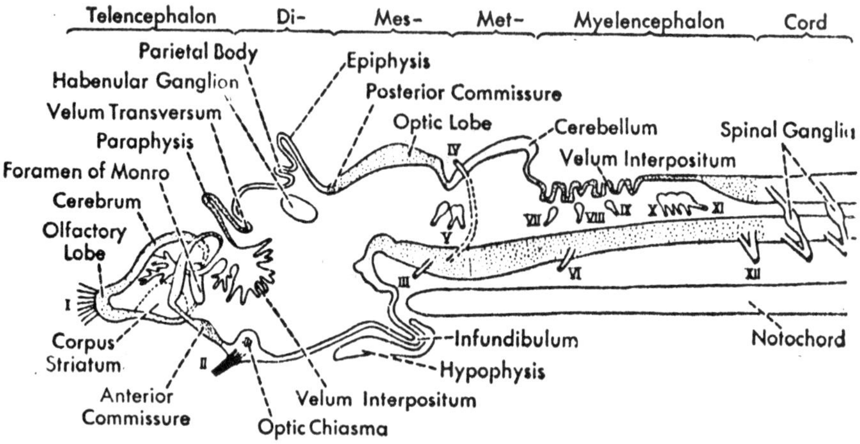

Fig. 1.11. Sagittal diagram through a vertebrate brain, showing the five general regions and the variations in thickness of the brain wall. Based upon the brain of a cyclostome. Telencephalon, mesencephalon, and myelencephalon stippled; other parts in outline.

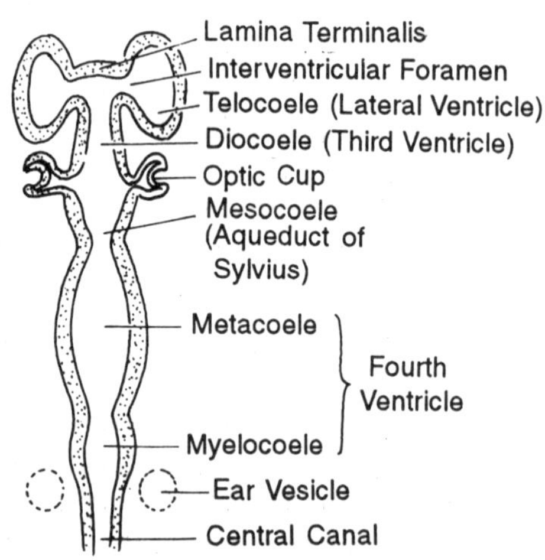

Fig. 1.12. Frontal diagram to show the cavities of the brain.

the dorsal side just behind the invaginated choroid plexus. The anterior of these evaginations, near the junction of the cerebral hemispheres and the diencephalon, is the *parietal organ,* which is particularly developed in certain reptiles, while the posterior projection, the *epiphysis,* or *pineal "gland,"* appears in some stage of degeneration or elaboration in practically all vertebrates.

A ventral median evagination of the floor of the diencephalon, the *infundibulum,* has already been mentioned. It joins a glandular upgrowth from the roof of the mouth to form the *hypophysis.*

The *optic stalks* extending out from the sides of the diencephalon in early embryonic life are also evaginations.

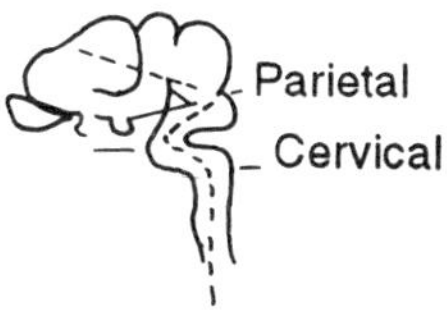

Fig. 1.13. Diagram showing the flexures of the brain.

(d) *Bendings.*— In cyclostomes and other lower vertebrates the parts of the brain retain their primitive tandem arrangement, but with the onrush of growth and the ultimate confining limits of the skull, it becomes necessary for the brain stem to bend and fold to accommodate itself to more compact quarters. The bends, or flexures, of the brain are typically three: (1) the *parietal flexure* in the region of the mesencephalon; (2) the *cervical flexure* near the junction of the medulla and the cord, and (3) the *pontine flexure* between these two. The first two flexures bend ventrally while the third bends in the opposite direction, thus tending to kink the brain stem together like a compressed accordion.

Ventricle

With the differentiation of the neural tube into brain and spinal cord, its original cavity becomes modified to form the ventricles of the brain and the central canal of the cord. When the telencephalon develops into the paired cerebral hemispheres, the cavity extends into those structures as the lateral ventricles, or ventricles I and II. The cavity of the diencephalon is then known as the third ventricle. Each lateral ventricle communicates with the third ventricle by means of an opening, the *interventricular foramen,* or *foramen* of Monro. In higher vertebrates a narrow canal extends posteriorly from the third ventricle through the mesencephalon and is referred to as the *cerebral aqueduct,* or *aqueduct of Sylvius.* In lower forms the cerebral aqueduct may be considerably expanded on either side and the term *optic ventricles,* or *mesocoele,* is then applied. Posteriorly the cerebral

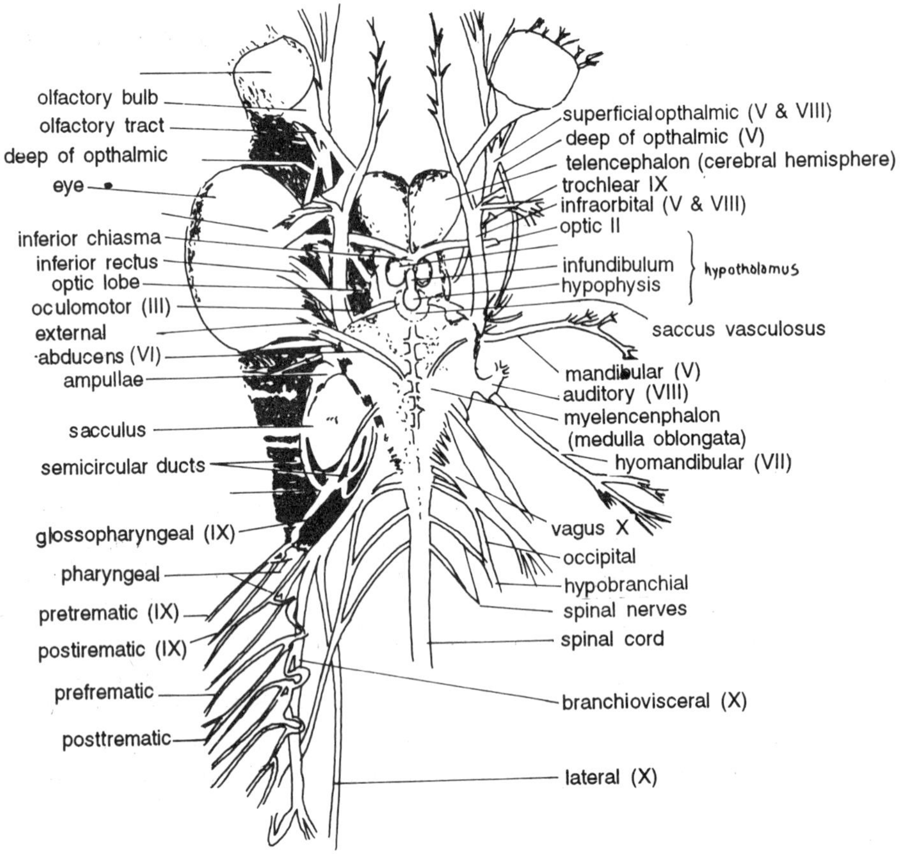

Fig. 1.14. Ventral view of brain, sense organs, and cranial nerves of *Squalus acanthias.*

aqueduct communicates with the enlarged cavity of the rhombencephalon, or the fourth ventricle. In numerous lower forms the anterior part of the fourth ventricle becomes modified into a chamber, the *metacoele*, extending into the cerebellum. The portion of the fourth ventricle within the medulla oblongata is then referred to as the *myelocoele*. It is continued posteriorly as the *central canal* of the spinal cord.

As development of the brain continues, its walls become thickened with nervous tissue except in two regions where only the epithelial ependymal layer is retained. These regions include the anterior part of the roof of the diencephalon and the roof of the medulla oblongata. In each region a fusion of the roof with a highly vascular membrane, the pia mater, forms a *tela choroidea*. Folds from the tela choroidea project into the third and fourth ventricles and are known, respectively, as the anterior and posterior choroid plexuses. The ependymal layer lining the choroid plexus region is referred to as the *choroid plexus epithelium*.

Lymphlike cerebrospinal fluid is contained within the cavities of brain and spinal cord and circulates through the ventricles and central canal. It passes out of these cavities through openings, to be mentioned later, to bathe the entire central nervous system. The choroid plexuses are important in forming the cerebrospinal fluid.

2

Brain

As stated in the previous chapter that central nervous system is the part of nervous system present along the central axis of the body and it includes brain and spinal cord. Brain is the controlling centre and is divided into the following parts:

(1) Prosencephalon (Fore brain)

  (a) Olfactory lobes

  (b) Cerebrum

  (c) Diencephalon

(2) Mesencephalon (Mid brain)

  (a) Optic lobes

(3) Rhombencephalon (Hind brain)

  (a) Cerebellum

  (b) Medulla oblongata.

The Brain Stem

There is some disagreement among various authors as to which structures constitute the brain stem. For the purposes of this text, the following structures will be discussed under this heading: the medulla oblongata, the pons, the mesencephalon (midbrain), and the diencephalon, including the thalamus and its subdivisions, as well as the hypothalamus.

All of the cranial nerves are attached to the brain stem, excepting the olfactory nerve and the spinal portion of the accessory nerve.

The Medulla Oblongata. The medullary region of the brain stem is an extremely important physiologic center for the initiation and coordination of many involuntary (vegetative) reflexes essential to the maintenance of life.*

---

* The medulla oblongata once was called the "bulb," and the term "bulbar" referred to this part of the brain stem; these terms now are obsolete.

The medulla is superficially continuous with the spinal cord and it extends anteriorly about 2.5 cm. to the caudal region of the pons. The central canal of the spinal cord is continuous within the medulla, but this channel expands dorsally at the obex into the large cavity of the fourth ventricle. The roof of the fourth ventricle, the choroid plexus, is made up of a thin sheet of ependyma and pia mater.

Externally, the pyramids form two longitudinal ridges on the ventral surface of the medulla on each side of the anteromedian fissure. These structures contain the pyramidal (corticospinal) tracts; the decussation of these fibers terminates the fissure caudally.

The ventrolateral sulcus contains the several roots of the hypoglossal nerve (XII). The dorsolateral sulcus, also continuous with that of the cord, contains roots of the spinal accessory nerve (XI), the vagus (X), and the glossopharyngeal nerve (IX). Swellings laterally between these sulci represent the olivary body or eminence, and the superior olivary nucleus lies within the medulla in this region of the brain stem.

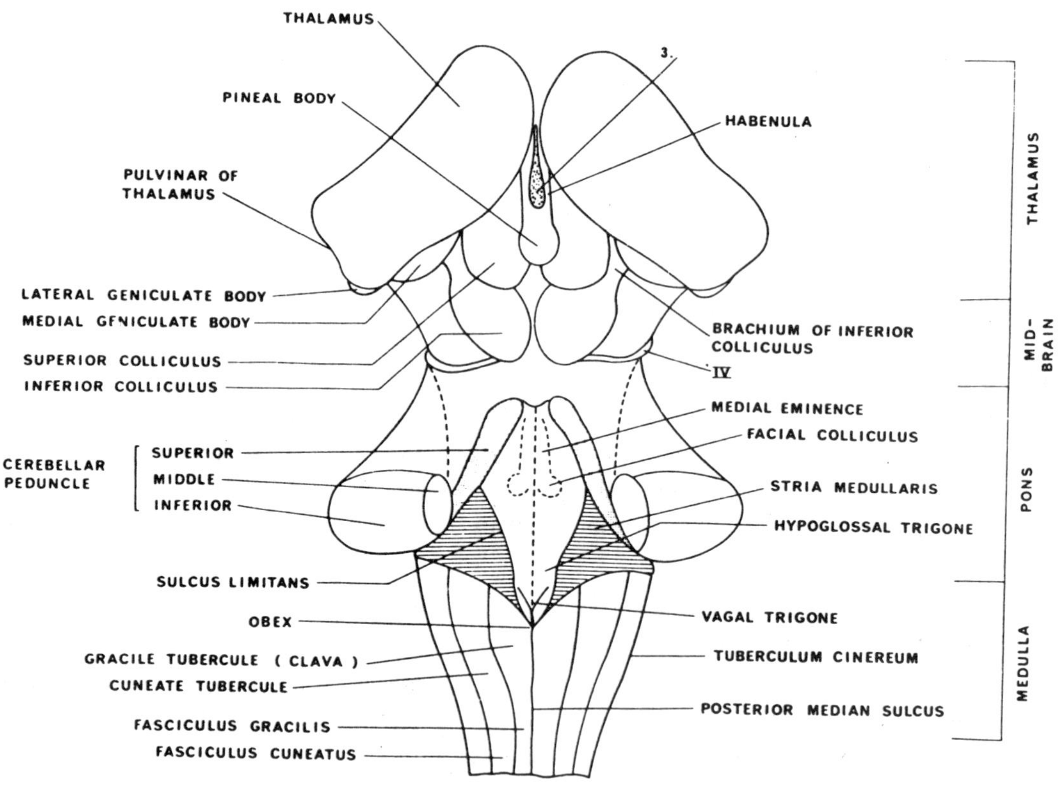

Fig. 2.1. The gross anatomic features of the brain stem from the dorsal aspect. 3 = third ventricle.

The dorsal aspect of the medulla presents two low ridges, the fasciculi gracilis and cuneatus. The nuclei within these tracts are marked respectively by small protuberances, the clava and cuneate tubercle. The restiform bodies or inferior cerebellar peduncles form two prominent ridges extending along the sides of the fourth ventricle. In the floor of the fourth ventricle two pairs of swellings are present; their margins taper to a point caudally, and meet in the median sulcus in a region known as the calamus scriptorius. The lateral ridges of this structure are called the vagal trigone; the medial ridges constitute the hypoglossal trigone. The facial colliculus lies rostral to the stria of the fourth ventricle, and the continuation of this ridge anteriorly is the median eminence. A groove on the lateral margins of these ridges, the sulcus limitans, demarcates the sensory and motor areas of the medulla.

Internally, several of the long nerve fiber tracts from the spinal cord pass directly through the medulla unchanged in position relative to each other; however, others undergo rearrangement within this region of the brain stem.

Within the lower half of the medulla, the central canal is surrounded by a central gray area. This contains the diffuse cells and fibers of the reticular formation, which extends through medulla, pons, and mesencephalon. The pyramidal tracts decussate in the most ventral part of the medulla. Dorsally, the fasciculi cuneatus and gracilis terminate in their respective nuclei; their axonic processes then arch downward and cross in the midline in the decussation of the medial lemniscus. Dorsolaterally, the spinal tract and spinal nucleus of the trigeminal nerve (V) are found.

Within the upper half of the medulla is located the inferior olivary nucleus. Many efferent fibers from this region cross and join spinocerebellar fibers in the inferior cerebellar peduncle, whereas other olivocerebellar fibres enter the peduncle without undergoing decussation.

Three symmetric paired areas are found in the dorsal region of the medulla near the floor of the fourth ventricle. These longitudinal columnar structures consist of the nucleus of the hypoglossal nerve (XII), the dorsal motor nucleus of vagus (X), and the vestibular nuclei (VIII) which receive afferent fibers from the vestibular branch of the auditory nerve (VIII).

The nucleus ambiguus is found in the ventro-lateral portion of the reticular formation, and its fibers pass into the inferior cerebellar peduncle together with other fibers of the vagus. The solitary tract, an isolated longitudinal fiber bundle, also is present in the reticular formation; it contains afferent fibers of the vagus nerve (X). The adjacent nucleus is called the nucleus of the solitary tract.

The lateral spinothalamic tract lies ventro-lateral to the nucleus ambiguus. In this region also are found two large fiber bands which contain the medial longitudinal fasciculus, and the tectospinal and vestibulospinal tracts, the remainder being the medial lemnisci.

Associated with the medulla are four cranial nerves which will be considered individually.

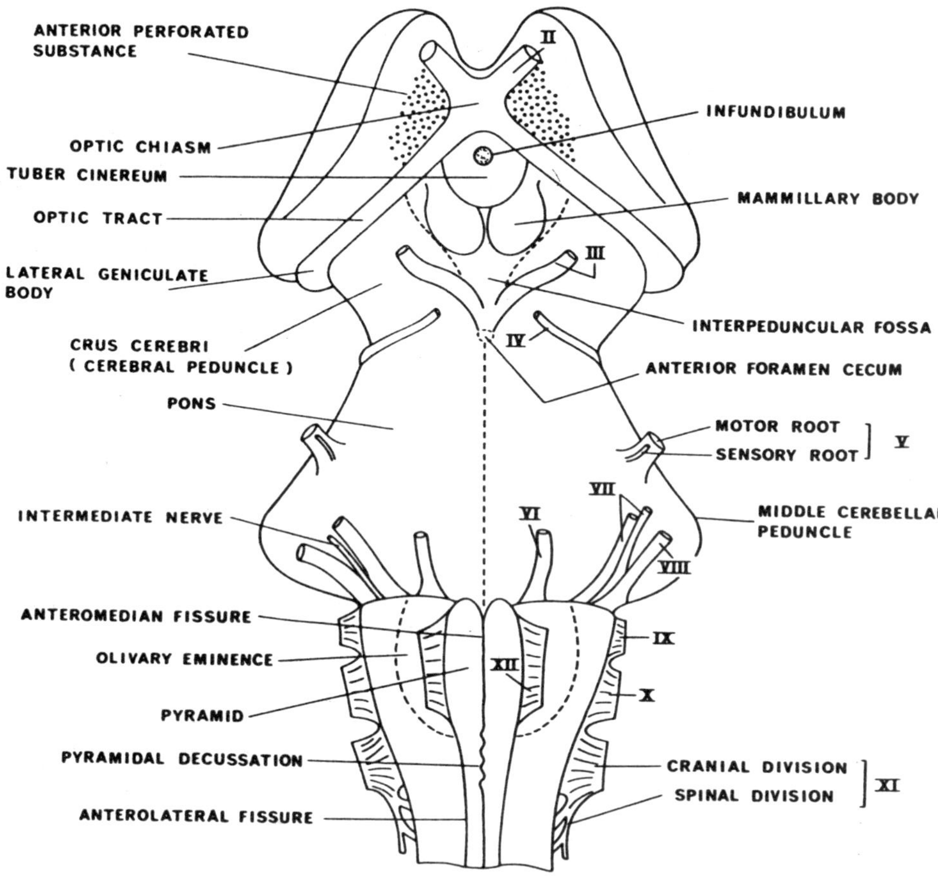

Fig. 2.2. The gross anatomic features of the brain stem from the ventral aspect.

The Hypoglossal Nerve (XII). The hypoglossal nerve contains some general somatic afferent (GSA) proprioceptive fibers from the lingual muscles. The nerve cell bodies that give rise to these GSA fibers are diffused. The hypoglossal nerve also is the motor nerve of the tongue muscles. The general somatic efferent (GSE) fibers of the hypoglossal nerve originate in cells of the hypoglossal nucleus (nucleus ambiguus) of the medulla described above (Fig. 2.4).

The Spinal Accessory Nerve (XI). There are two discrete components to the spinal accessory nerve. First, the spinal root contains GSA fibers that terminate in proprioceptors within the neck musculature. These fibers arise from cervical spinal cord segments (C-1 through C-5), ascent through the foramen magnum, and join the second component of XI, the bulbar root, from the medulla. The bulbar fibers run with the spinal fibers for a short distance, then join the vagus nerve and course together with the vagus to terminate with the vagal fibers.

The spinal branch of XI, which consists of special visceral efferent (SVE) fibers, descends in the neck and terminates in the sternomastoid and trapezius muscles. Thus, the spinal division of this nerve actually is a loop of nerve from the brachial plexus and not a true cranial nerve.

The Vagus Nerve (X). The vagus nerve is complex and is made up of both sensory and motor divisions; this nerve also makes important contributions to the cranial division of the parasympathetic nervous system.

The two sensory ganglia of the vagus lie outside of but near the medulla, strung in series on the roots of the vagus nerve like two elongated beads on a string: These are the superior (or jugular) ganglion and the inferior (or nodose) ganglion. GSA fibers from the skin in back of the ear and the posterior wall of the external auditory meatus pass through the auricular branch of the vagus to the superior ganglion.

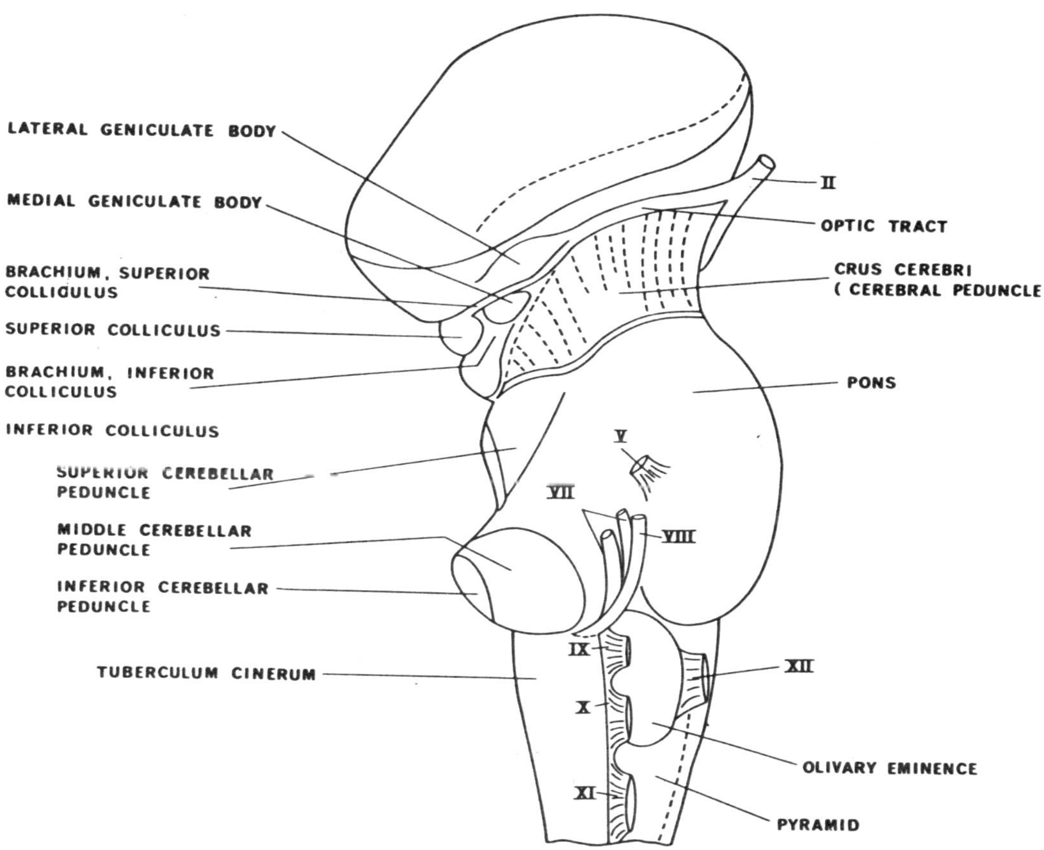

Fig. 2.3. The gross anatomic features of the brain stem from the right lateral aspect.

General visceral afferent (GVA) fibers from the pharynx, larynx, trachea, esophagus, and the thoracic as well as the abdominal viscera conduct impulses centrally to the inferior ganglion of the vagus or else pass on the nucleus solitarius via the appropriate branches of the vagus. These branches include the pharyngeal, superior and recurrent laryngeal, cardiac, bronchial, and esophageal nerves.

Special visceral afferent (SVA) fibers from diffusely located taste buds in the vicinity of the epiglottis also pass to the inferior (nodose) ganglion of the vagus.

The vagal motor nuclei in the medulla include the dorsal motor nucleus, the salivatory nucleus (also associated with the glossopharyngeal nerve), and the nucleus ambigus. The latter, found as a column of cells within the reticular formation, contributes bronchiomotor neurons to both the glossopharyngeal as well as vagus nerves, and its axons innervate the voluntary muscles of the soft palate, larynx, and pharynx as SVE preganglionic fibers.

General visceral efferent (GVE) preganglionic fibers, which arise from neurons in the dorsal motor nucleus of the vagus, provide motor innervation to thoracic structures and the smooth muscle of the abdominal viscera as far as the level of the splenic flexure of the colon.

The postganglionic fibers of both SVE and GVE fibers originate in the terminal ganglia. It should also be remembered that in the medullary region afferent and efferent branches do not form separate dorsal and ventral roots as in the spinal cord, but enter and emerge from the brain stem together.

The Glossopharyngeal Nerve (IX). The glossopharyngeal nerve is related intimately to the vagus and both nerves share common intramedullary nuclear origins and connections, as well as similar functional components; consequently the glossopharyngeal nerve contains both sensory and motor components.

GSA fibers of IX innervate a small cutaneous area back of the ear; the cell bodies of these sensory neurons lie within the superior ganglion and run together with vagal fibers in the auricular branch of the vagus. The axons terminate centrally in the spinal trigeminal nucleus.

GVA nerve fibers of the glossopharyngeal nerve, whose cell bodies lie within the inferior ganglion, enter the fasciculus solitarius and terminate in the solitary nucleus. These fibers convey pain, tactile, and thermal sensations from the mucous membranes of the posterior tongue region, tonsils, and eustachian tubes. More abundant SVA fibers transmit sensory impulses from taste buds on the posterior third of the tongue via the lingual nerve.

An important SVA branch of IX, the carotid sinus nerve which innervates the carotid sinus, is important in the regulation of blood pressure. Centrally, this nerve sends collaterals to the dorsal motor nucleus of the vagus; preganglionic fibers then pass from this vagal nucleus to terminate in ganglion cells located within the atria of the heart. Postganglionic axons then innervate the atrial muscle as well as the sinoatrial and atrio-ventricular nodes.

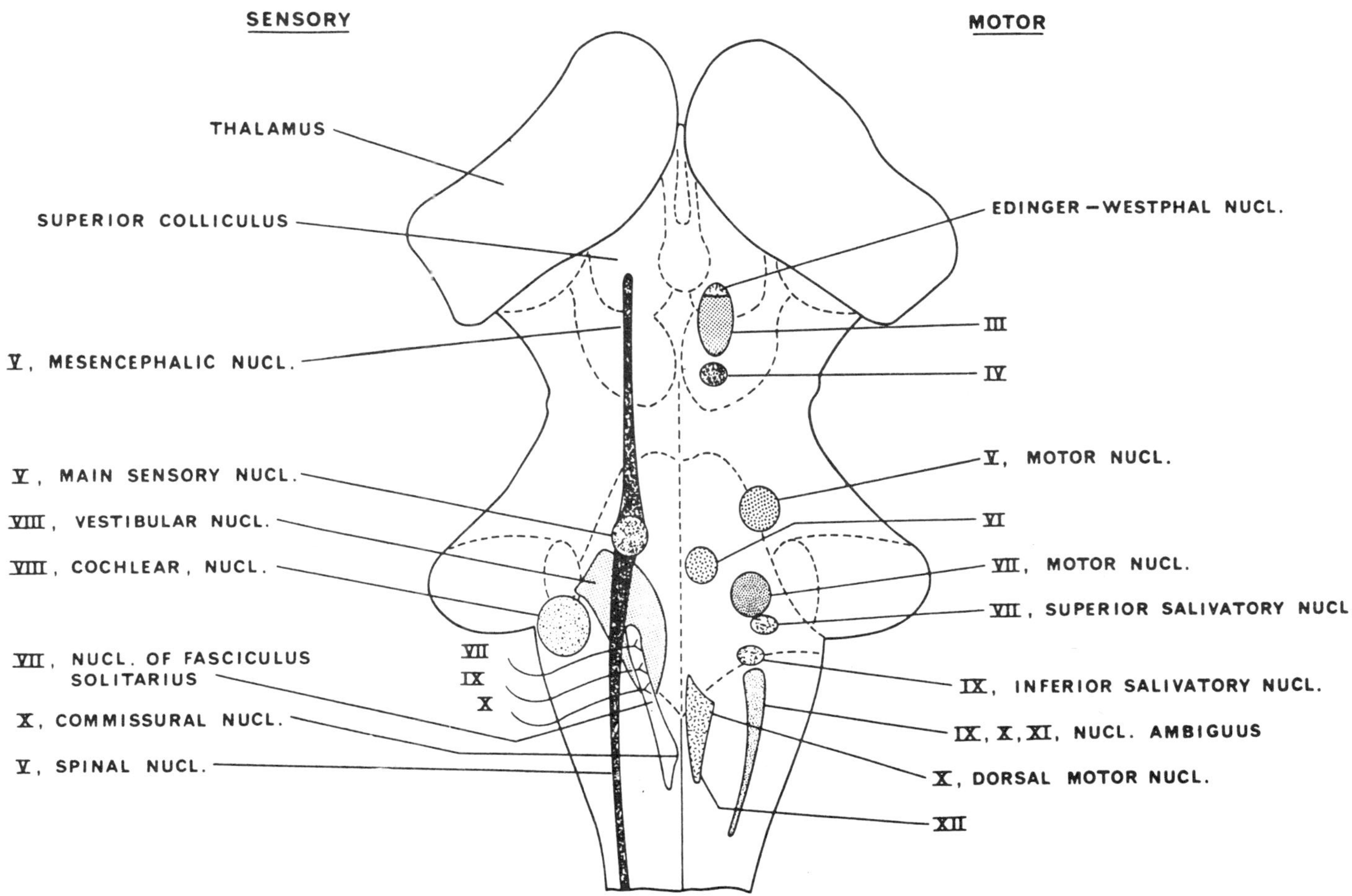

Fig. 2.4. Dorsal view of brain stem illustrating general locations of the sensory (on left) and motor (on right) nuclei of the cranial nerves.

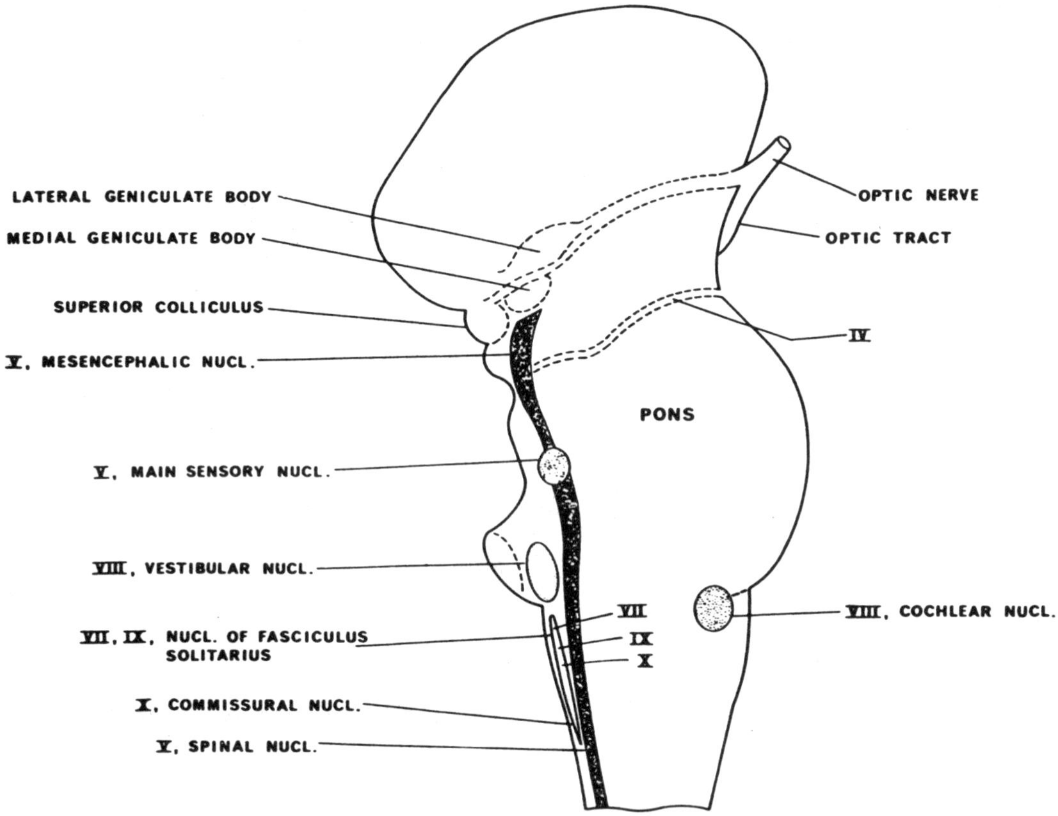

Fig. 2.5. Lateral view of brain stem showing locations of the sensory nuclei for cranial nerves IV through X. Dorsal aspect of brain stem is to the left in the figure.

Preganglionic GVE fibers of IX arise from the inferior salivatory nucleus, enter the tympanic plexus as the tympanic nerve, and then run in the lesser petrosal nerve to terminate within the otic ganglion. Postganglionic fibers originating within the otic ganglion transmit motor impulses which regulate secretion of the parotid salivary glands. A small component of IX, containing SVE preganglionic fibers, arises from the nucleus ambiguus to innervate the stylopharyngeus muscle via the stylopharyngeal nerve.

The pharyngeal branch of the glossopharyngeal nerve, which originates in the nucleus ambiguus, enters the pharyngeal plexus together with branches of cranial nerves X and V; thence motor fibers are sent to the voluntary pharyngeal muscles that are involved in the various reflexes listed below. Afferent impulses are conveyed in cranial

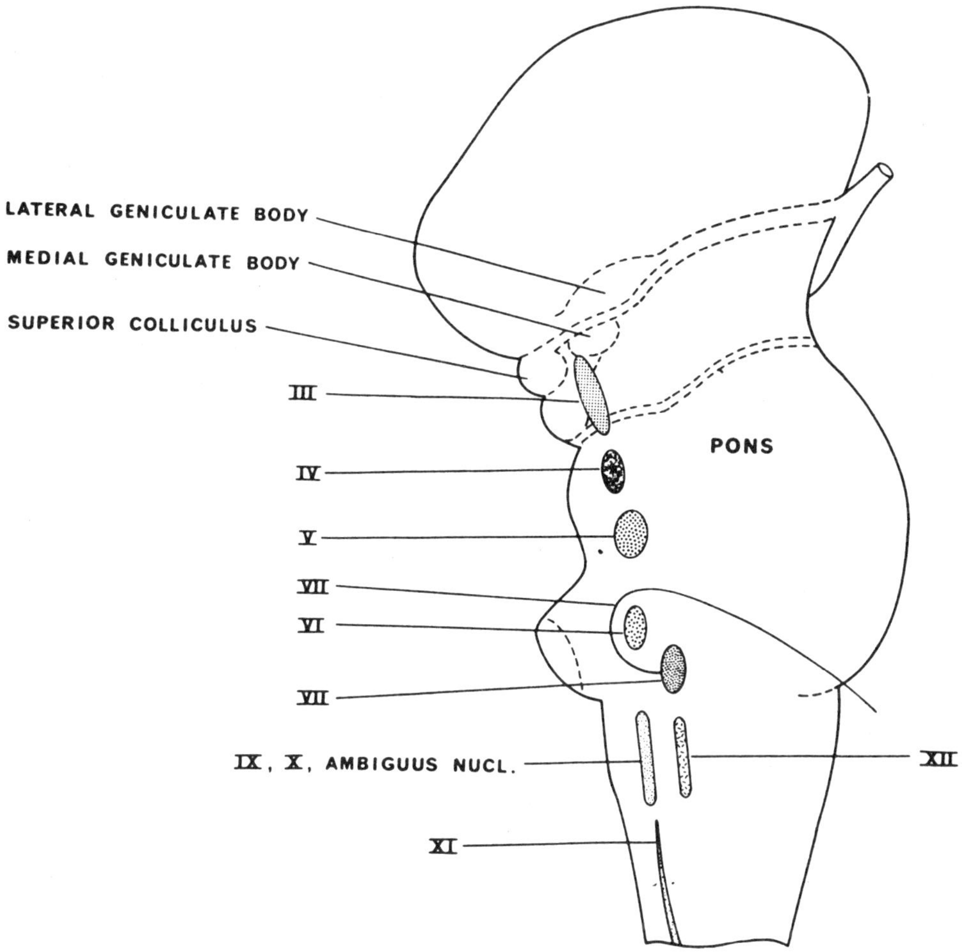

Fig. 2.6. Lateral view of brain stem showing the motor nuclei of cranial nerves III through XII. Dorsal aspect of brain stem is to the left in the figure.

nerves IX and X from both oral and respiratory mucosa, in addition to the proprioceptive impulses that arise from the various striated muscles involved.

Within the medulla oblongata also are found several neuroanatomically nonspecific "centers" which are involved in the functional integration of several complex and physiologically important reflexes. The afferent and efferent nerves which transmit impulses governing these reflexes involve pathways in the "vagal system" (or complex) of nerves; that is, portions of VII, IX, X, and XI. The reflexes listed here, among others, will be discussed fully in relation to the specific organ system (or systems) with which they are associated: (1) cardiac, vasomotor, carotid sinus, and carotid body reflexes, the respiratory and cough reflexes, the swallowing, gag, and vomiting reflexes.

The Pons. The pons (or pons varolii) contains a number of fiber tracts which relay impulses to both lower spinal centers as well as to higher brain centers. The pons also contains the sensory and motor nuclei of cranial nerves V through VIII.

Anatomically the pons consists of a very large mass of nerve cells, called the pontine nuclei, which is situated rostral to the medulla (Fig. 2.3). The cerebral peduncles are located anteriorly to the pons, whereas the pyramids emerge from its lower (or caudal) margin.

Externally, the ventral surface of the pons exhibits a thick band of transverse fibers which constitute the pons itself. The abducens nerve (VI) exits from the basal sulcus of the pons at its caudal border near the pyramids.

The aforementioned transverse fibers form compact lateral bundles, the middle cerebellar peduncles, and these fibers attach the pons to the cerebellum lying above it.

The small triangular region bounded by the middle cerebellar peduncle (or brachium pontis), the cerebellum, and the upper medulla is called the pontocerebellar angle, and both the facial nerve (VII) as well as the acoustic nerve (VIII) emerge from the brain stem in the region. The trigeminal nerve (V), one of the largest of the cranial nerves, is located in the brachium pontis near the middle of the lateral aspect of the pons.

The triangular rostral floor of the fourth ventricle is composed of the dorsal surface of the pons. Two bands which traverse the sides of this triangular region are the superior cerebellar peduncles (brachia conjunctive). A thin layer of tissue, the medullary velum, completes the roof of the fourth ventricle.

Internally, the pons exhibits two major subdivisions, dorsally the tegmentum, and ventrally the basilar portion. The roof of this part of the brain stem, which overlies the cavity of the fourth ventricle, has become functionally specialized and anatomically enlarged to form the cerebellum.

Within the central caudal region of the basilar portion of the pons are found the pyramidal (or corticospinal) tracts, surrounded by the gray matter of the pontine nuclei. The axons of these nuclei form transverse fiber bands which cross dorsally as well as ventrally to enter the pyramidal tracts, and these fibers also enter the middle cerebellar peduncle where they course to the cerebellar cortex.

In transverse contact with the basilar portion of the pons is the medial lemniscus. The medial longitudinal lemniscus remains near the midline in the floor of the fourth ventricle; this band of fibers contains the tectospinal, the tectobulbar, and the vestibulomesencephalic tracts.

Within the dorsal subdivision of the pons, the tegmentum, the trapezoid body is found as a ventral band of decussating fibers. A small ovoid nucleus, the superior olive, lies dorsolateral to the trapezoid body.

Just dorsal to the superior olive and medial to the nucleus of the spinal root of the trigeminal nerve (V) is found the motor nucleus of the facial nerve (VII). Prior to emerging from the brain stem, the fibers of VII form a loop, the genu of the facial nerve, and along its course this nerve passes just caudal to the nucleus of the abducens nerve (VI).

Vestibular nuclei are present in the lateral portions of the floor of the fourth ventricle. At this level of the brain stem the individual nuclei are called the lateral and superior vestibular nuclei instead of medial and spinal (inferior), as these nuclei are called in the medulla.

In sections made at the lower level of the pons at its junction with the cerebellum, the following paired cerebellar nuclei usually are seen. For convenience these nuclei may be summarized here:

1. *The fastigial nuclei* are situated in the midline on the roof of the fourth ventricle near the vermis. Their afferent fibers arise in the flocculonodular lobe of the cerebellum. Efferent fibers run to the vestibular nuclei in the fastigiobulbar tract.

2. *The globose nuclei* are small groups of cells located immediately lateral to the fastigial nuclei. Afferent fibers course to these nuclei from the paleocerebellum. Efferent fibers from the globose nuclei pass to the red nucleus via the superior cerebellar peduncle.

3. *The emboliform nuclei* are elongated cellular masses found between the globose and dentate nuclei. Their afferent and efferent fibers are similar to the globose nuclei.

4. *The dentate nuclei* are the largest, most lateral of the cerebellar nuclei. Afferent fibers reach this structure from the paleocerebellar and neocerebellar cortex. Efferent fibers run to the red nuclus and the ventrolateral nucleus of the thalamus via the superior cerebellar peduncle.

In the middle region of the pons the basilar portion widens and thickens, while the pyramidal tracts become dispersed into separate fascicles. The longitudinal corticopontine tracts intermingle with the pyramidal fibers in this region; these important motor fibers descend from the frontal, temporal, parietal, and occipital lobes of the cerebral cortex to synapse with cells of the pontine nuclei.

Within the dorsolateral portion of the tegmentum lie two oval nuclei: the superior sensory nucleus of the trigeminal nerve (V) is situated laterally, while the motor (masticator) nucleus of the trigeminal nerve is located medially. Small branches of this nerve run dorsally as the mesencephalic root of V, whereas trigeminal fibers emerging from the surface of the pons pass through the middle cerebellar peduncle.

The four cranial nerves associated with the pons now may be discussed individually:

The Vestibulocochlear Nerve (VIII). The vestibulocochlear nerve contains only special somatic afferent (SSA) fibers; it is composed of two main divisions, the cochlear and auditory.

The cochlear division of VIII arises from sensory cells located within the cochlear duct of the inner ear. The cochlear nerve originates from the bipolar neurons of the

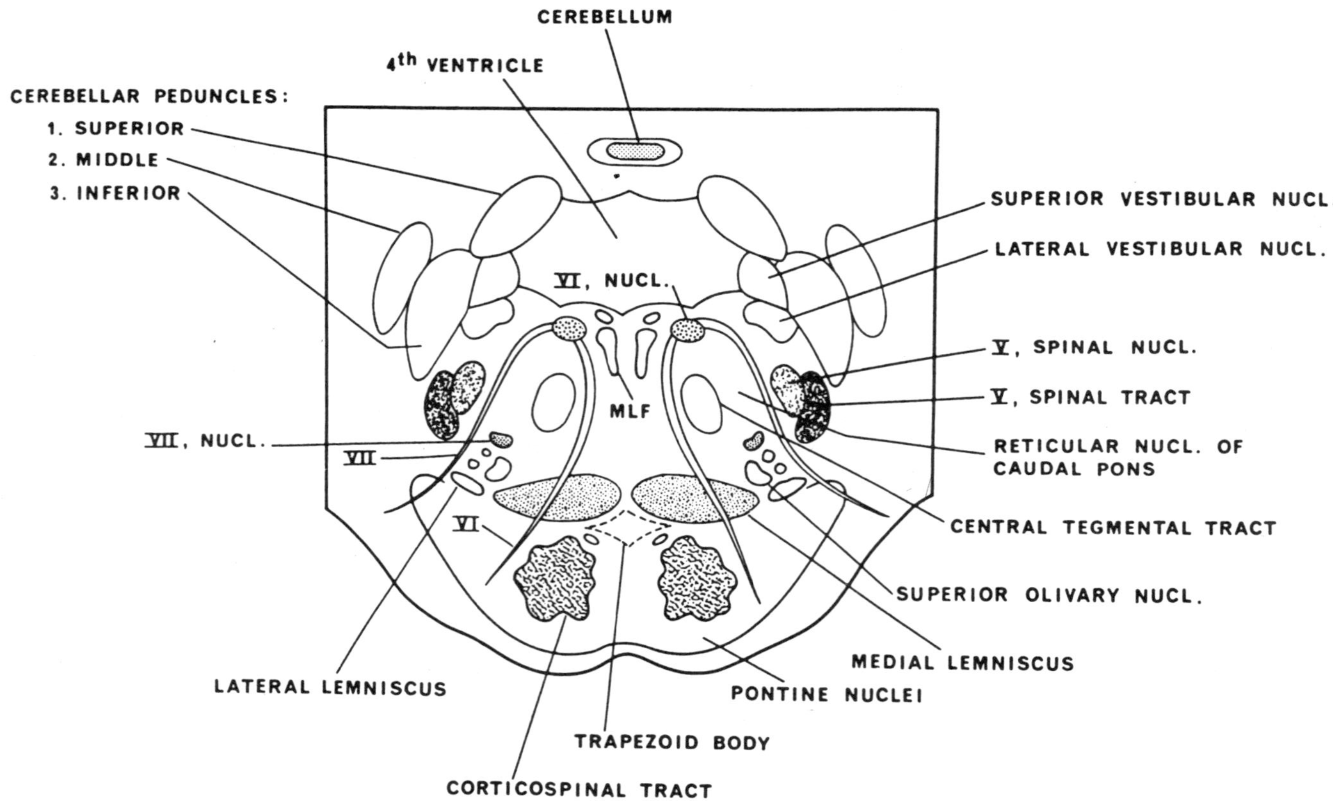

Fig. 2.7. The pons in cross section at the level of the abducens nucleus. The dorsal region (i.e., the tegmentum) contains the reticular formation, ascending and descending tracts, as well as cranial nerve nuclei. The ventral region contains large bundles of corticofugal fibers, the pontine nuclei, and transverse pontine fibers which constitute the middle cerebellar peduncle. MLF = medial longitudinal fasciculus; NUCL = nucleus. The cranial nerves and their nuclei are indicated by Roman numerals.

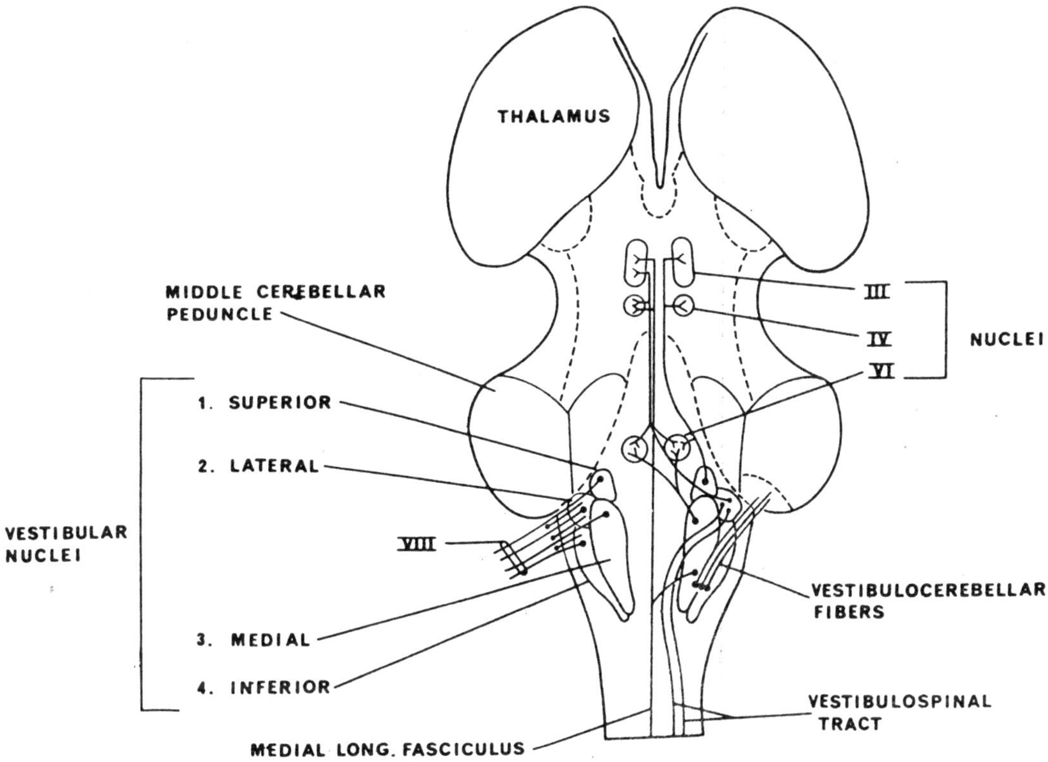

Fig. 2.8. The central connections and some projections of the vestibular nuclei on a dorsal view of the brain stem.

spiral ganglion, and the central processes of these cells terminate within the cochlear nuclei of the medulla.

The vestibular branch of VIII forms the vestibular nerve. The peripheral branches of this nerve receive proprioceptive impulses from hair cells located within the maculae of the utricle and saccule as well as the cristae of the three semicircular canals of the inner ear. The bipolar neurons of the vestibular nerve originate in the vestibular ganglion of the upper medulla-pontine region.

Further details of the neuroanatomic connections and functions of the vestibulocochlear nerve will be presented subsequently in relation to its roles in the maintenance of equilibrium as well as hearing.

The Facial Nerve (VII). The facial nerve has four major components: First, general visceral afferent (GVA) fibers which originate in the geniculate ganglion and receive impulses related to deep sensations from the facial region; these impulses are conducted in fibers which are components of the nervous intermedius. Second, special visceral afferent (SVA) fibers pass centrally from peripheral exteroceptors (taste buds) that are located on the anterior two-third of the tongue. Their dendrites originate in neurons whose cell bodies are located in the geniculate ganglion, and pass to the tongue via the intermediate and lingual nerves as well as the chorda tympani. The central axons terminate in the nucleus solitarius. Third, general visceral efferent (GVE) fibers of VII or preganglionic parasympathetic fibers, which are components of the nervus intermedius. These fibers originate in the superior salivatory nucleus and synapse with postganglionic neurons in the submandibular and pterygopalatine ganglia. Fourth, special visceral efferent (SVE) fibers arise from nerve cell bodies in the motor nucleus of VII. These innervate the muscles of the scalp and face, including the platysma, stylohyoid, and posterior digastric muscles.

The special visceral efferent division of VII is considered to be the facial nerve proper, and this nerve subserves all movements concerned with facial expression, and through its motor action on the orbicularis oculi muscles, the facial nerve also closes the eyelids.

The Abducens Nerve (VI). The abducens nerve has general somatic afferent (GSA) fibers which receive impulses from proprioceptive and organs located within the lateral rectus muscles of the eyes. General somatic efferent (GSE) fibers, arising in the abducens nucleus, provide motor innervation to the lateral rectus muscles.

The Trigeminal Nerve (V). The trigeminal nerve has two functional components. First, GSA fibers receive impulses from exteroceptors that are located within the skin of the face, orbit, and scalp as well as in the mucous membranes of the mouth and nasal cavity. The neurons of this portion of V arise in the semilunar ganglion. Proprioceptive fibers of the trigeminal nerve receive impulses from neuromuscular spindles located within the muscles involved in mastication; the cell bodies of these fibers are located within the mesencephalic nucleus of the trigeminal nerve.

SVE fibers from the masticator (or motor) nucleus in the lateral tegmentum of the pons enter the mandibular branch and portis minor of the trigeminal nerve to innervate the temporal, masseter, and medial as well as the lateral pterygoid muscles in addition to the tensor veli palatini, tensor tympani, mylohyoid, and the anterior belly of the digastric muscles.

The Mesencephalon or Midbrain. The midbrain forms a short junction between the pons and diencephalon. Within the midbrain, the small cerebral aqueduct connects the third and fourth ventricles.

Externally, the lower ventral surface of the mesencephalon is made up of two bundles of fibers, the basis pendunculi cerebri or crura cerebri which are separated by the deep interpeduncular space or fossa. At its junction with the cerebral hemisphere above, each peduncle of the crura cerebri is traversed by the optic tract. Caudally, the peduncles run directly into the basilar portion of the pons, and contain the corticospinal, corticopontine, and corticobulbar tracts. These descending (motor) fiber tracts pass from the cerebral cortex to the pons and they form the longitudinal fasciculus of that structure. The oculomotor nerves (III) emerge from each side of the interpeduncular fossa and appear at the surface at the transverse groove between midbrain and pons.

The dorsal surface of the midbrain has four rounded protuberances, the corpora quadrigemina. The pair of rostral elevations are called the superior calliculi, whereas the smaller caudol pair are the inferior colliculi. The trochlear nerves (IV) exit just posterior to the inferior colliculi.

Internally, the midbrain is divided into three regions: the ventrolateral portion or basis pedunculi (crus cerebri); the tegmentum, similar to the pontine tegmentum; and the tectum or roof, which lies just above the cerebral aqueduct and forms the quadrigeminal plate.

Within the lower half of the midbrain, each crus cerebri contains in its central portion the pyramidal tract, on each side of which lie corticopontine fibers. The substantia nigra, a pigmented (brownish) area of gray matter, lies between the peduncles and the tegmentum (Fig. 2.9).

Centrally, the tegmentum contains the decussation of the superior cerebellar peduncle. The medial lemniscus is found more laterally in this region of the brain stem, and its outer border is adjacent to the fibers of the lateral spinothalamic tract. Dorsal to the spinothalamic fibers, the lateral lemniscus contains the ascending fibers of the special sensory pathway that is involved in hearing. A nucleus of the inferior colliculus lies beneath each of these structures in the tectal region. Fibers that arise within the inferior colliculus, as well as those of the lateral lemniscus, run to the medial geniculate body by way of the brachium of the inferior colliculus. Consequently this brachium is the pathway whereby sensory impulses arising in the cochlea are transmitted from the midbrain to their specific relay nucleus in the thalamus.

Both the rubrospinal and tectospinal tracts originate within the mesencephalon. The cell bodies of each rubrospinal tract lie within the red nucleus of the mesencephalic tegmentum. Crossed fibers from the superior cerebellar peduncle pass into as well as around this nucleus; some of these cerebellar fibers terminate within the red nucleus, whereas others pass rostrally to the thalamus. The tectospinal tract arises from the nucleus of the superior colliculus. Both of these tracts undergo decussation near their points of origin in the midbrain. The rubrospinal tract crosses in the ventral tegmental decussation (decussation of Forel), whereas the tectospinal tract crosses the midline in the dorsal tegmental decussation (fountain decussation of Meynert).

The relationships between the midbrain and the two cranial nerves which originate within this region of the brain stem are as follows.

The Trochlear Nerve (V). The nucleus of the trochlear nerve is situated near the medial longitudinal fasciculus and ventral to the central gray matter in the region of the inferior colliculus. This cranial nerve contains general somatic afferent (GSA) fibers

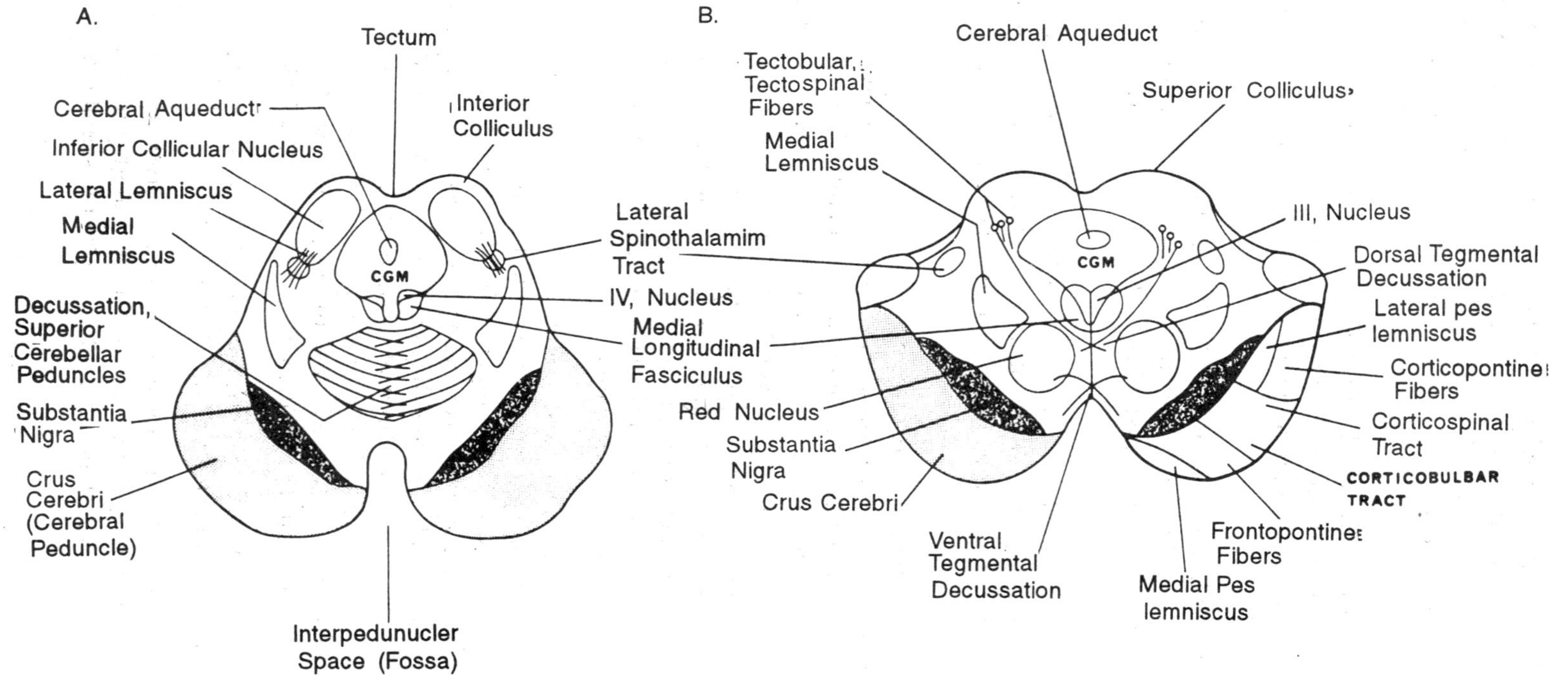

Fig. 2.9. A. Transverse section of the midbrain at the level of the inferior colliculi, CGM = central gray matter. **B.** Transverse section through the midbrain at the level of the superior colliculi. The particular regions of the cerebral peduncle are indicated within the heavy outline on the right side of this figure.

which innervate the proprioceptive neuromuscular spindles in the superior oblique muscle. General somatic efferent (GSE) fibers arise in the trochlear nucleus and provide motor innervation to the superior oblique muscle of the eye.

The Oculomotor Nerve (III). The nuclear complex of the oculomotor nerve is situated ventrally in the central gray matter adjacent to the medial longitudinal fasciculus. The root fibers of this cranial nerves pass through and around the red nucleus, then converge at their exit within the interpeduncular fossa.

The oculomotor nerve contains GSA fibers which transmit proprioceptive impulses from the ocular muscles (i.e., the superior, middle, and inferior rectus muscles and the

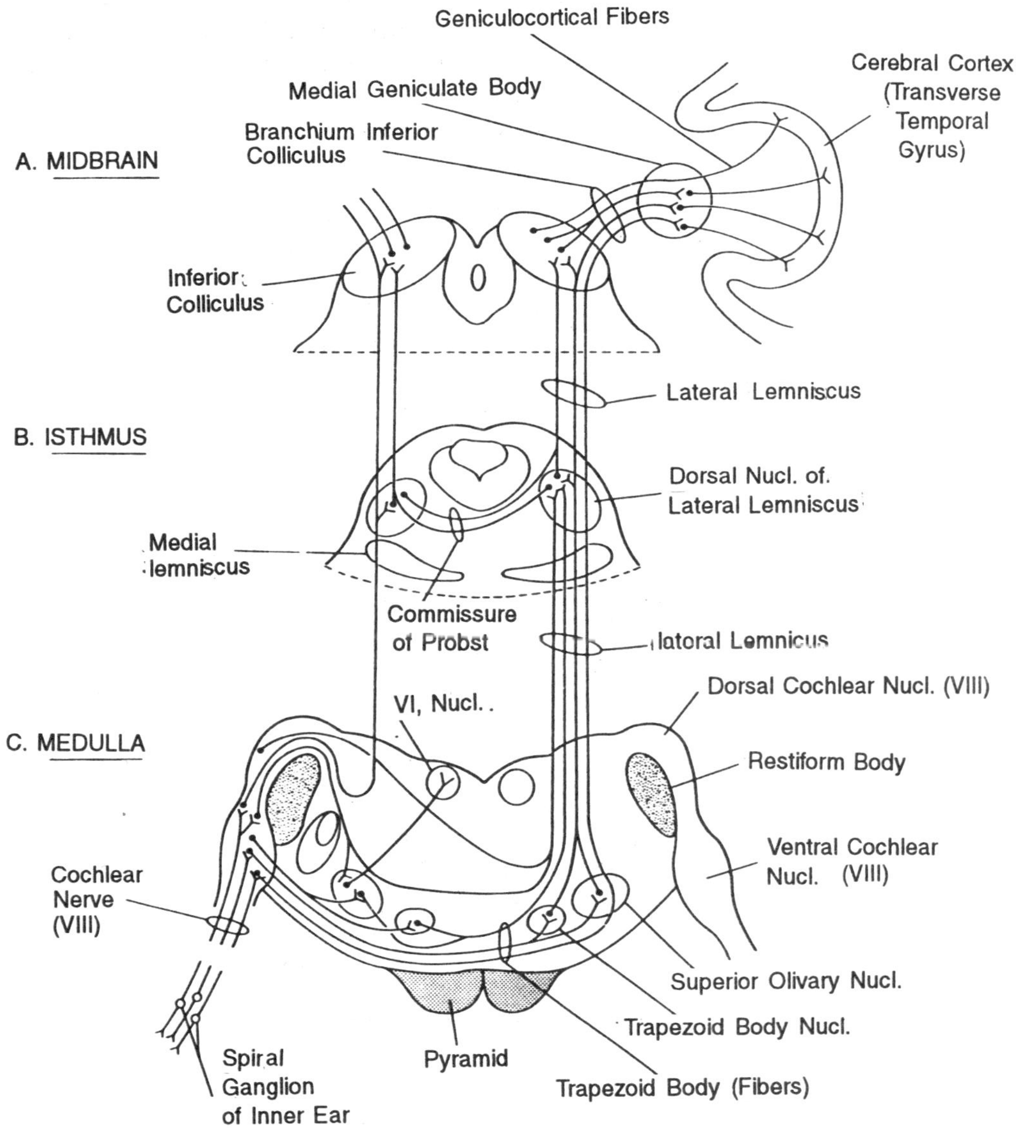

Fig. 2.10. The auditory pathway.

inferior oblique muscle). GSE fibers of the oculomotor nerve arise in the oculomotor nucleus and provide motor innervation for the same four pairs of ocular muscles. The parasympathetic component of III consists of preganglionic general visceral efferent fibers which arise in the accessory oculomotor nucleus (Edinger-Westphal nucleus) and which terminate in the ciliary ganglion.

The Diencephalon. The diencephalon forms the rostral end of the brain stem, and this structure consists of an oval mass of gray matter that is situated deep within the brain ventral and caudal to the frontal lobes of the cerebral hemispheres. The transitional region between the Mesencephalon and diencephalon is shown in Figure 2.11, whereas a cross section of the brain at the level of the diencephalon is presented in Figure 2.12. The fibers of the internal capsule demarcate the diencephalon laterally from the basal ganglia. Ventrally, the diencephalon extends from the optic chiasma to the mamillary bodies, which are included in this part of the brain stem. The choroid plexus of the third ventricle forms the roof of the diencephalon, and the two diencephalic halves are separated by the slitlike cavity of this ventricle.

Functionally the diencephalon provides a vital integrative and relay center for impulses passing between the cerebral cortex and the more caudal regions of the brain stem. Consequently, the diencephalon is associated closely with somatic as well as visceral sensory and motor functions. The sensory pathways of the lower centers of the brain stem as well as the reticular arousal system synapse at this level of the brain stem before they transmit (i.e., project) sensory impulses onward to the cerebral cortex. Furthermore,

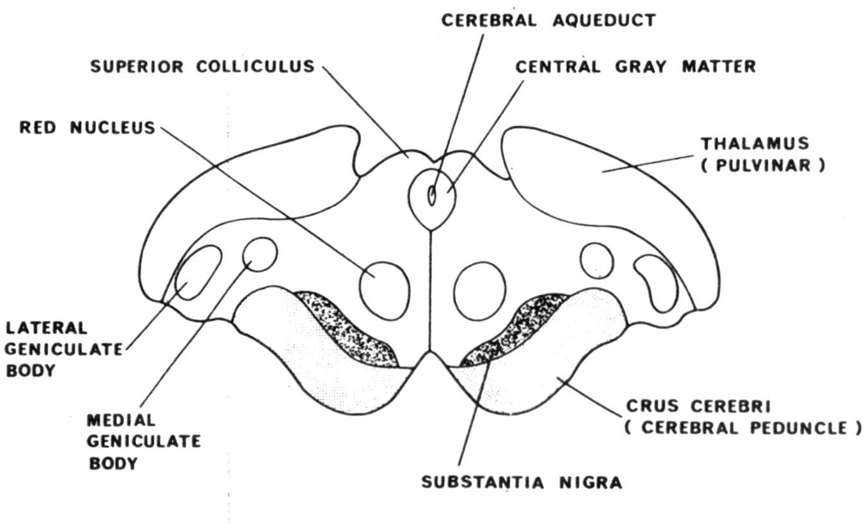

Fig. 2.11. Cross section of the midbrain at the mesencephalic-diencephalic level.

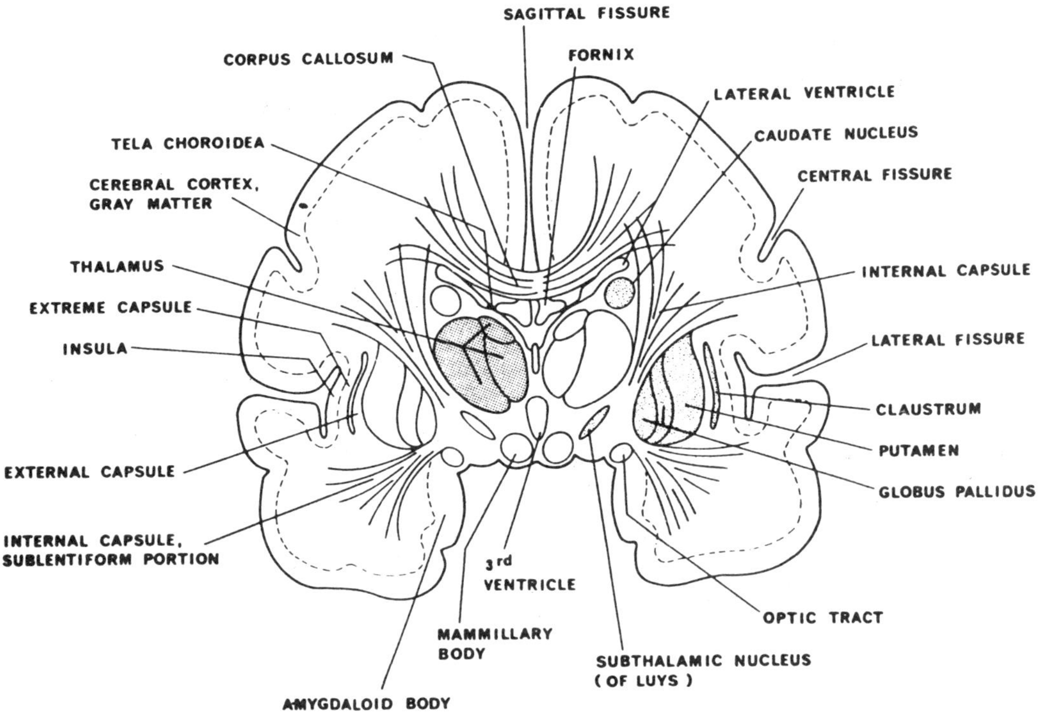

Fig. 2.12. Frontal section through the brain at the level of the diencephalon. The putamen and globus pallidus together make up the corpus striatum.

portions of the visceral sensory and visceral motor systems, in addition to the extrapyramidal system, are interconnected functionally within the diencephalon.

Anatomically, the diencephalon is divided into the epithalamus, thalamus proper (or dorsal thalamus), hypothalamus, and subthalamus.

The Epithalamus. The epithalamus is the most dorsal division of the diencephalon and is composed of the pineal body, the habenula, the habenular commissure, the posterior commissure, and the striae medullaris.

The pineal body (epiphysis) is a small mass of tissue that projects on a stalk from the dorsal roof of the diencephalon in the vicinity of the posterior commissure. The pineal body, or pineal gland, is composed principally of glial cells, although some parenchymal cells, presumably secretory in function, also are present.

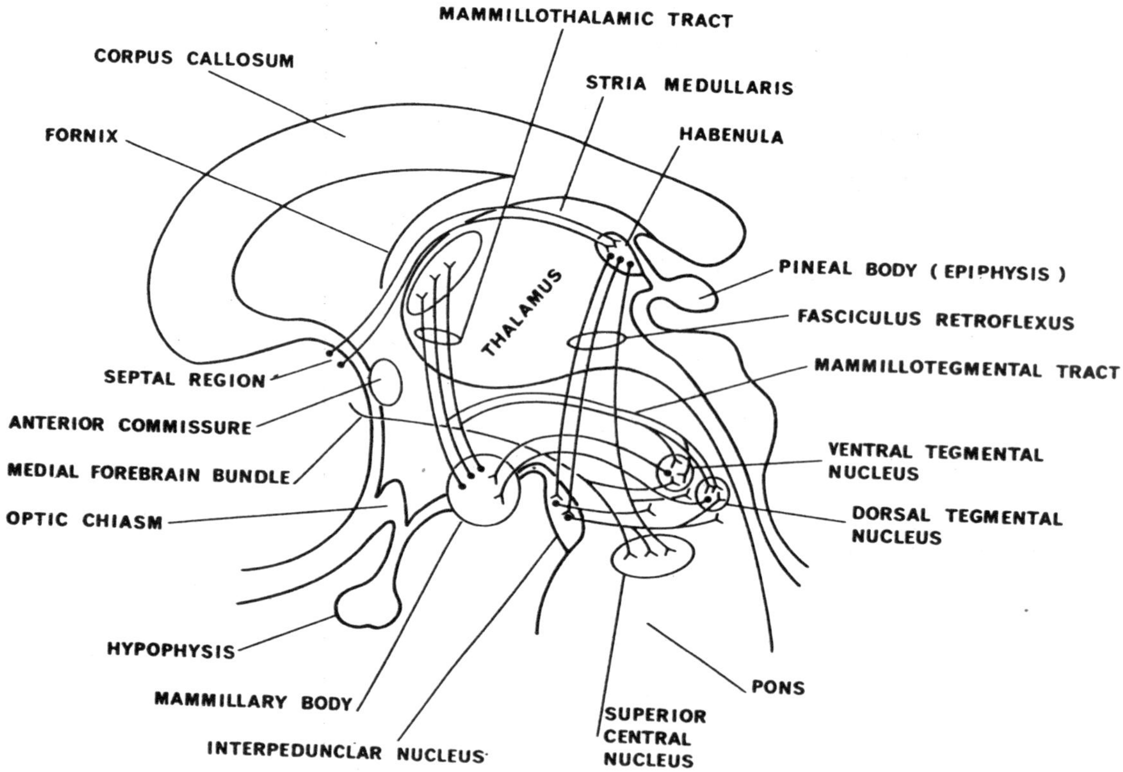

Fig. 2.13. The limbic pathways that interconnect medial midbrain structures to the telencephalon and diencephalon.

The habenular trigone is a small concavity located just forward of each superior colliculus. The trigone region contains the habenular nuclei; these nuclear structures are connected by nerve fibers to the striae medullaris and are interconnected with each other by fibers of the habenular commissure. Afferent fibers to the habenular nuclei originate from the olfactory and septal nuclei as well as in the lateral hypothalamus, and these fibers are carried in the striae medullaris. The habenulopeduncular tract (retroflex tract of Meynert, fasciculus retroflexus) carries efferent fibers that originate within the habenula and terminate in the intrapeduncular nucleus of the midbrain. From here, postsynaptic fibers descend to synapse once again in the nuclei of certain cranial nerves. The habenular nuclei thus appear to be relay stations for olfactory impulses.

The posterior commissure is located ventrally to the base of the pineal body, and this structure consists of a small mass of decussating nerve fibers of the superior colliculi or tectum which traverse the midline on the dorsal side of the cerebral aqueduct (or aqueduct of Sylvius), and which are involved in the visual reflex.

The Thalamus. The thalamus proper functions as a vital way station for the receipt of sensory impulses which arise within receptors that are located throughout the body (with the exception of olfactory impulses). From the thalamus, this broad range of sensory information is relayed or projected to appropriate areas of the cerebral cortex. In addition, the thalamus integrates and transmits nerve impulses to subcortical areas of the brain and receives afferent impulses that originate within the cerebral cortex, cerebellum, and basal ganglia.

The thalamus is the dorsal portion of the diencephalon and it is composed of two lateral avoid masses of gray matter that are joined together in the midline by the massa intermedia, a short isthmus of gray matter. Each lateral half of the thalamus is embedded deeply within the corresponding cerebral hemisphere, and is, bounded laterally by the internal capsule and medially by the wall of the third ventricle. The roof of the thalamus is formed by the choroid plexus of the third ventricle.

The rostral (or anterior) end of the thalamus is relatively narrow and lies close to the midline. This region delimits the posterior end of the interventricular foramen. The caudal end of the thalamus is somewhat larger, and its medial portion is called the pulvinar. The pulvinar overhangs the superior colliculi. An oval swelling, the lateral geniculate body, is located in this region. Note also in these figures the location of the medial geniculate body. Along the dorsolateral surface of the thalamus runs a groove known as the terminal sulcus which contains a band of fibers, the stria terminalis, which was discussed in the previous section.

The medial surface of the thalamus forms the lateral wall of the third ventricle, and here the aforementioned massa intermedia connects the medial surfaces of each half of the thalamus.

The term thalamic radiation indicates the tracts of nerve fibers that emerge from the lateral surface of the thalamus to enter the internal capsule, thence to terminate in the cerebral cortex. The external medullary lamina, located on the lateral surface of the thalamus adjacent to the internal capsule, is a layer of myelinated fibers. The internal medullary lamina is a vertical partition of white matter which bifurcates anteriorly and thus divides the gray matter of the thalamus into anterior, medial, and lateral portions.

The thalamus contains a large number of individual nuclei whose anatomic and functional relationships are exceedingly complex. Consequently there is some disagreement among various authorities as to the nomenclature, classification (anatomic as well as functional), and subdivisions of the various thalamic nuclei.

By definition, a specific thalamocortical nucleus is one which receives anatomically well-defined afferent nerve fibers and which is connected to a clearly delineated area of the cerebral cortex by well-defined efferent thalamic tracts. Included within this category

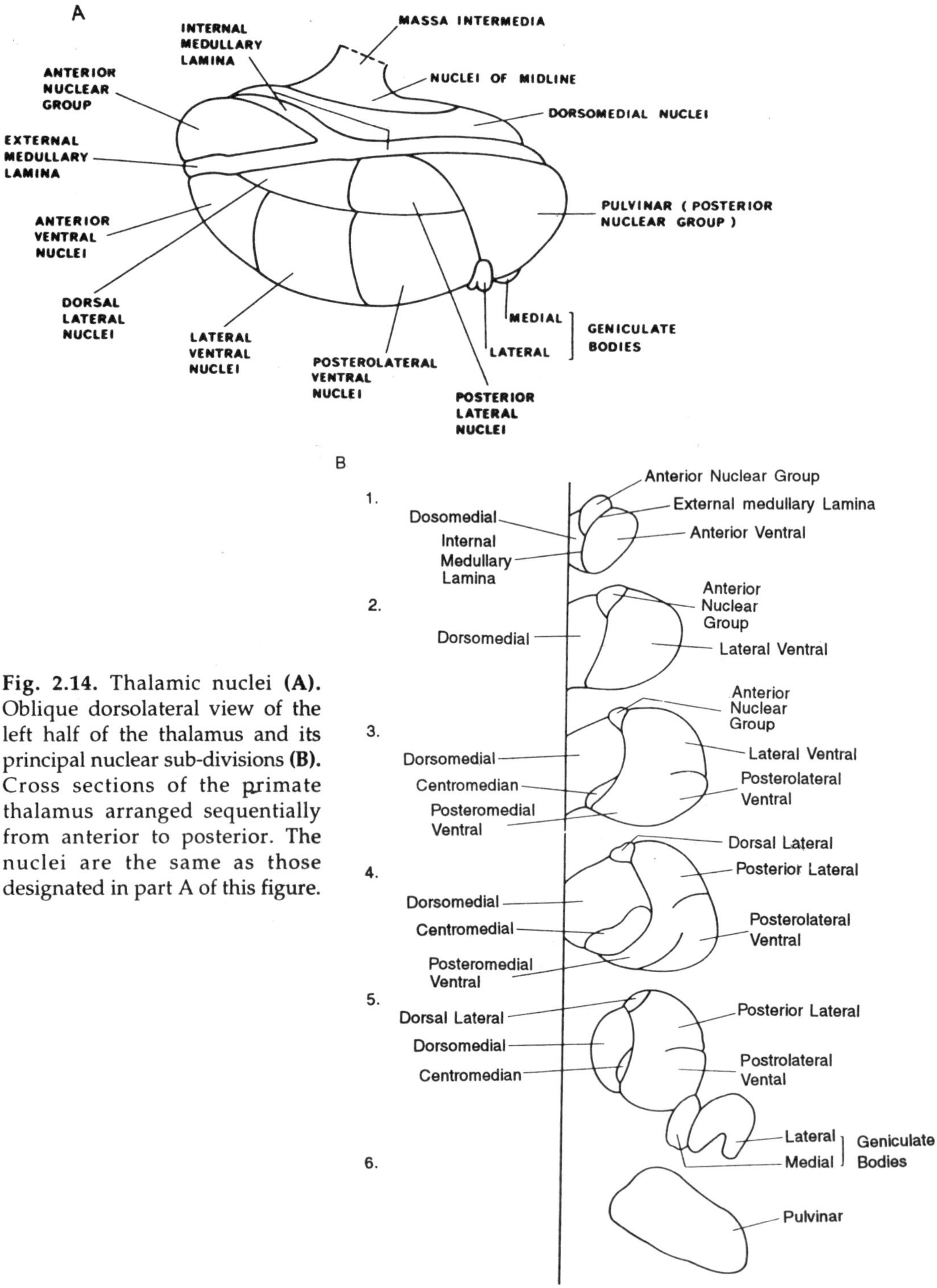

Fig. 2.14. Thalamic nuclei **(A).** Oblique dorsolateral view of the left half of the thalamus and its principal nuclear sub-divisions **(B).** Cross sections of the primate thalamus arranged sequentially from anterior to posterior. The nuclei are the same as those designated in part A of this figure.

are the principal thalamic sensory relay nuclei (e.g., certain of the lateral nuclear group as well as the medial and lateral geniculate bodies).

The nonspecific projections nuclei of the thalamus in contrast to the specific projection nuclei have less well-defined afferent and efferent connections, anatomically speaking. For example, the midline and medial nuclear groups are assigned to the category of nonspecific projection nuclei. The majority of the nonspecific nuclei also are considered to fall within a subcortical classification as they do not project to the cortex or their cortical projection has not been determined (e.g., the midline, centromedian, and reticular nuclei).

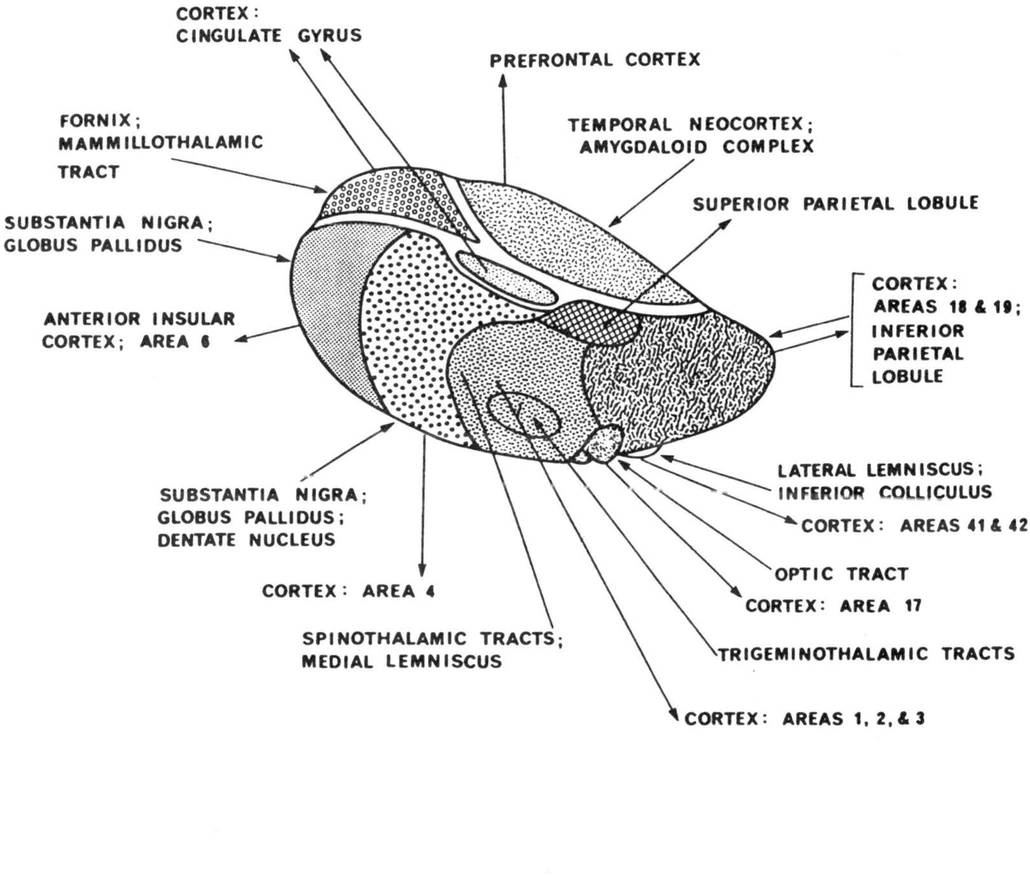

Fig. 2.15. Major thalamic projections to the cerebral cortex. The majority of cortical areas reciprocally project fibers back to the thalamic nuclei whence they receive fibers, however not all of these have been indicated. The shadings used in this figure correspond to those in Figure 2.17, and thus indicate which regions of the thalamus project to which specific cortical areas.

Table 2.1
Principal Thalamic Nuclei

Neuroanatomic Classification	*Functional Classification*	*Principal Connections Afferent Fibers*	*Efferent Fibers*	*General Function(s)*
1. Anterior Nuclei		From hypothalamus via mammillothalamic tract (of Vicq d'Azyr); higher order olfactory neurons	To cingulate gyrus of cerebral cortex	Part of circuit involved in limbic system (qv); convey olfactory impulses
a. Anteromedial	Nonspecific projection			
b. Anterodorsal	Nonspecific projection			
c. Anteroventral	Nonspecific projection			
2. Midline Nuclei				
a. Cell groups beneath lining of wall, 3rd ventricle	Nonspecific projection	From spinothalamic, trigeminothalamic tracts, medial lemniscus, reticular formation, other thalamic nuclei, hypothalamus	To hypothalamus and cortex (few to anterior rhinencephalon); basal ganglia (?); other thalamic nuclei	Center for integrating crude visceral and somatic sensations
b. Massa intermedia	Nonspecific projection			
3. Medial Nuclei				
a. Scattered cells in internal medullary lamina (intralaminar nuclei)	Nonspecific projection	From prefrontal cortex, septal areas, basal ganglia, and other thalamic nuclei	To prefrontal cortex	Integrate somatic and visceral sensory impulses before projecting this information to cortex. Association center for synthesis of crude somatic sensations.
b. Dorsomedial	Nonspecific projection	From thalamic nuclei, prefrontal cortex, basal ganglia	To prefrontal cortex	
c. Centromedian	Nonspecific projection	From putamen, caudate nucleus, other thalamic nuclei	To basal ganglia, other thalamic nuclei (?)	Intrathalamic integrating center (?)
4. Lateral Nuclei				
a. Anterior ventral	Nonspecific projection	From globus pallidus via thalamic fasciculus	To corpus striatum; cortex (frontal lobe)	

(Contd.)

Neuroanatomic Classification	Functional Classification	Principal Connections Afferent Fibers	Efferent Fibers	General Function(s)
b. Lateral ventral	Specific projection	From cerebellum via superior cerebellar peduncle; globus pallidus via thalamic fasciculus	To cerebral cortex (pre-motor areas) via posterior limb of internal capsule	Part of circuit involved in voluntary motor functions
c. Posterolateral ventral	Specific projection	Termination of spinothalamic tracts, medial lemniscus	To sensory areas of cortex (postcentral gyrus) via post limb of internal capsule	Relay sensory impulses from trunk and limbs
d. Posteromedial ventral	Specific projection	Termination of secondary trigeminal and taste fibers		Relays sensory impulses from face
e. Dorsal lateral	Specific projection	From other thalamic nuclei; parietal lobe of cerebral cortex	To cerebral cortex (parietal lobe)	Primary sensory relay nuclei
f. Posterior lateral	Specific projection			
g. Reticular	Nonspecific projection	From entire cerebral cortex, other thalamic nuclei, reticular formation of brain stem	To other thalamic nuclei; tegmentum of midbrain	Functions controversial
5. Posterior Nuclei				
a. Pulvinar	Specific projection	From other thalamic nuclei, cerebral cortex (parietal, temporal, occipital lobes)	To cerebral cortex (parietal, temporal, occipital lobes)	Integrates auditory, visual, somatic impulses (?)
b. Medial geniculate	Specific projection	From brachium of inferior colliculus	To auditory cortex via sublenticular portion of internal capsule (bilateral projection)	Audition
c. Lateral geniculate	Specific projection	From optic tract (cranial nerve II)	To ipsilateral striate cortex via retrolenticular portion of internal capsule	Vision

Alternatively, the thalamic nuclei have been classified as relay nuclei, association nuclei, and nuclei that are connected principally with other subcortical areas (i.e., the diffuse conducting or projection system). The relay nuclei are the ventral groups of thalamic cells which transmit impulses to the cerebral cortex, e.g., the anterior ventral, the lateral ventral, and the posterolateral nuclei as well as the medial and lateral geniculate bodies. The association nuclei have afferent as well as efferent fiber connections with the cerebral cortex; however, no other specific ascending or descending connections are present. Included among the association nuclei are the anterior nuclear group, as well as the pulvinar, dorsal lateral, and posterior lateral nuclei. The subcortical nuclei of the diffuse conducting system include those nuclei which are located within the internal medullary lamina as well as upon the extreme lateral or medial aspects of the thalamus; e.g., the midline nuclei, the centromedian nucleus, and the reticular nuclei. These regions are termed diffuse projection nuclei because stimulation of any one of the thalamic areas

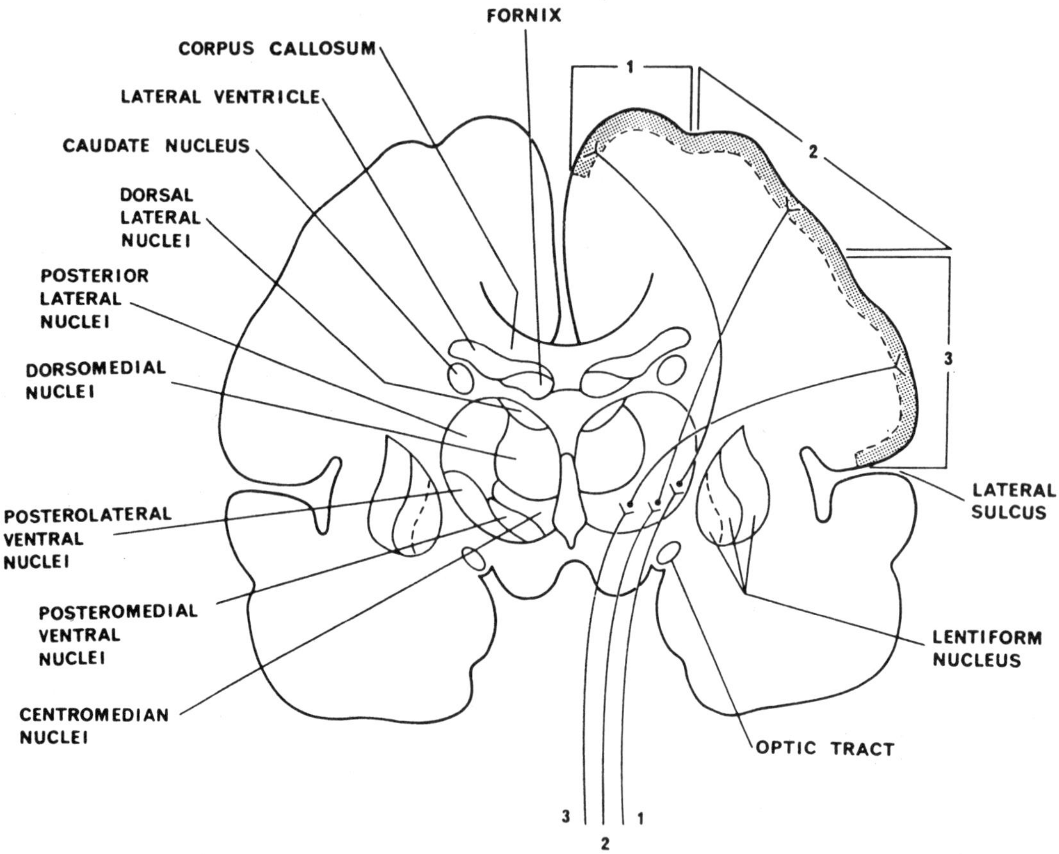

Fig. 2.16. The sensory tracts and their terminations in the lateral region of the thalamus as well as the fiber projections from these nuclei to the somesthetic cortex via the internal capsule. 1. Sensory fibres from lower extremity project to leg area of cortex. 2. Sensory fibers from upper extremity project to arm area of cortex. 3. Secondary trigeminal area projects to face area of cortex. Note that a snatial orientation of all fiber pathways is maintained at all levels of the nervous system.

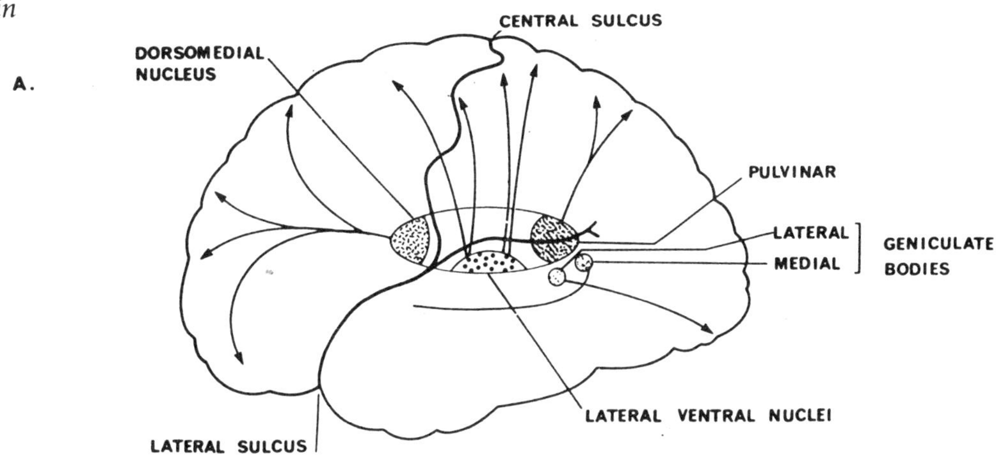

Fig. 2.17. A. The principal thalamocortical projections.

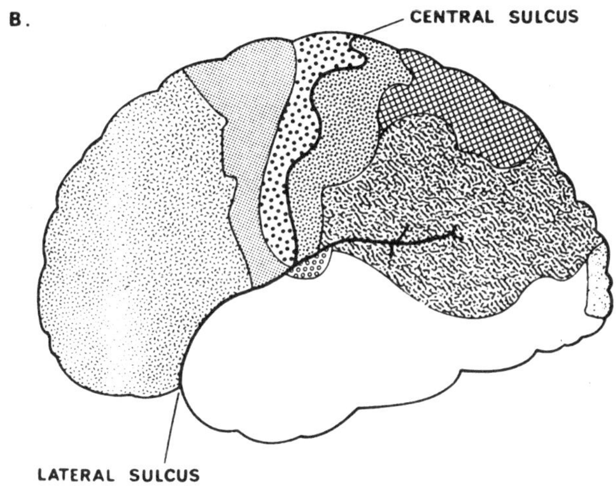

Fig. 2.17. B. Lateral surface of the left cerebral hemisphere indicating the cortical projection areas of the thalamic

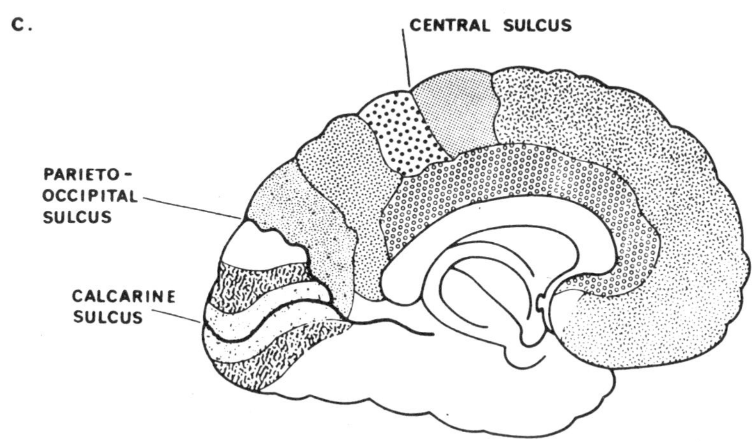

Fig. 2.17. C. Same, but viewed from the medial surface of the left hemisphere.

listed above causes a widespread conduction of impulses to the cerebral cortex together with recruitment and alerting of the subject. Consequently these diffuse projection nuclei are considered by some investigators to represent the thalamic portion of the ascending reticular activating system.

The functional attributes of the thalamus will be considered in somewhat greater however; it should be reiterated here that the thalamus serves as the major relay station for afferent impulses that arise in all sensory end organs throughout the body (excepting the olfactory end organs). Furthermore, the thalamus is the center in which integration of many sensory impulses takes place, and this region of the diencephalon appears to be related to the synthesis of visceral and crude somatic sensations which are perceived at the conscious level. In particular, the dorsomedial nuclei are believed to function as an association center for these crude sensations and also to provide the loci where sensations are integrated into subjective feelings that are either pleasant or unpleasant. The thalamus also appears to play a vital role in the integration and coordination of visceral as well as somatic motor responses. The ventromedial portion of the thalamus, including the reticular formation and the intralaminar nuclei, participate together with the reticular formation of the brain stem in the alerting and arousal responses.

Lastly, the lateral geniculate body of the thalamus is a critical relay station for visual impulses that arise within the retina of the eye and which are transmitted via this thalamic nucleus to the visual cortex. The visual pathway is depicted in Figure and discussed in greater detail in connection with the visual reflex. Similarly, the medial geniculate body has an essential physiologic role in the process of hearing, and the role of this nucleus also will be considered in further Chapter.

The Hypothalamus. Anatomically, the hypothalamic region of the diencephalon lies ventral to the hypothalamic sulcus and forms the floor as well as portions of the inferior lateral walls of the third ventricle. The following structures are included in the hypothalamus. First, the mamillary bodies are a pair of white masses that lie inferior to the gray matter which comprises the floor of the third ventricle. Second, the tuber cinereum forms a prominence immediately rostral to the mamillary bodies. Third, the infundibulum is a hollow columnar process that projects downward from the tuber cinereum to the posterior lobe of the hypophysis or pituitary gland. Fourth, is the optic chiasm.

As shown in Figure 2.20, the infundibulum continues into the neural or posterior lobe of the hypophysis. Collectively, the median eminence, the infundibulum, and the neural lobe of the pituitary gland comprise the neurohypophysis.

Each lateral half of the hypothalamus can be divided into an anterior supraoptic region, a tuberal region which lies just behind the supraoptic region, and a posterior mamillary region. The preoptic area is situated between the optic chiasm and the anterior commissure.

The hypothalamic nuclei are classified into four principal groups. First, the anterior nuclear group includes the paraventricular and supraoptic nuclei. Second, the lateral nucleus is composed of the lateral portion of the tuber cinereum. Third, the middle part

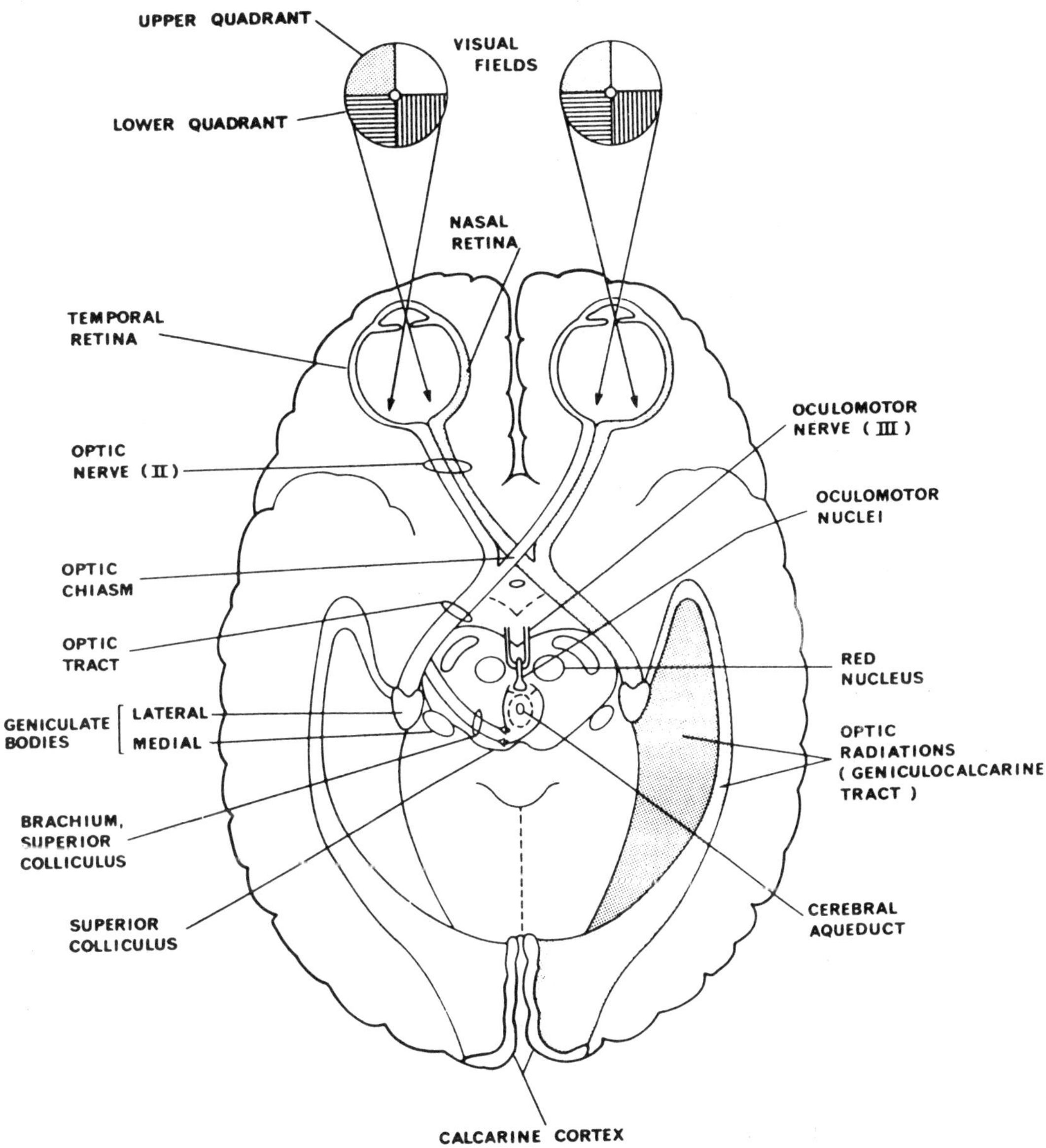

Fig. 2.18. The visual pathway as seen from the ventral aspect of the brain. Note particularly the pathways taken by the fibers of the optic nerves after they undergo partial decussation in the optic chiasm (shaded and unshaded areas).

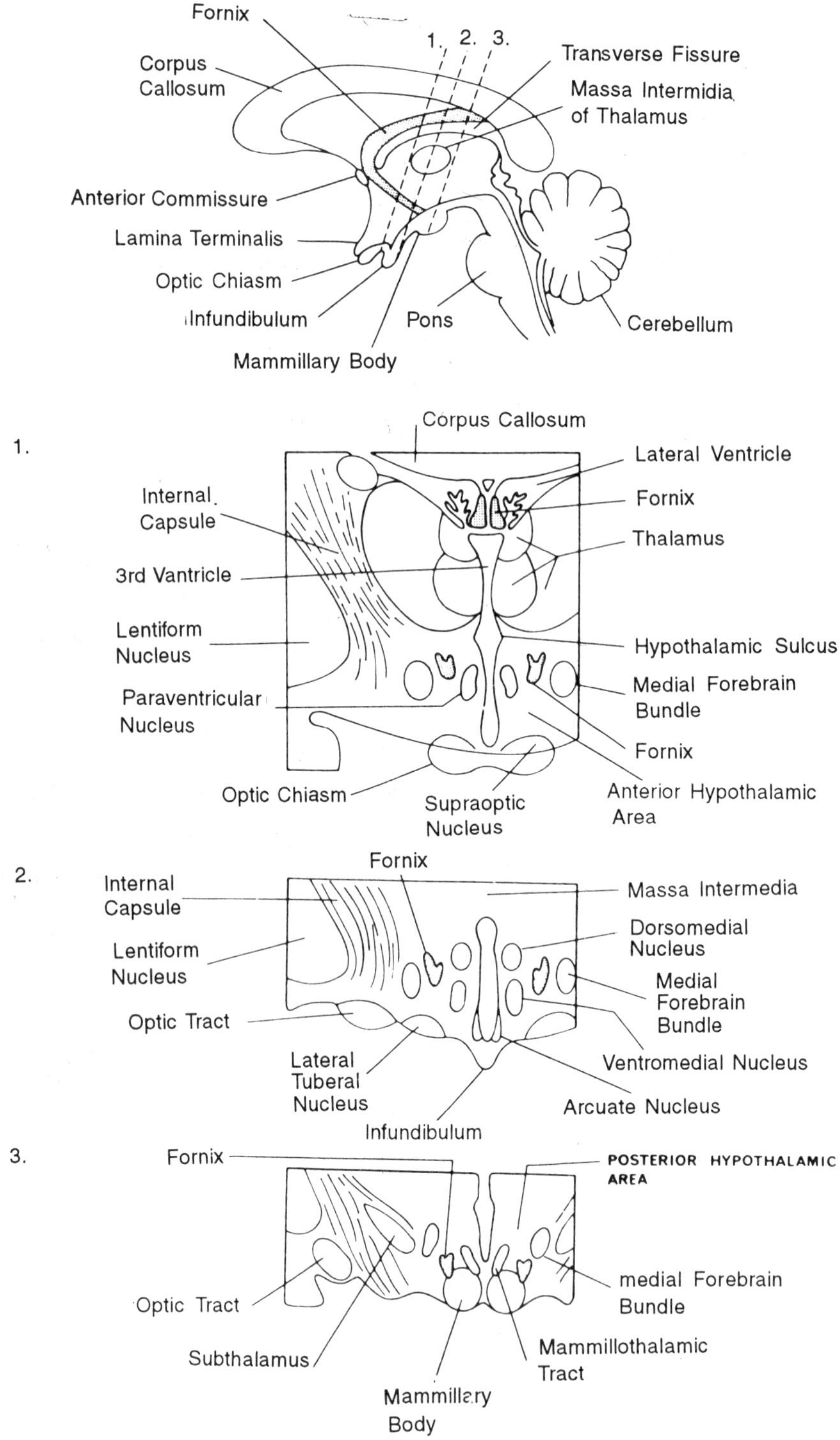

Fig. 2.19. At top, sagittal section through brain stem indicating the relationship of the hypothalamus to adjacent brain structures. Cuts 1, 2, and 3, indicated by dashed lines, are shown in transverse section in the three lower drawings. In all instances, the fornix has been shaded to facilitate comparison of the specific hypothalamic and other structures at each level.

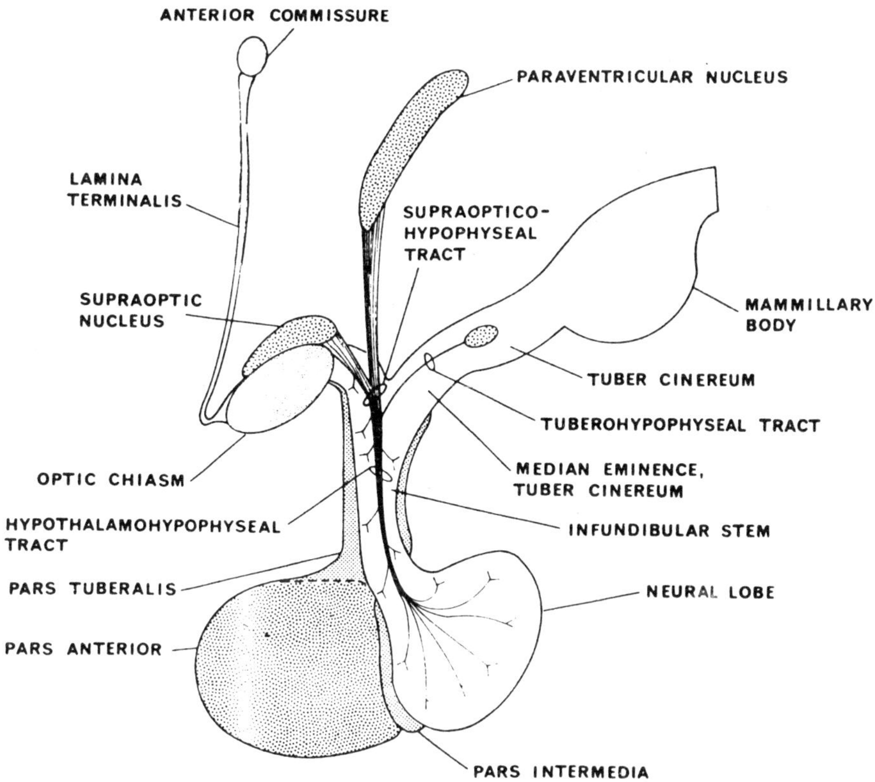

Fig. 2.20. Sagittal section through the hypophysis and hypothalamus illustrating the origins and distribution of the hypothalamohypophyseal tract.

of the hypothalamus contains the ventromedial nucleus. Fourth, the posterior nuclei include the medial and lateral mamillary nuclei. The cell bodies of the medial mamillary nucleus comprise the protuberance of the mamillary body.

The principal afferent and efferent connections of the hypothalamus to other brain structures are summarized in Table 2.2 an depicted in Figures 2.13, 2.20, and 2.22.

Functionally, the hypothalamus integrates a number of rather straightforward visceral reflexes and it also participates in the regulation of several more complex behavioral and emotional responses. The physiologic regulatory processes that are mediated by the hypothalamus are summarized in Table 2.3, and the particular roles of this structure in each of these processes will be discussed in context throughout the remainder of this book.

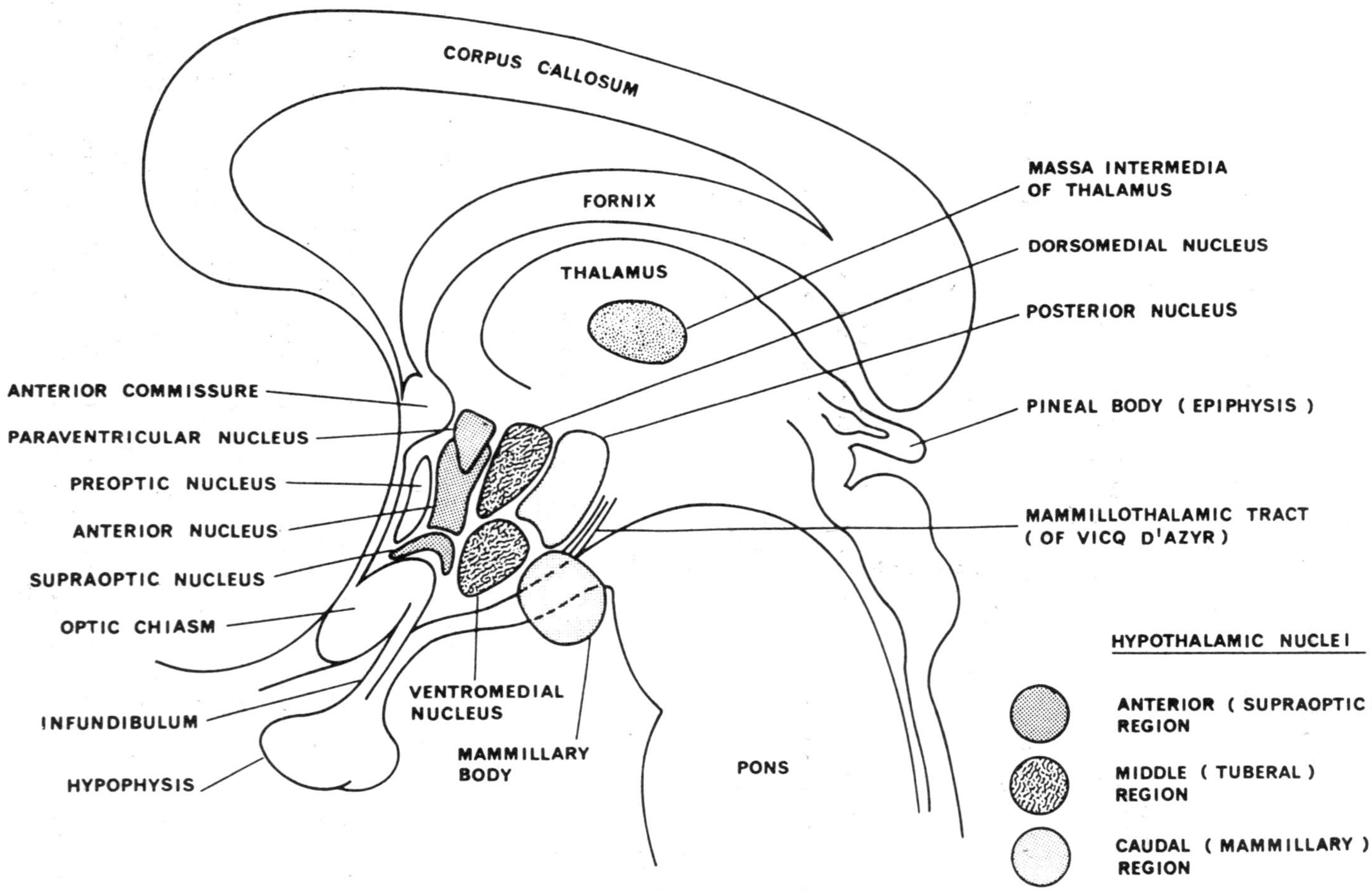

Fig. 2.21. Relationships among the medial hypothalamic nuclei. The shading code used for the three hypothalamic regions is given in the inset to the lower right of the figure.

Table 2.2
Major Afferent and Efferent Hypothalamic Connections

Name	*Remarks*
A. Afferent Pathways	
1. Medial forebrain bundle	Connects septal (or medial) olfactory area of brain with preoptic and hypothalamic areas. Also contains efferent (descending) fibers which connect hypothalamus to midbrain. Several hypothalamic nuclei involved, particularly the ventromedial nucleus.
2. Thalamohypothalamic fibers	From medial and midline thalamic nuclei.
3. Fornix	Connects hippocampus to anterior hypothalamus and mammillary nuclei; possibly others. Efferent fibers may be present. Largest fiber system of hypothalamus.
4. Stria Terminalis	Connects amygdala to hypothalamus.
5. Inferior mammillary peduncle	Connects tegmentum of midbrain with hypothalamus.
6. Pallidohypothalamic fibers	From lenticular nucleus to ventromedial hypothalamic nucleus.
7. Retinohypothalamic fibers	Fibers of optic nerve enter hypothalamus from optic chiasm.
B. Efferent Pathways	
1. Hypothalamohypophyseal tract (composed of supraoptico-hypophyseal and paraventriculo-hypophyseal tracts)	Connects supraoptic nuclei to infundibulum and neuro-hypophysis.
2. Mammillotegmental tract	Connects hypothalamus with reticular formation in tegmentum of midbrain.
3. Mammillothalamic tract (of Vicq d'Azyr)	Connects mammillary nuclei with anterior thalamic nuclei.
4. Periventricular system (includes dorsal fasciculus of Schütz)	Connects hypothalamus with midbrain; efferent fibers to spinal cord. Some afferent fibers from sensory pathways also present.
5. Tuberohypophyseal tract	Connects tuberal region of hypothalamus with neuro-hypophysis.

The Subthalamus. The ventral thalamus or subthalamus is the brain tissue which lies between the tegmentum of the midbrain and the dorsal thalamus. The hypothalamus is located medially and rostrally to the subthalamus, whereas the internal capsule is situated laterally. Caudally, the red nucleus and substantia nigra extend into the subthalamic region. The subthalamic nucleus (or subthalamic body of Luys) extends caudally to the lateral part of the red nucleus.

The subthalamic nucleus receives afferent fibers from the globus pallidus and thus forms a component of the efferent pathway from the corpus striatum. Located rostrally

Table 2.3
Hypothalamic Functions

Function	*Afferent Impulses to Hypothalamus*	*Hypothalamic Area Responsible for Integration of Function*
1. Control of Endocrine Secretion		
a) Catecholamines	Emotional stimuli, presumably via limbic system	Dorsomedial and posterior hypothalamus
b) Vasopressin	Osmoreceptors	Supraoptic nuclei
c) Oxytocin	Mechanoreceptors in external genitalia, breast, uterus	Paraventricular nuclei
d) Thyrotropin (thyroid stimulating hormone, TSH)	Thermoreceptors; others (?)	Anterior hypothalamus and anterior median hypothalamic eminence
e) Adrenocorticotropic hormone (ACTH)	Emotional stimuli via limbic system; reticular formation; anterior hypophyseal as well as hypothalamic receptor cells responsive to blood corticoid level; others (?)	Middle portion, median hypothalamic eminence
f) Follicle stimulating hormone (FSH), luteinizing hormone (LH)	Hypothalamic cells responsive to blood estrogen level	Posterior median hypothalamic eminence
g) Prolactin	Tactile receptors in breast	Posterior median hypothalamic eminence (inhibits secretion)
h) Somatotropin (growth hormone, GH)	Receptors unknown	Anterior median hypothalamic eminence
2. Thermoregulation	Cold receptors in skin; thermosensitive hypothalamic cells responsive to blood temperature	Anterior hypothalamus responsive to heat; posterior hypothalamus responsive to cold (thermo-regulatory centers)
3. "Appetitive" Functions		
a) Thirst	Osmoreceptors	Lateral superior hypothalamus
b) Hunger	Cells responsive to rate of glucose utilization ("glucostats")	Ventromedial hypothalamic satiety center; ventrolateral hypothalamic hunger center; limbic components also
c) Sexual behavior	Cells responsive to blood estrogen or androgen levels among others	Anterior ventral hypothalamus; in male, pyriform cortex also
4. Defense Reactions		
a) Fear, rage	Special sense organs, neocortex	Diffuse; in hypothalamic and limbic system

to the red nucleus are the fields of Forel, whose cells may represent a forward extension of the reticular nuclei. The fields of Forel contain fibers of the globus pallidus which are designated H (ventromedial fibers), H_1 (dorsomedial fibers), or H_2 (ventrolateral fibers).

Functionally the subthalamus is integrated with the extrapyramidal system and hence will be discussed in this context.

The Reticular Formation of the Spinal Cord and Brain Stem; The Reticular Activating System. The central region of the upper spinal cord and brain stem consists of a poorly defined, diffuse mass of interconnected nerve fibers and cells that are known as the *reticular formation*. The large number of small neurons that comprise this phylogenetically primitive formation are not organized anatomically into discrete tracts or fasciculi. Rather, the neurons that comprise the reticular formation are arranged as complex, intertwining networks containing many nuclei of uncertain function. Consequently these nuclei will not be discussed here.

The reticular formation extends in an uninterrupted fashion from the upper spinal cord through the medullary tegmentum and pons to terminate within the thalamic region of the diencephalon. Thus the reticular formation includes the hypothalamus, the subthalamus, and the ventromedial portion of the thalamus (including the intramedial nuclei), as well as the thalamic reticular nucleus.

The reticular system receives many afferent collaterals from the long ascending (sensory) spinal tracts as well as from the visual, olfactory, auditory, and trigeminal nerve systems. Additional afferent inputs to the reticular formation arise within the cerebellum, basal ganglia, rhinencephalon, and cerebral cortex. Consequently the reticular formation provides a polysynaptic pathway for sensory impulses of all types. In turn, nonspecific efferent fiber pathways from the reticular formation conduct impulses into the higher brain centers, in particular to all regions of the cerebral cortex, as well as caudally into the spinal cord.

Functionally the reticular formation is one of the most important regulatory system that is located within the central nervous system. The reticular formation of the spinal cord and brain stem provides the neurologic substrate for the so-called *reticular activating system* (RAS). The activity of this system makes possible the alert, conscious (waking) state, whereas a diminution of RAS activity results in the unconscious (or sleeping) state. Thus the RAS exerts a marked influence upon the electric activity of the cerebral cortex. Furthermore, the RAS is concerned intimately with such fundamental processes as maintaining attention; the development of various emotional states and conditioned reflexes; learning; the regulation of skeletal muscle tone and activity; the regulation of visceral functions such as respiration, cardiac rate, vasomotor tone, and gastrointestinal functions; the control of certain endocrine secretions (which in turn regulate the metabolic rate); the regulation of body temperature; and the modulation of sensory inputs from exteroceptors throughout the body.

The particular functions of the RAS enumerated above will be discussed in context subsequently, but it should be stressed here that this system provides a complex, multisynaptic pathway which receives afferent impulses from all exteroceptors and

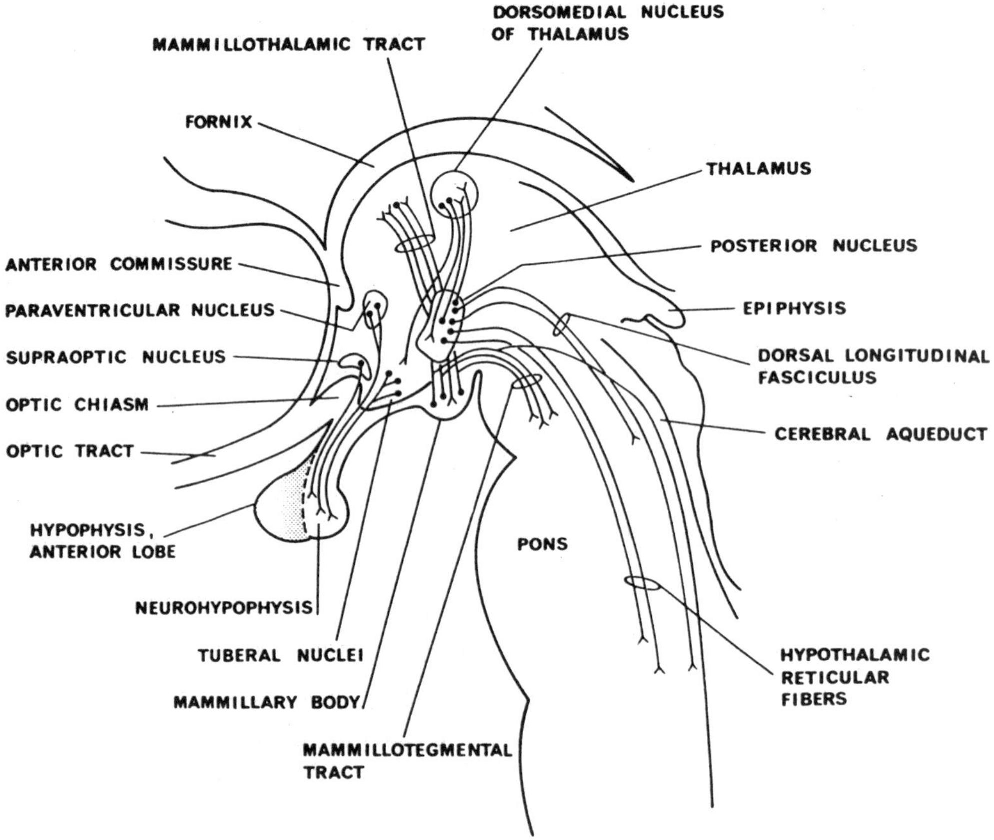

Fig. 2.22. The major efferent hypothalamic pathways.

interoceptors. The large extent to which convergence of these impulses takes place within the RAS in turn tends to abolish any specificity insofar as the particular modalities of sensation are concerned. Consequently the RAS is functionally nonspecific in contrast to the specific neural pathways that are stimulated by only one kind of sensory input.

From a physiologic standpoint, most of the reticular formation, hence the RAS, is excitatory. In particular, the excitatory regions of the reticular formation are located within the pons, mesencephalon, and diencephalon. The lateral portions of the medullary reticular formations are also excitatory. Collectively these regions are termed the *bulboreticular facilitory area*. On the other hand, a small region of the reticular formation that is located within the ventromedial medulla is primarily inhibitory; therefore this part of the RAS is called the *bulboreticular inhibitory area*.

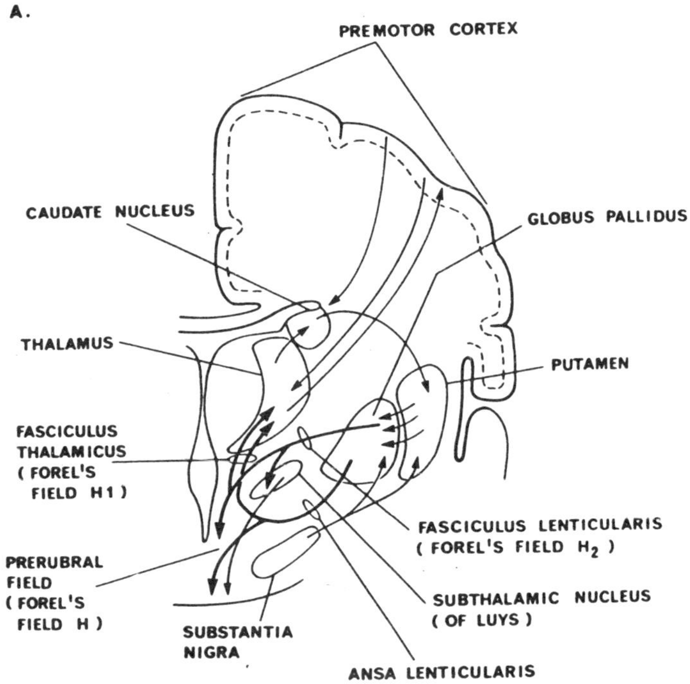

Fig. 2.23. A. Major interconnections of the subthalamus and corpus striatum.

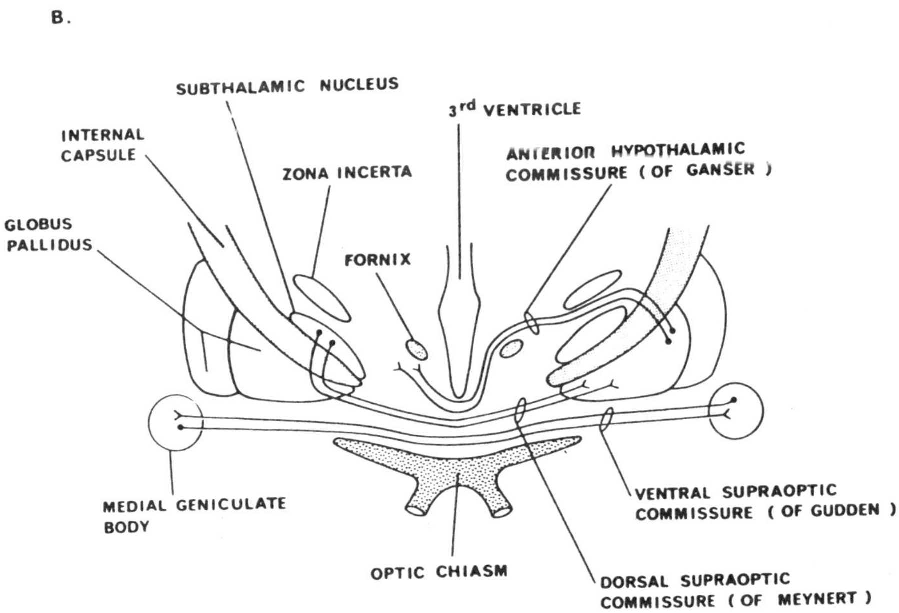

Fig. 2.23. B. The anterior hypothalamic and supraoptic commissures in cross section.

A.

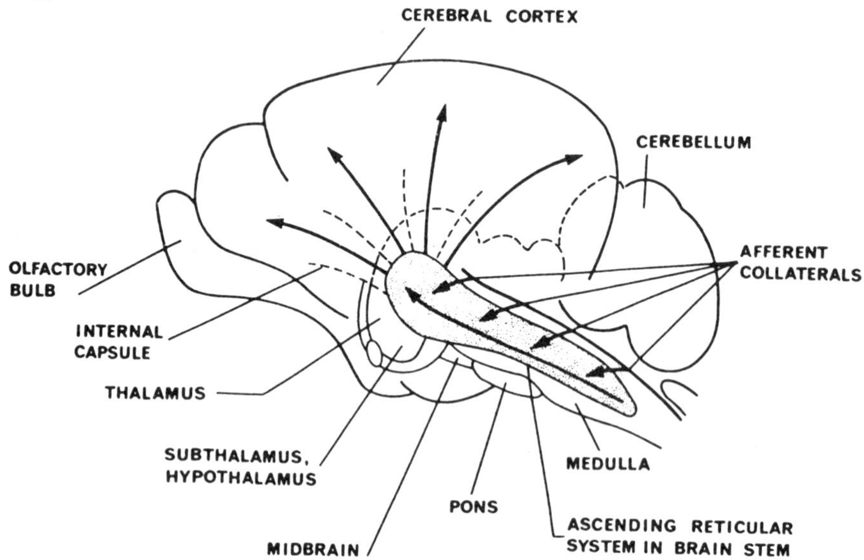

Fig. 2.24. A. Ascending reticular activating system (RAS) of cat brain. Impulses converge on the RAS via afferent collaterals from specific neural pathways, thereby producing excitation of the RAS which in turn evokes nonspecific excitation of the entire cerebral cortex.

B.

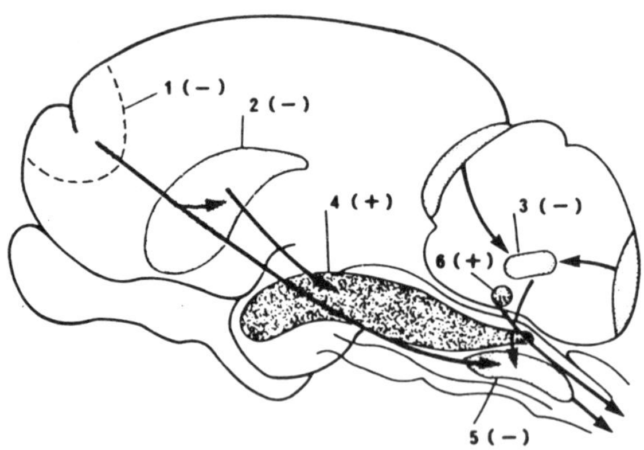

Fig. 2.24. B. Descending suppressor, or inhibitory (—), and facilitory, or excitatory (+), systems (light shading) that act upon the reticular formation of the cat brain. 1. Corticomedullaryreticular pathway. 2. Caudatospinal pathway. 3. Cerebelloreticular pathway. 4. Reticulospinal pathway. 5. Reticulospinal pathway. 6. Vestibulospinal pathway. 1, 2, 3, and 5. exert suppressor effects upon the activity of the reticular formation, whereas 4. and 6. provide facilitatory mechanisms.

Normally the bulboreticular facilitory area generates and transmits nerve impulses spontaneously; i.e., the neurons are inherently capable of generating repetitive impulses. However, in the normal conscious individual inhibitory neural inputs are constantly bombarding the bulboreticular facilitory area, and these inhibitory impulses arise within such structures as the cerebral cortex and basal ganglia. Therefore the intrinsic patterns of activity within the facilitory part of the RAS are reduced considerably.

The Cerebellum

The cerebellum performs a critical, albeit subconscious, role in the control of reflex skeletal muscle tone, in the maintenance of posture and equilibrium, and in the coordination and control of all voluntary muscular activities.

The cerebellum consists of a large and highly organized accumulation of neurons that is located above the medulla and pons and covered posteriorly by the cerebral hemispheres. The cerebellum is attached to the brain stem on each side of the midline by three large bundles of nerve fibers, the superior, middle, and inferior cerebellar peduncles. Thus an abundance of afferent as well as efferent connections are present between the cerebellum, brain stem, spinal cord, and cerebral hemispheres. The cerebellum is separated from the overlying cerebral hemispheres by a horizontal sheet of dura mater called the tentorium cerebelli.

The principal gross subdivisions of the cerebellum are the paired lateral cerebellar hemispheres and the median vermis. The principal lobules and fissures that subdivide the cerebellum anatomically.

The flocculonodular lobe, which appears first during embryogenesis, is demarcated by the postnodular and posterolateral fissures from the remainder of the cerebellum which is known as the corpus cerebelli. The flocculonodular lobe, also called the archicerebellum to indicate the early phylogenetic appearance of this region, is connected principally to vestibular structures. The anterior lobe, pyramis, and uvula collectively make up the paleocerebellum. The paleocerebellum is the region within which mainly proprioceptive and interoceptive impulses are received from the head and body in general. Except for the pyramis and uvula, the posterior lobe is known as the neocerebellum, and this region of the cerebellum developed most recently from a phylogenetic standpoint and concurrently with the cerebral cortex. Therefore extensive neural connections are present between the neocerebellum and cortex via the corticopontile system.

When viewed grossly in cross section, the cerebellum is seem to have an outer gray cortex that surrounds an inner core of white matter within which are embedded four pairs of nuclei. These structures are the dentate, emboliform, globose, and fastigial nuclei. As the emboliform and globose nuclei have similar connections, these structures are known together as the nucleus interpositus.

Upon microscopic examination, the cerebellar cortex is seen to be composed of two layers, an outer molecular layer and an inner granular layer.

Fig. 2.25. Gross anatomy and major divisions of the cerebellum.

A.

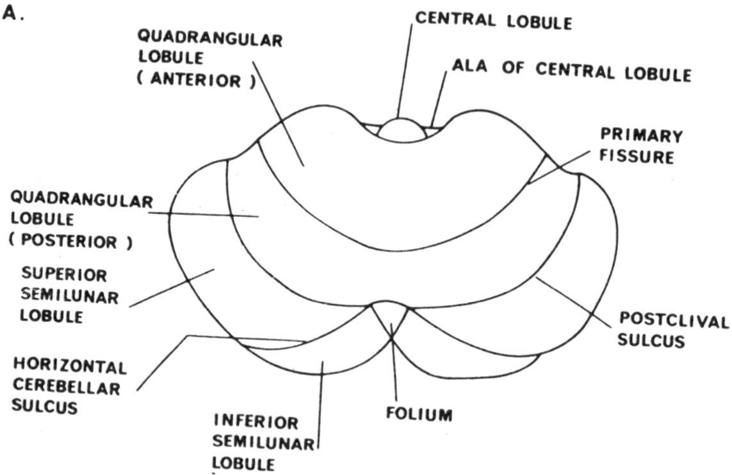

Fig. 2.25. A. Superior surface

B.

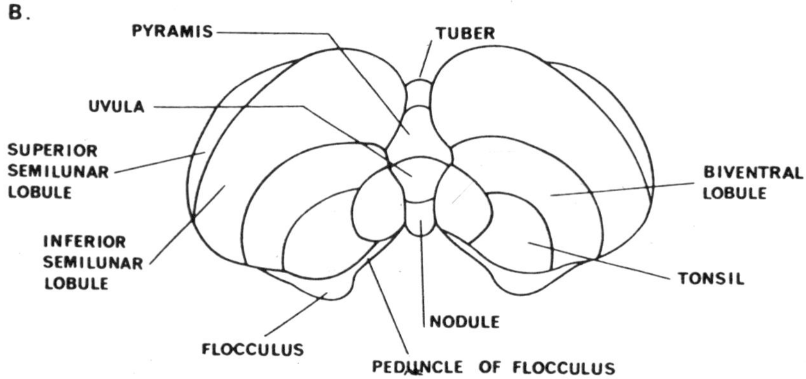

Fig. 2.25. B. Inferior surface.

C.

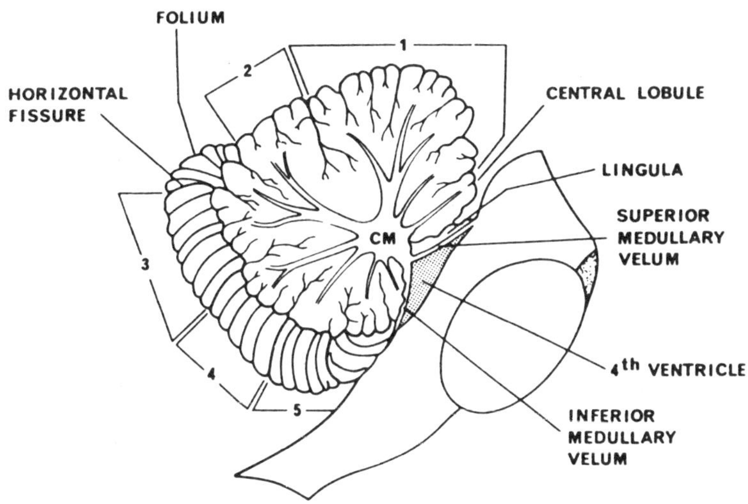

Fig. 2.25. (C) (Cont.) Sagittal section to indicate the lobules of the vermis. 1. Culmen. 2. Declive. 3. Tuber. 4. Pyramis. 5. Uvula. CM = central white matter.

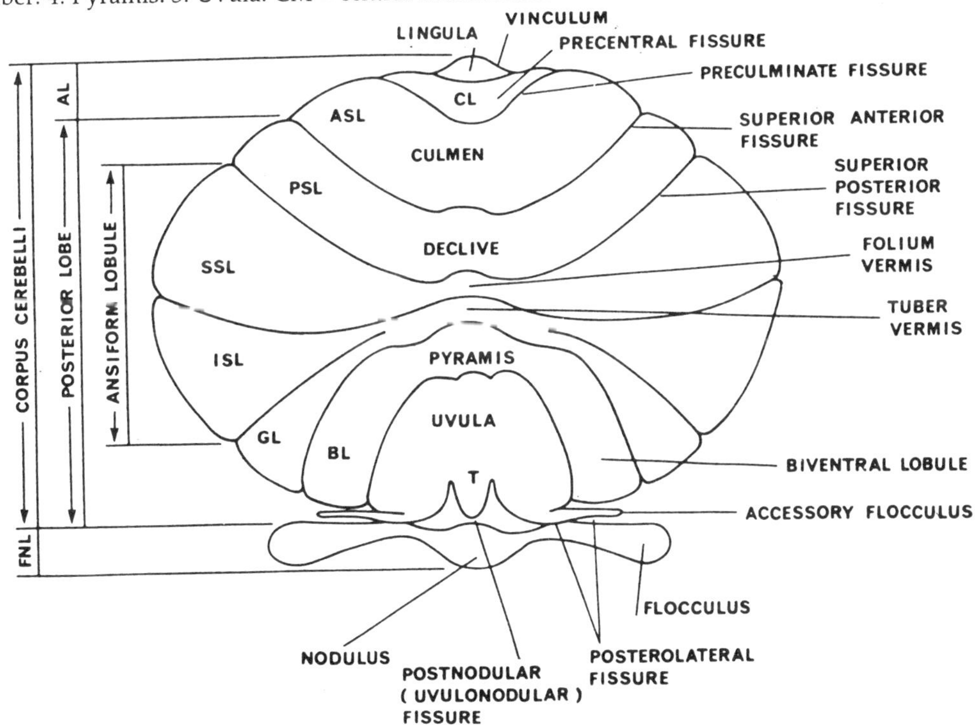

Fig. 2.25. Major gross divisions of the cerebellum. AL = anterior lobe; FNL = flocculonodular lobe; CL = central lobule; ASL = anterior semilunar lobule; PSL = posterior semilunar lobule; SSL = superior semilunar lobule; ISL = inferior semilunar lobule; GL = gracile lobule; BL = biventral lobe; T = tonsil.

The outer *molecular layer* contains an abundance of neural processes whose cell bodies are located deeper within the cerebellum; consequently many synapses are present in this region of the cerebellar cortex. Deep within the molecular layer are many so-called basket cells whose axons pass above the Purkinje cells and emit many collaterals, the most obvious being those which form synaptic networks (baskets) about the Purkinje cells. The Purkinje cells in turn are relatively large neurons that are located in a single layer deep within the molecular layer. Functionally, the Purkinje cells are the efferent

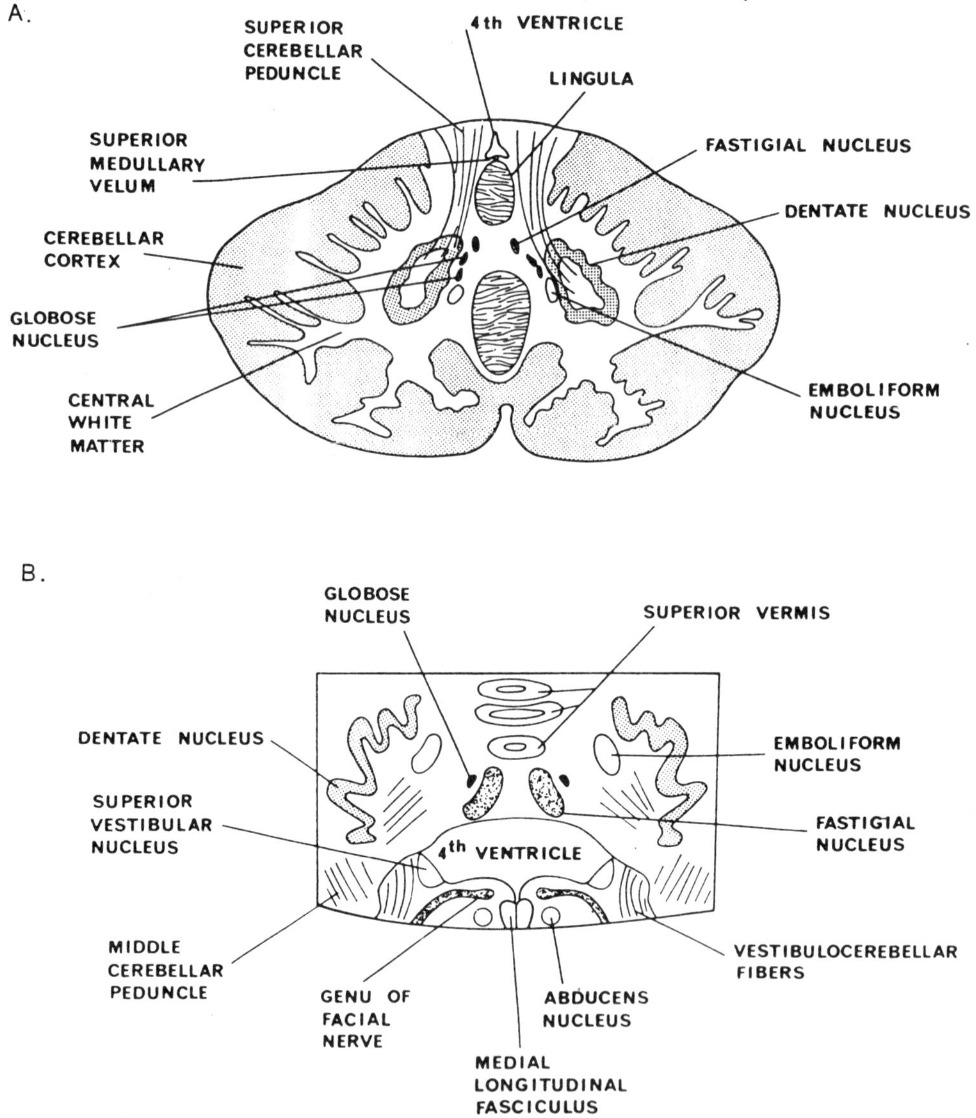

Fig. 2.27. A. Cerebellum in horizontal section to illustrate the relationship between the cortical gray matter (shaded around periphery) and the centrally located nuclei within the white matter. B. Frontal section through the cerebellum at a level similar to that of the abducens nucleus of the pons to illustrate the relationships among the cerebellar nuclei.

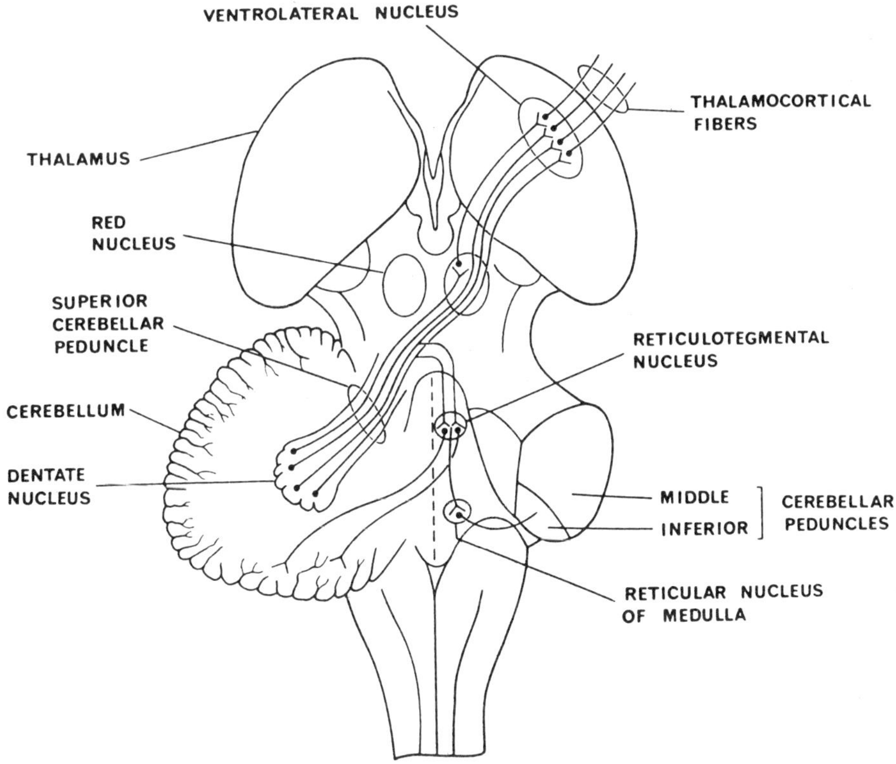

Fig. 2.28. The efferent fibers which project from the dentate nucleus of the cerebellum.

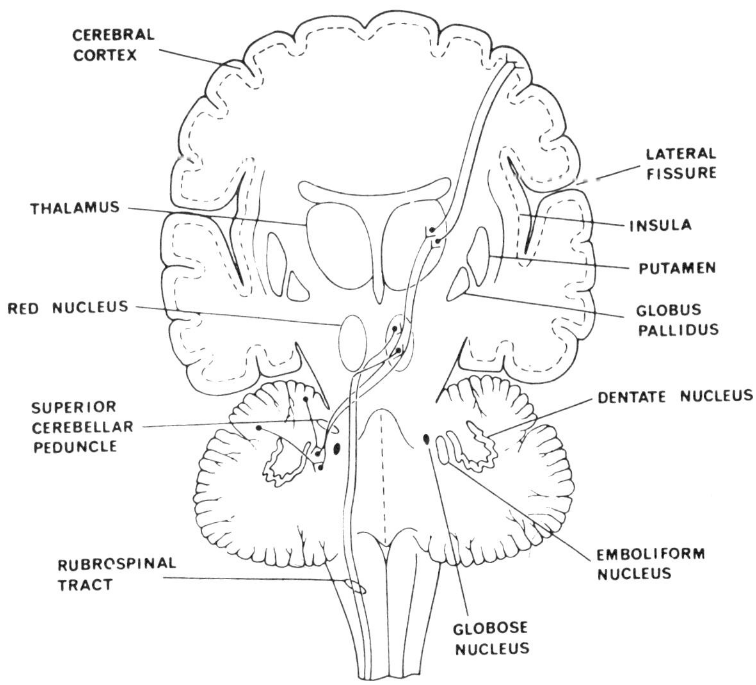

Fig. 2.29. The efferent projections from the emboliform nucleus of the cerebellum to the red nucleus.

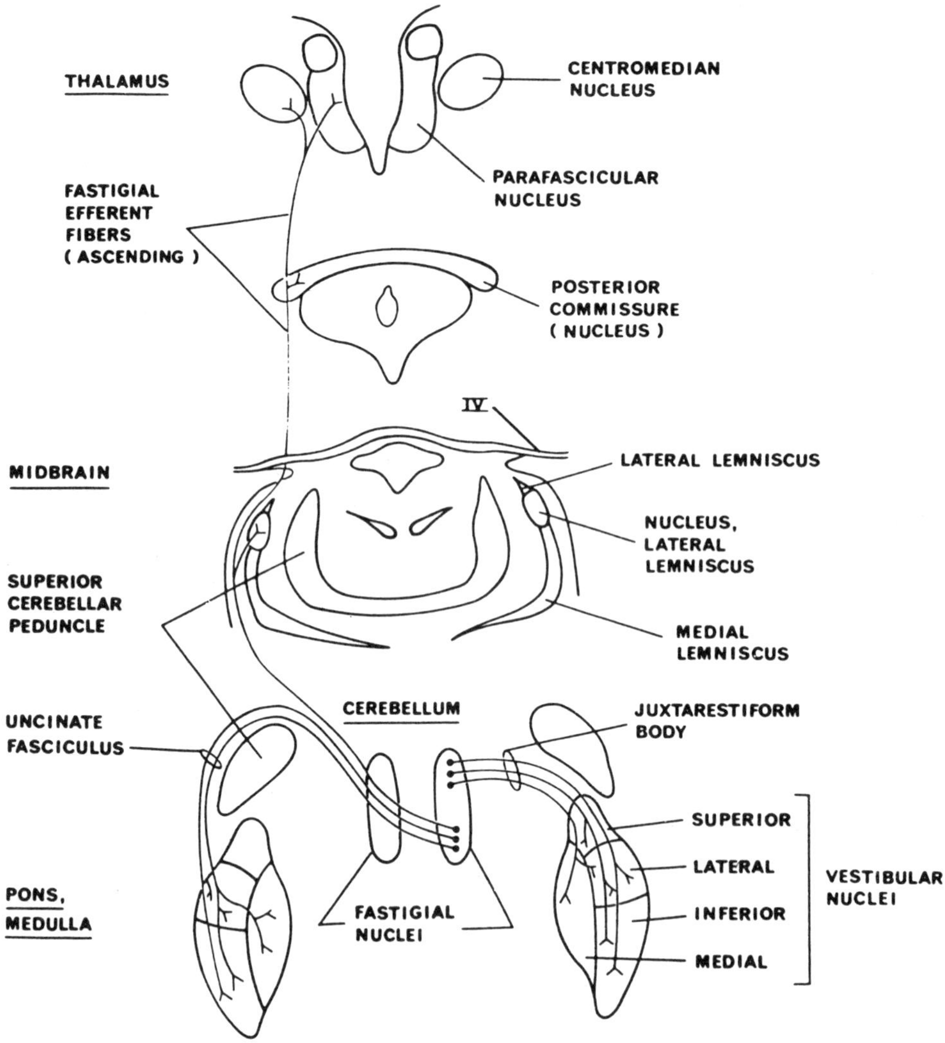

Fig. 2.30. The ascending and descending efferent fiber projections from the fastigial nucleus of the cerebellum. IV = trochlear nerve.

neurons of the cerebellar cortex, and their axons pass to the cerebellar nuclei. Some of the recurrent axons that arise from these neurons appear to terminate upon other Purkinje cells.

The *granular layer* of the cerebellar cortex contains many small, densely packed cells, the so-called granule cells. Several short, curved dendrites are present on these cells. The axons of the granule cells are longer than the dendrites and they project into the molecular layer, there to undergo bifurcation into layers of parallel fibers. The parallel

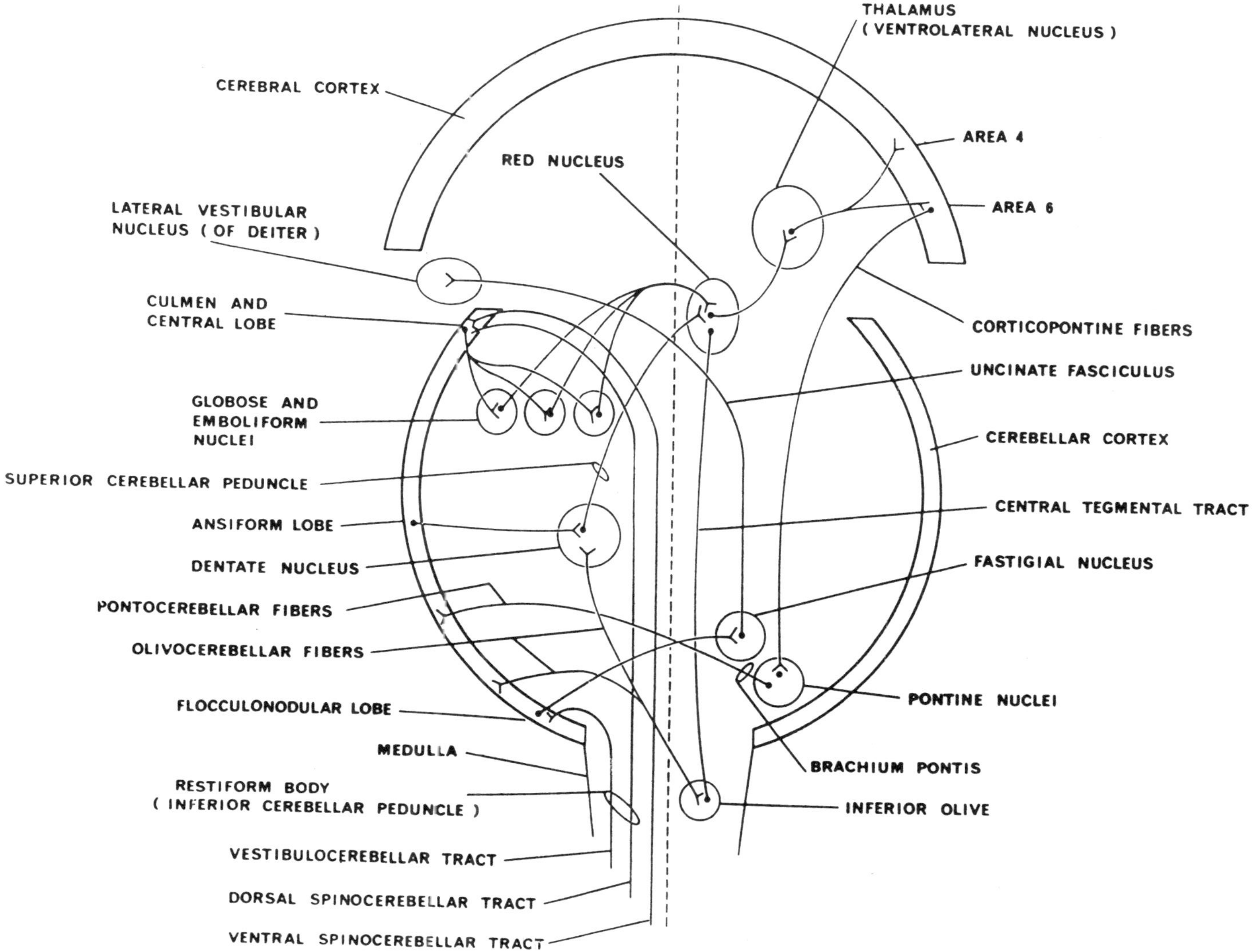

Fig. 2.31. Highly schematic diagram illustrating the principal afferent and efferent cerebellar connections. Unicinate fasciculus = hook bundle of Russell.

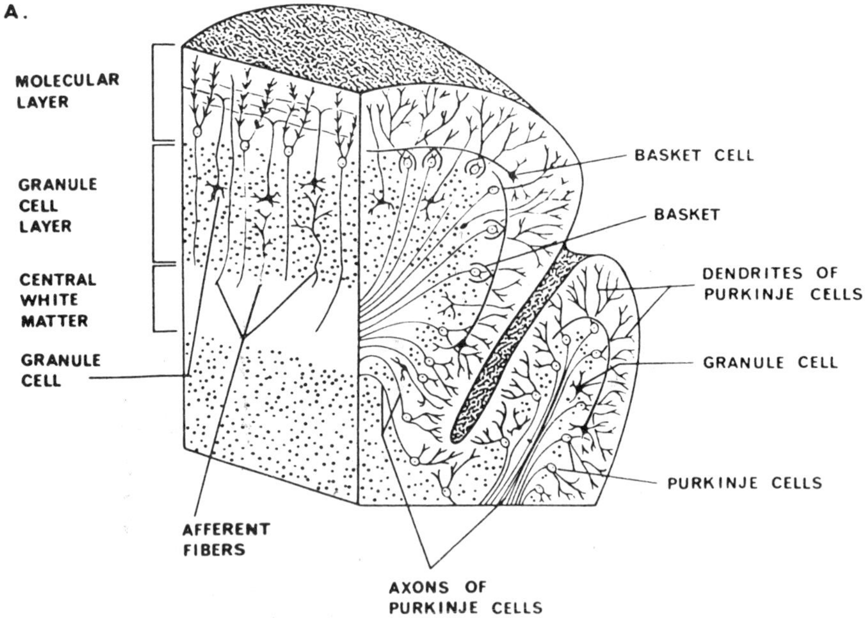

Fig. 2.32. A Microanatomy of the cerebellar cortex. **A.** Longitudinal section of a single cerebellar folium on left and cross sections of two adjacent folia on right illustrating the principal cell layers and synaptic connections.

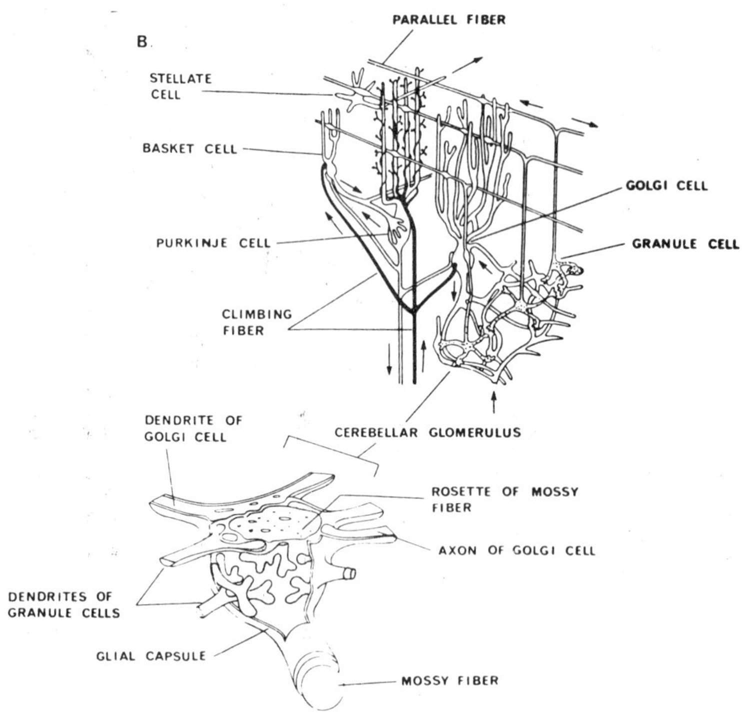

Fig. 2.32. B. Interconnections among cerebellar neurons. Inset at the bottom shows a cerebellar glomerulus in greater detail.

fibers then synapse upon the spines located on the dendritic processes of the Purkinje cells. The anatomic relationship between the parallel fibers of the granule cells and the dendrites of the Purkinje cells underlies the physiologic properties of spreading (or diffusion) of impulses as well as convergence of impulses within the cerebellar cortex, as one parallel fiber may make synaptic contact with the dendrites of several hundred Purkinje cells.

Table 2.4
Cerebellar Nuclei and Their Connections

Nucleus	*Afferent Fibers From*	*Efferent Fibers To*
Dentate	Neocerebellar portion of posterior lobe; anterior lobe	Superior cerebellar peduncles, red nucleus, ventrolateral nucleus of thalamus
Emboliform	Paleocerebellum	Red nucleus via superior cerebellar peduncle
Globose	Paleocerebellum	Red nucleus via superior cerebellar peduncle
Fastigial	Flocculonodular lobe	Vestibular nucleus via the uncinate fasciculus (hook bundle of Russell)

The superior cerebellar peduncle (or brachium conjunctivum) passes from the white substance of the upper medial portion of the cerebellar hemisphere and then enters the lateral wall of the fourth ventricle. Thence the major portion of this fiber tract ascends to decussate in its entirety within the midbrain at the level of the inferior colliculi beneath the cerebral aqueduct. The superior cerebellar peduncle contains three principal fiber tracts. First, efferent dentatorubral fibers pass from the dentate nucleus to the contralateral red nucleus and thalamus. Second, the ventral spinocerebellar tract (afferent) enters the cerebellum from the spinal cord, and then terminates in the cortical region of the paleocerebellum. Third, the uncinate fasciculus contains efferent fibers that arise within the fastigial nucleus and terminate in the lateral vestibular nucleus (of Deiter) after traversing the superior cerebellar peduncle.

The middle cerebellar peduncle (or brachium pontis) consists of fibers that originate within the pontine nuclei and run to the contralateral neocerebellum via this peduncle.

The inferior cerebellar peduncle (or restiform body) emanates from the lateral walls of the fourth ventricle and ascends to enter the cerebellum in the region intermediate to the superior and middle cerebellar peduncles. The inferior cerebellar peduncle contains five major tracts. First, the olivocerebellar tract consists of fibers that arise within the opposite inferior olivary nucleus, and which pass to the cortex of the cerebellar hemisphere as well as the vermis. Second, the dorsal spinocerebellar tract contains afferent fibers from the spinal cord that run to the cerebellar cortex (anterior lobe) as well as to the pyramis of the paleocerebellum. Third, the dorsal external arcuate fibers (afferent) pass from the nuclei of the funiculus gracilis and cuneatus of the medulla. Fourth, the ventral external arcuate fibers run from the arcuate and lateral reticular nuclei of the medulla to the cerebellum via the inferior cerebellar peduncle. Fifth, the vestibulocerebellar tract passes from the vestibular nuclei to the flocculonodular lobe of the cerebellar cortex.

The general functions of the cerebellum may be localized to some extent on the basis of various types of experimental and clinical study.

The phylogenetically ancient archicerebellum functions to keep the body oriented in space, i.e., is concerned with the maintenance of equilibrium. Afferent impulses that arise within the labyrinth of the inner ear enter the flocculonodular lobe of the cerebellar cortex via the vestibulocerebellar pathways. Thence these impulses are transmitted to the fastigial nucleus, and efferent impulses pass by way of the uncinate fasciculus (or hook bundle of Russell) to the lateral vestibular nucleus (or Deiter). The flocculonodular lobe thus is concerned primarily with vestibular mechanisms.

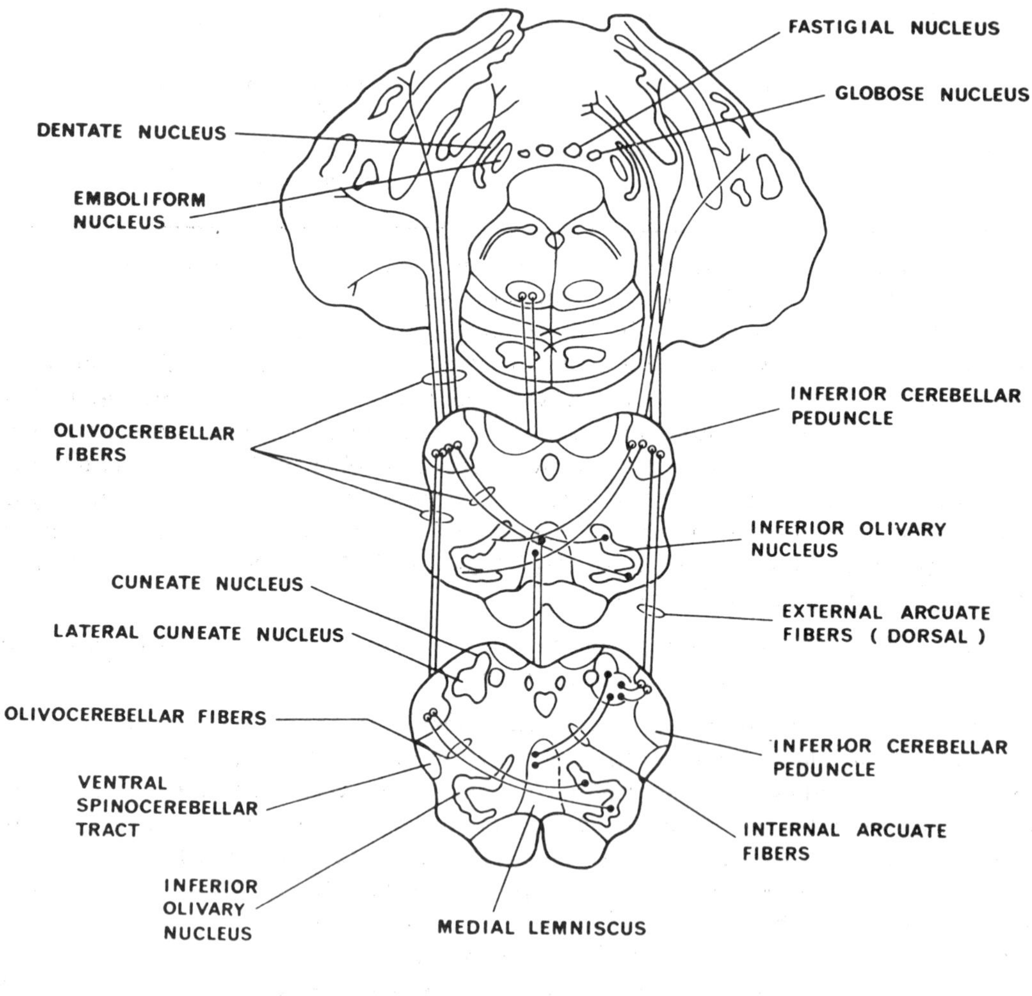

Fig. 2.33. The connections between the lateral nucleus, the olivary nucleus, and the cerebellum.

The paleocerebellum regulates contraction of the antigravity or postural muscles of the body as well as those concerned with movement and the maintenance of equilibrium. Thus afferent impulses from the extensor muscles, for example, are transmitted via the spinocerebellar tracts of the culmen and central portions of the cerebellar cortex, and from these regions impulses are conducted to the globose and emboliform nuclei. Ultimately, the impulses pass via the superior cerebellar peduncle to the red nucleus.

The neocerebellum functions to check (or brake) discrete voluntary movements, particularly those involving delicate movements of the hands. Afferent impulses are transmitted from the precentral motor cortex to the ansiform region of the neocerebellar cortex via the pontocerebellar tracts. From this part of the cerebellum, the impulses are relayed to the dentate nucleus. Thence the impulses pass to the red nucleus and thalamus via the superior cerebellar peduncle, and ultimately return to the premotor areas of the cerebral cortex.

In conclusion, the cerebellum receives a broad range of sensory information from end organs that are located throughout the body, and this information is coordinated and integrated within the cerebellum itself. Thence, and following appropriate synthesis, the modified (i.e., facilitated or inhibited) impulse patterns are projected (or transmitted) from the cerebellum to motor centers that are located within the spinal cord, brain stem, and cerebral cortex. In this manner the activity of the motoneurons that innervate the skeletal muscles of the body is controlled by the cerebellum. The neural circuits that involve the cerebellum and other central nervous structures, and which underlie the control of complex muscular activities, are excellent examples of feedback loops (or servomechanisms).

The Cerebrum and Related Structures

The cerebrum is by far the largest anatomic region of the human brain, and it contains the highest (or functionally most sophisticated) neural centers to be found in the central nervous system. The cerebrum is so voluminous that it occupies the larger part of the cranial cavity of the skull and covers the cerebellum and brain stem.

Anatomically the cerebrum is divided into two lateral cerebral hemispheres by the longitudinal cerebral fissure, and this sagittal fissure is occupied by a projection of dura mater known as the flax cerebri. The two cerebral hemispheres are joined together by a large mass of white nerve fibers, the corpus callosum. The corpus callosum is the white central commissure which crosses the longitudinal cerebral fissure.

Caudally the cerebral hemispheres are connected to lower brain centers by the continuous nerve fibers of the internal capsule and cerebral peduncle.

Deep within each cerebral hemisphere are embedded several large masses of gray matter collectively known as the basal ganglia.

The pertinent neuroanatomic features of the cerebral hemispheres and basal ganglia together with a number of their important functional correlates now may be considered. In this regard, the various anatomic levels within the central nervous system at which certain functions become integrated. The reader will note in this table that the cerebral

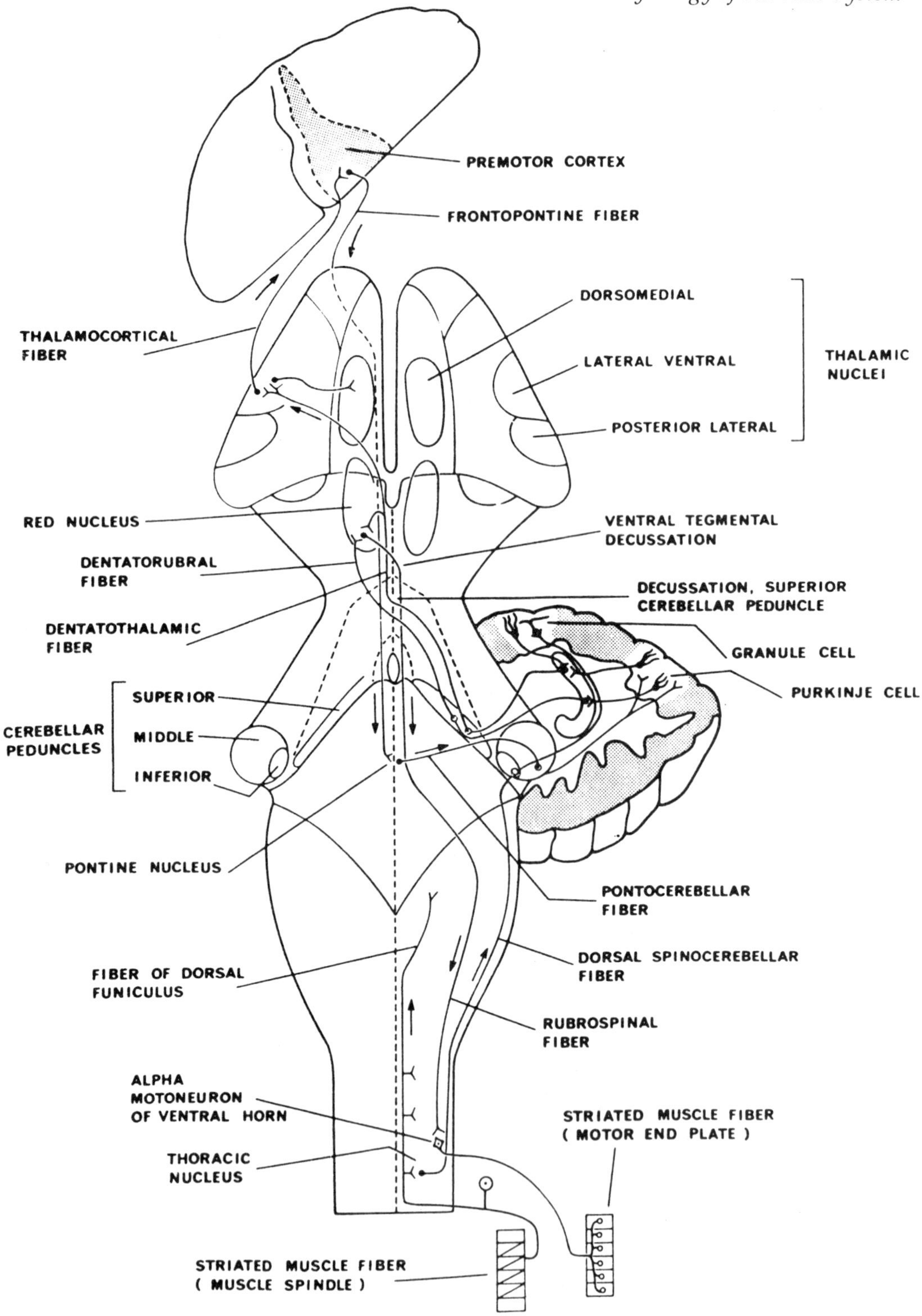

Fig. 2.34. Some of the neural circuits which underlie the coordination of complex motor activity.

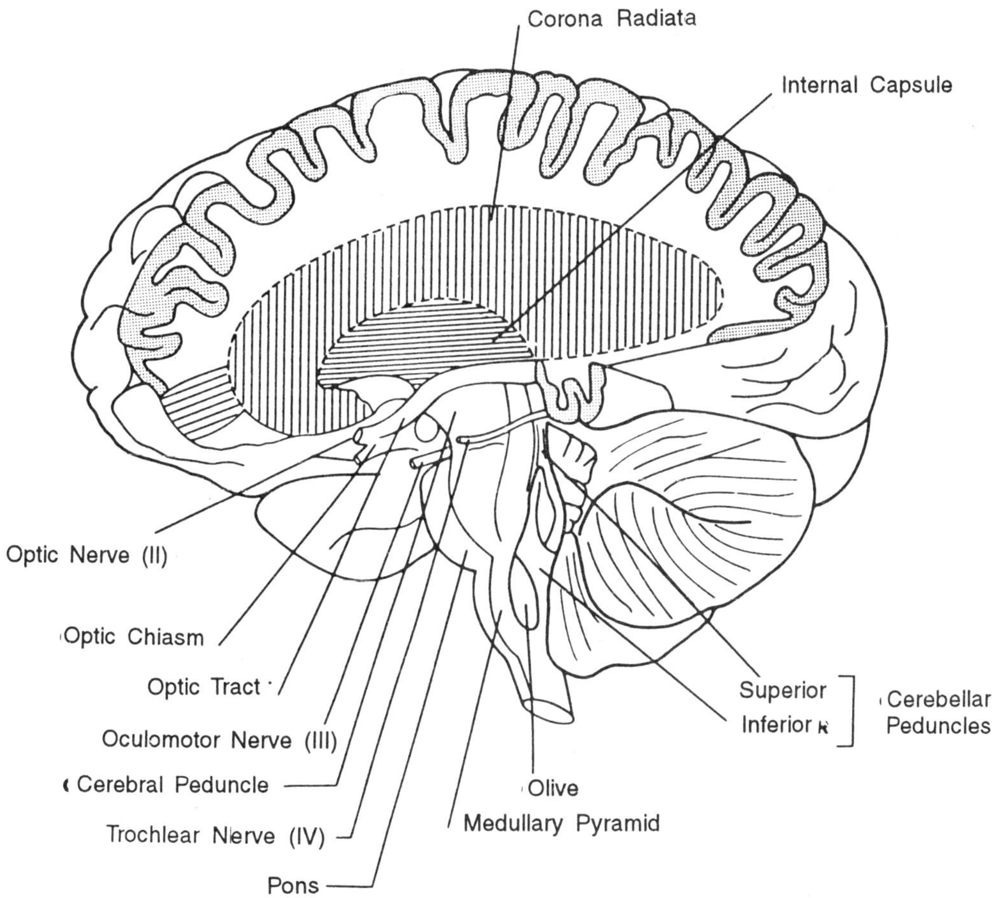

Fig. 2.35. Relationships among the cerebrospinal fibers and other regions of the brain. The stippled area represents the cut gray matter of the cerebral cortex.

cortex provides the ultimate neural region wherein the so-called higher functions of the human nervous system take place.

The Cerebral Hemispheres

Gross Anatomy. Upon gross inspection, the surfaces of the cerebral hemispheres are seen to be covered with a number of elevated convolutions (or gyri) which are separated by furrows known as fissures (or sulci).

Each cerebral hemisphere can be divided into several general regions, the frontal, parietal, occipital, and temporal lobes, as well as the insula and rhinencephalon.

The *frontal lobe* extends from the most anterior portion of each hemisphere to the central sulcus (or fissure of Rolando) posteriorly, and is delimited inferiorly by the lateral cerebral fissure (or fissures of Sylvius) on the dorsolateral surface. The frontal

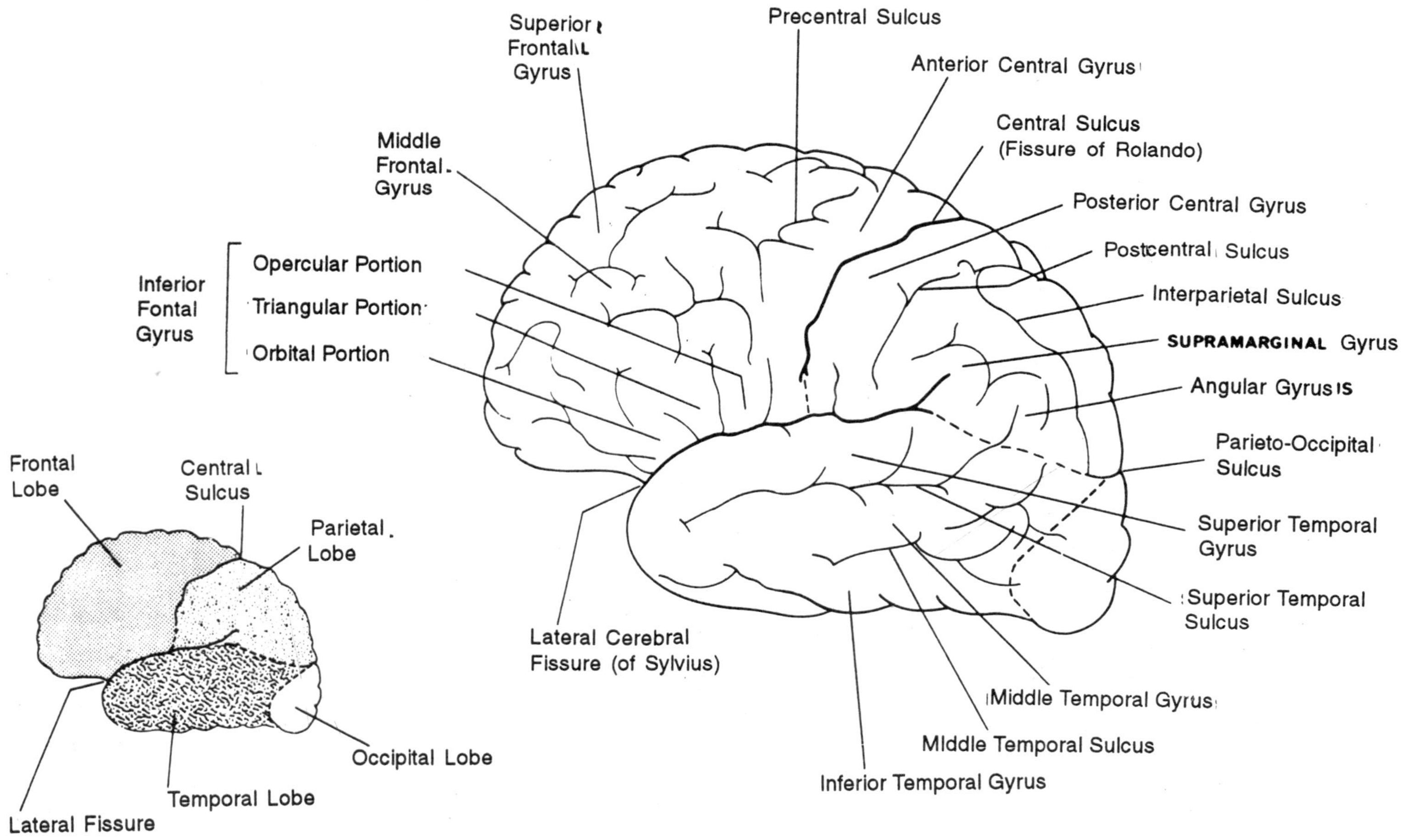

Fig. 2.36. Gyri and sulci of the left cerebral hemisphere as viewed from superolateral surface. The dashed lines indicate the principal lobes of the cerebral hemisphere as indicated by shaded areas in the small diagram inset at the lower left of the figure.

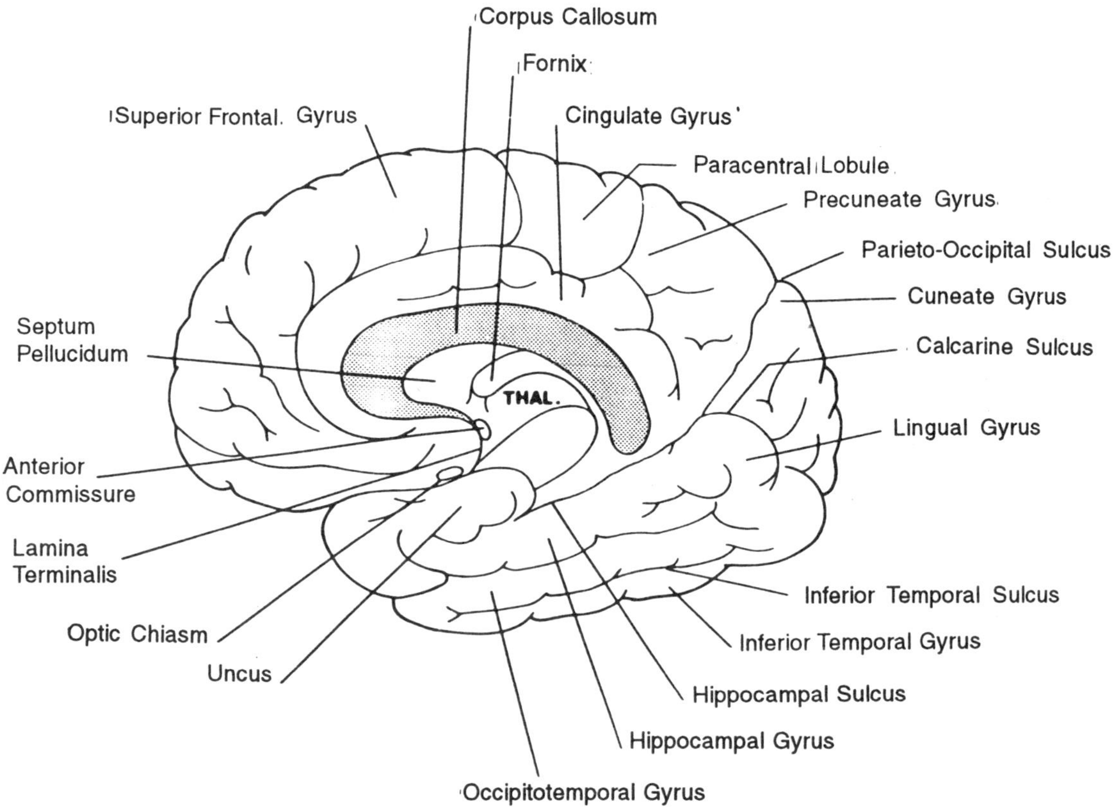

Fig. 2.37. Principal gyri and sulci seen on the medial surface of the left cerebral hemisphere. THAL = thalamus.

lobe includes the superior, middle, and inferior frontal gyri, as well as the orbital and the cingulate gyri. The gyrus rectus (or straight gyrus) also is part of the frontal lobe.

The *parietal lobe* includes the region between the central sulcus and the parieto-occipital fissure, and extends laterally to the lateral cerebral fissure. The superior and inferior parietal lobules as well as the supramarginal, angular, and postcentral gyri are the subdivisions of the parietal lobe.

The *occipital lobe* is roughly pyramidal in shape and this region lies behind the parietooccipital fissure. The occipital lobe is divided into superior and inferior gyri, and this lobe also contains the cuneus as well as the lingual and fusiform gyri.

The *temporal lobe* is located inferior to the lateral cerebral fissure (of Sylvius), and reaches posteriorly to the level of the parieto-occipital fissure. The superior, middle, and inferior temporal gyri as well as the transverse temporal gyrus (Heschl's gyrus) are included in the temporal lobe. In addition, the hippocampal gyrus and its hook-shaped anterior portion (the uncus) also is a part of the temporal lobe.

The *insula* (or island of Reil) is located deep within the lateral fissure (of Sylvius), and can be seen by moving apart the upper and lower edges of this fissure. The insula consists of several short gyri as well as a posterior long gyrus.

The *rhinencephalon* ("nose brain") is a phylogenetically ancient region of the cerebral hemisphere, and it includes those parts of the brain that are involved in the perception of olfactory stimuli, among other functions. The ovoid olfactory bulb rests upon the ethmoid bone (cribriform plate) where it receives olfactory nerves from the olfactory region of the nasal cavity. The olfactory tract* divides posteriorly into the lateral olfactory stria which then enters the uncus of the hippocampal gyrus, and the medial olfactory stria which runs medially and to the subcallosal gyrus adjacent to the inferior part of the corpus callosum. The pyriform area of the rhinencephalon includes the anterior portion of the hippocampal gyrus, the uncus, and the lateral olfactory gyrus.

The rhinencephalon also includes the subcallosal and supracallosal gyri, the medial and lateral longitudinal striae which lie along the upper surface of the corpus callosum, and the hippocampus. The hippocampus is composed principally of gray matter and this structure runs the length of the floor of the lateral ventricle where it becomes continuous with the supracallosal gyrus in the splenium region of the corpus callosum. The fornix is a curved fiber tract that emerges from the hippocampal formation. A white layer called the alveus is found upon the ventricular surface of the hippocampus, and this structure contains nerve fibers that lead from the dentate fascia (a thin layer of cortex located upon the upper surface of the hippocampus) and the hippocampus proper. Fibers pass from the alveus to the medial surface of the hippocampus to form the fimbria. The fimbria consist of a flat band of white nerve fibers which rise beneath the splenium of the corpus callosum, bend forward above the thalamus, and thus form the crus of the fornix. The two lateral crura of the fornix are interconnected by the transverse fibers of the hippocampal commissure. Each crus lies adjacent to the underside of the corpus callosum and the two crura unite anteriorly, thereby forming the body of the fornix. The two columns of the fornix in turn arch downward and posteriorly, enter the anterior region of the lateral wall of the third ventricle, and there terminate in the mamillary bodies of the hypothalamus.

The anterior commissure is composed of a band of white nerves fibers that crosses the midline of the cerebrum to interconnect both cerebral hemispheres. The anterior commissure appears to have two distinct regions: The rostral part joins both olfactory bulbs, whereas the more caudal portion interconnects the pyriform areas of each cerebral hemisphere with the other.

---

* *Actually the olfactory nerve (cranial nerve I) is not a true nerve; rather it is a fiber tract of the brain.*

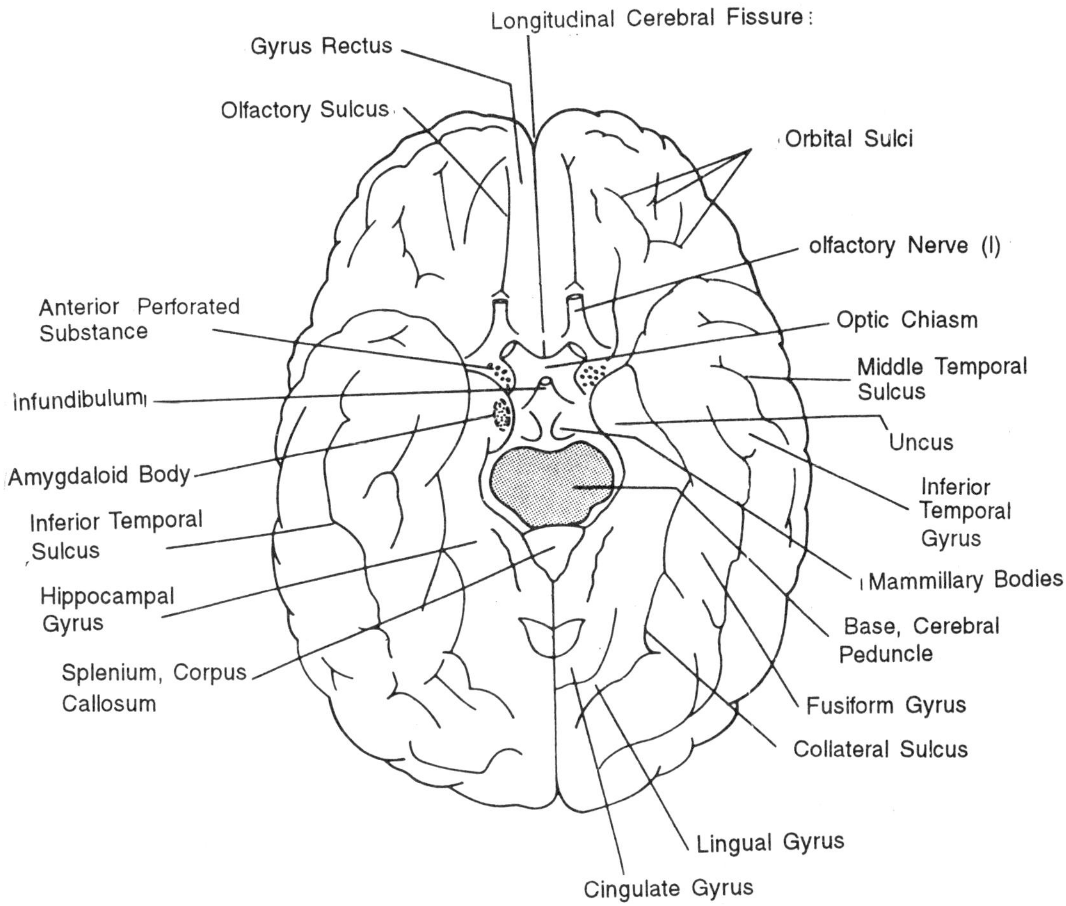

Fig. 2.38. Inferior surface of the cerebrum The anterior portion of the left temporal lobe has been removed in order to show the location of the amygdaloid body.

The septum pellucidum is a thin-walled partition which is located between the lateral ventricles and which is situated between the fornix and corpus callosum.

The White Matter. The white matter of the cerebral hemispheres is composed of a vast number of myelinated nerve fibers of various sizes as well as neuroglial elements. The core of each cerebral hemisphere includes three types of myelinated nerve fiber. Thus, transverse, projection, and association fibers are present.

Transverse Fibers. Transverse (or commissural) fibers provide interconnections between the two cerebral hemispheres. The largest tract of commissural fibers is the corpus callosum. The majority of the fibers present within the corpus callosum arise in various particular regions of one cerebral hemisphere and terminate in similar regions in

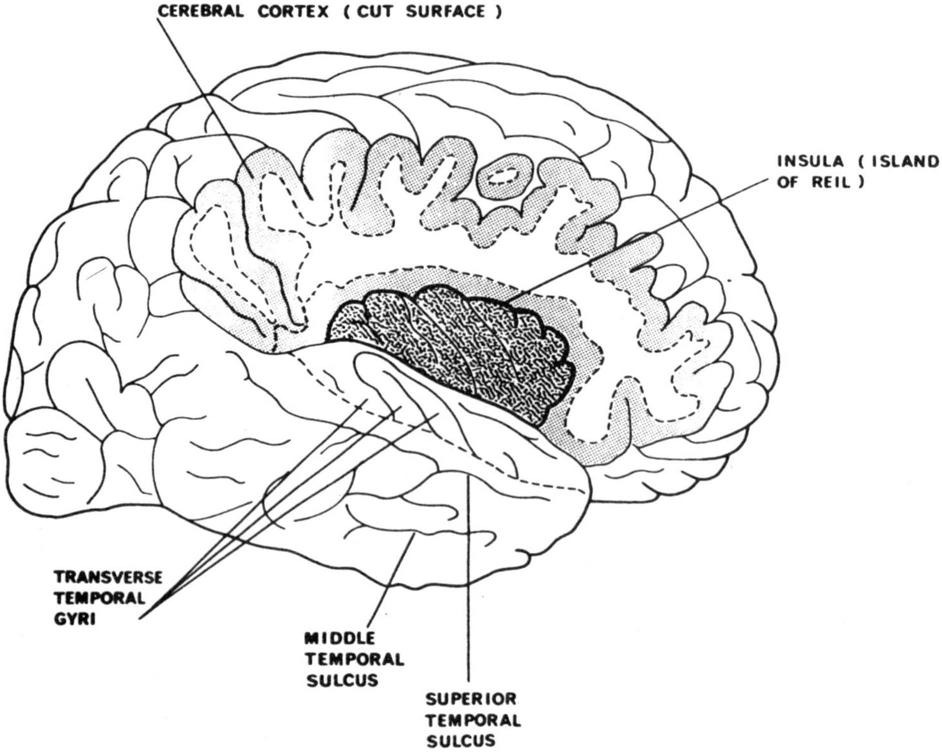

Fig. 2.39. Superior lateral aspect of the right cerebral hemisphere. The lower portions of the formal and parietal areas have been removed to show the superior of the temporal lobe (delimited by sloping dashed line in lower center of figure) and the insula (dark shading circumscribed by heavy black line).

the opposite hemisphere. The corpus callosum is a thick, bandlike, transverse structure which makes up the roof of the lateral ventricles as well as the roof of the third ventricle.

As noted earlier, the anterior commissure interconnects the two olfactory bulbs in its rostral portion; caudally the anterior commissure interconnects the paired pyriform areas of the rhinencephalon.

The hippocampal commissure unites the two hippocampal gyri.

Projection Fibers. Certain projection fibers of the white substance of the cerebral hemisphere traverse the corona radiata to enter the internal capsule, and these fibers serve to connect the cerebral cortex with lower regions of the brain as well as the spinal cord.

The principal afferent (or corticipetal) projection fibers include thalamic radiations from the several thalamic nuclei to specific areas of the cerebral cortex, the geniculocalcarine tract which arise in the lateral geniculate body and passes to the calcarine region of the cerebral cortex, and thalamic auditory fibers that arise within the medial geniculate body and radiate to Heschl's gyrus of the auditory cortex.

The efferent (or corticofugal) fibers originate within the cerebral cortex, and pass from this region to the thalamus, brain stem, and spinal cord. The corticobulbar and corticospinal tracts, which together comprise the pyramidal motor system of the body, originate from the motor cortex, thence proceed caudally via the internal capsule. The corticopontile tracts, which pass from the cerebral cortex to the pons, include the frontopontile tract and the temporopontile tract. The frontopontile tract originates within the frontal lobe of the cerebral cortex and runs to the pontine nuclei. The temporopontile tract originates in the temporal lobe of the cerebral cortex and also terminates in the pontine nuclei. Corticothalamic fibers course from the cerebral cortex to various thalamic nuclei, and the corticorubral tract connects the frontal lobe of the cerebral cortex to the red nucleus located within the midbrain. The fornix sends some projection fibers to the midbrain from their origins within the hippocampus.

Association Fibers. The association fibers of the white matter serve to connect various regions within the same cerebral hemisphere.

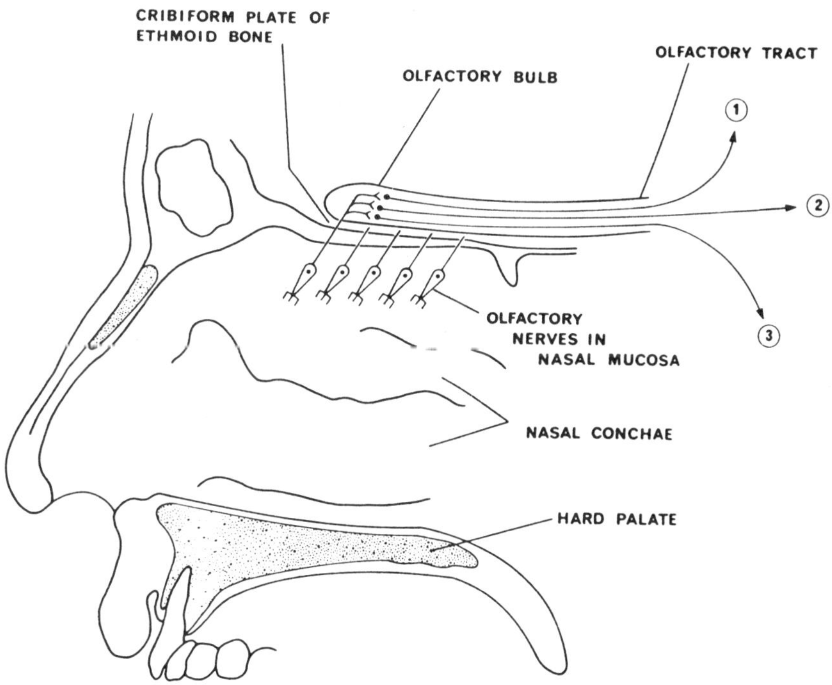

Fig. 2.40. Lateral view of the olfactory nerve. 1. Medial olfactory stria to contralateral olfactory bulb via anterior commissure. 2. Intermediate olfactory stria to anterior perforated substance and diagonal band. 3. Lateral olfactory stria to nuclei of amygdaloid complex (limbic system) and prepyriform cortex.

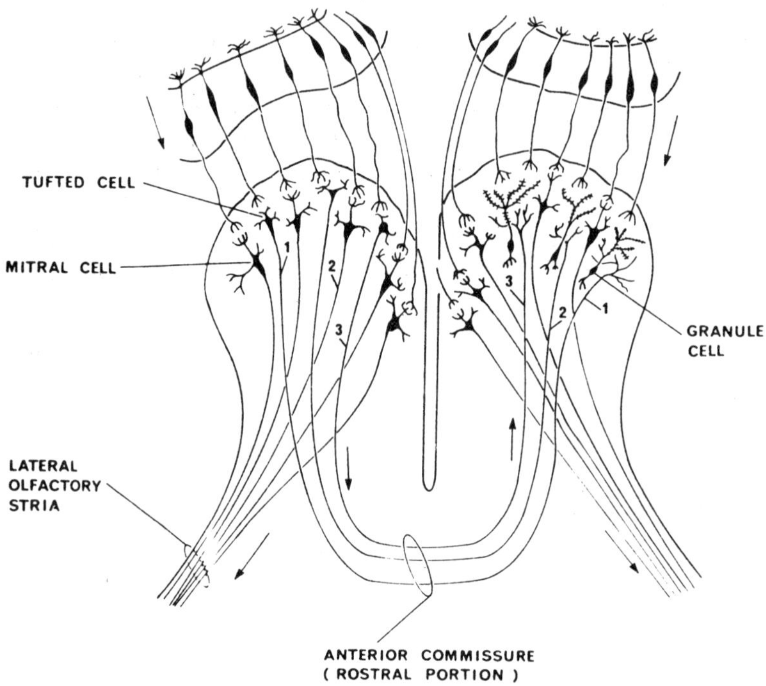

Fig. 2.41. The course of olfactory signals (arrows) from the olfactory mucous membrane to the olfactory cortex via the olfactory bulbs. The bipolar cells of the olfactory mucous membrane project axons into the olfactory bulb where their terminations synapse upon tufted and mitral cells forming structures called olfactory glomeruli. Axons of the mitral cells form the lateral olfactory stria (or tract), whereas the axons of the tufted cells (1, 2, 3) form the medial olfactory stria (or tract) that runs to the contralateral olfactory bulb via the anterior commissure. The granule cells are the elements upon which the fibers of the contralateral tufted cells terminate (3, 2, 1).

Short association (arcuate) fibers connect adjacent gyri. The deeper-lying short association fibers within the cortex are called intracortical fibers, whereas the short association fibers found immediately beneath the cerebral cortex per se are called subcortical fibers.

The long association fibers of the cerebral cortex, in contrast to the short association fibers, serve to connect more distant areas of the cerebral cortex. Six important tracts or bundles of long association fibers are found within each cerebral hemisphere. First, the

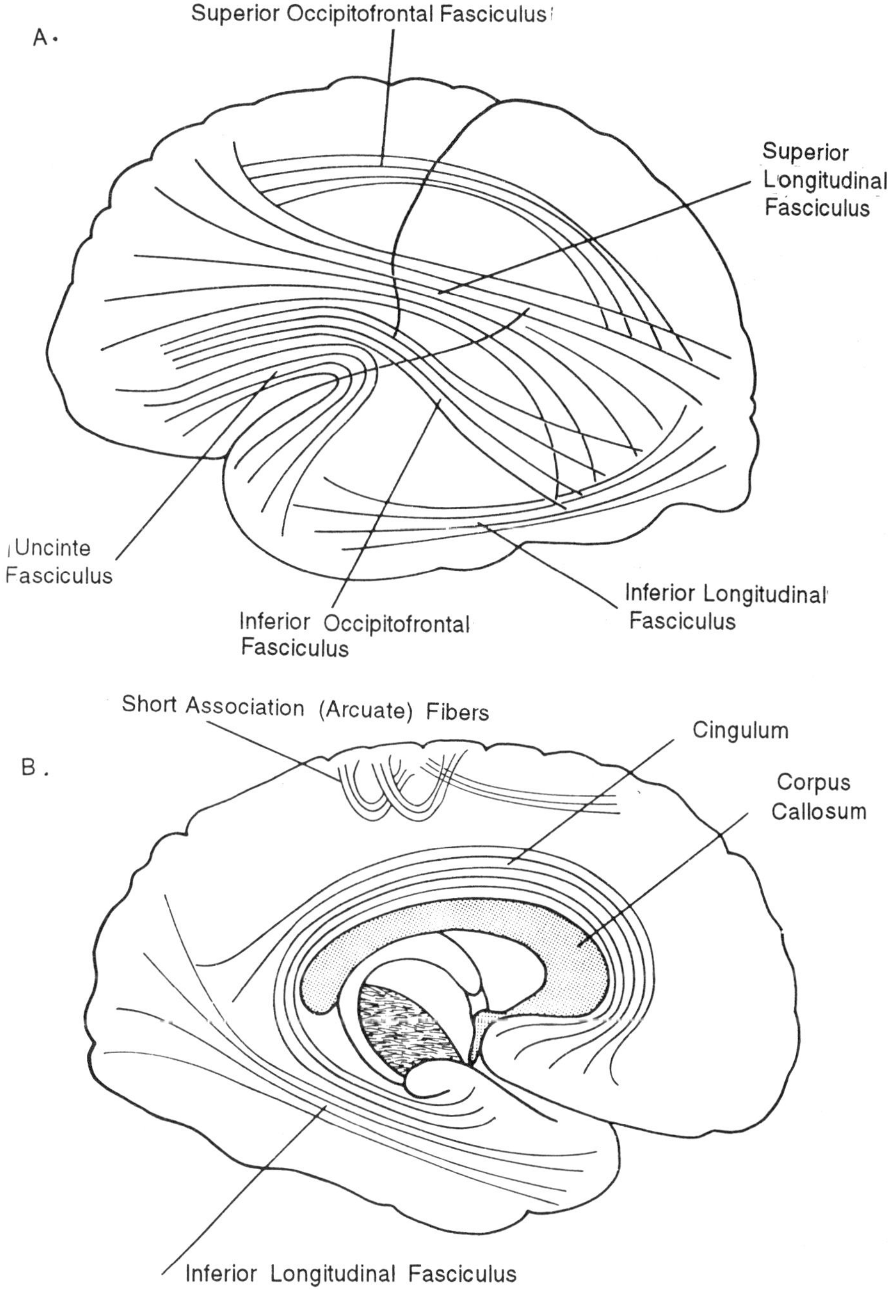

Fig. 2.42. Principal long and short association pathways of the cerebral hemispheres. **A.** Superior lateral view of left hemisphere **B.** Medial view.

superior longitudinal fasciculus connects certain regions of the frontal lobe with areas located in the temporal and occipital lobes. Second, the inferior longitudinal fasciculus connects the temporal and occipital lobes. Third, the occipitofrontal fasciculus courses dorsally from the frontal lobe, thereby connecting this structure with the occipital and

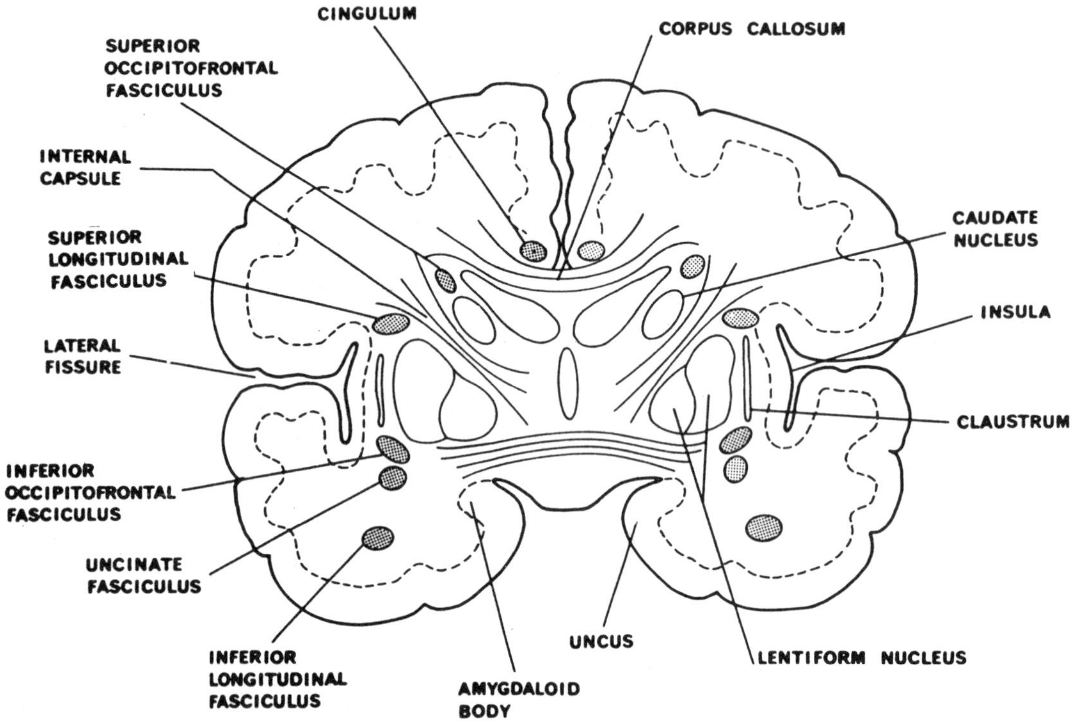

Fig. 2.43. Transverse section of brain illustrating the long association pathways (shaded areas).

temporal lobes. Fourth, the uncinate fasciculus connects the inferior gyri of the frontal lobe with the anterior temporal lobe. Fifth, the cingulum, which is found within the cingulate gyrus as a white strip, connects the anterior perforated substance of the rhinencephalon and the hippocampal gyrus. Sixth, the principal radiations of the fornix serve to connect the hippocampus to the mamillary body of the hypothalamus.

Histology and Cytoarchitecture of the Cerebral Cortex. The major functional region of the cerebral cortex is composed of a thin superficial layer of neurons and glial elements (gray matter) that ranges between 1.5 and 4.0 mm. in thickness, and which has a total surface area of roughly 2,000 cm^2. And yet this layer, which contains approximately 9 billion individual neurons and covers the surfaces of all of the convolutions of cerebrum, is responsible for all of the perceptive, integrative, and motor functions of the cerebral cortex.

The cerebral cortex is composed of a great morphologic variety of neural elements; however, these elements are highly organized into a remarkably constant laminar pattern over most cortical regions.

For purposes of discussion, the cerebral cortex frequently is divided into the phylogenetically ancient allocortex and more recently evolved isocortex. The allocortex includes those rhinencephalic structures that developed in relation to the sense of olfaction, and includes the hippocampus (or archipallium) and pyriform cortex (or paleopallium). The allocortex does not exhibit the characteristic six-layered organizational pattern of neural elements that is found in the isocortex. The isocortex (also called the neocortex or neopallium) forms by far the largest area of the human cortex, and this region exhibits six distinct histologic layers during some stage of ontogeny (Brodmann). Despite the fact that there is a nonuniform distribution of similar neural elements throughout the isocortex, nevertheless the typical lamination of neurons is present throughout this cortical region.

The six layers of the neocortex can be discerned in Nissl-stained sections of the cortex, and the laminar pattern seen in such preparations is said to represent the cytoarchitecture of the cortex.

Five principal types of neuron are found within the cerebral cortex:

First, *pyramidal cells* are the most abundant neural components of the cortex, and these elements range in diameter from approximately 10 to 100 μ. Pyramidal cells are classed as small, medium, large, and giant. The dendrite arises from the apex of the pyramidal cell body and runs toward the cortical surface, there to terminate in many branches. An abundance of smaller dendrites (basal dendrites) emerge from the base and sides of the pyramidal cell bodies and course into the adjoining cortical layers.

The giant pyramidal cells (of Betz), found in the primary motor projection cortex, give rise to axons which control voluntary movements of skeletal muscles on the contralateral side of the body.

Second, *satellite* (or *granule*) *cells* are small neural elements that range between 5 and 10 μ in diameter. The satellite cells have numerous branched dendrites which terminate near the cell from which they originate.

Third, *horizontal cells* are relatively small neural elements which have spindle-shaped cell bodies. The processes of the horizontal cells run for long distances in a direction parallel with the outer cortical surface.

Fourth, *cells of Martinotti* are small multipolar neurons that have a rounded or triangular shape, and whose processes terminate exclusively within the cortex. Cells of Martinotti are found in all cortical layers, and their axons pass toward the cortical surface, while their dendrites remify in all directions.

Fifth, *fusiform cells* are found principally within the deepest layer of the cortex, and their dendrites course into the upper cortical layers. The axons of the fusiform cells enter the white matter, but their termination and distribution are unknown.

The six layers of the neocortex are as follows, from without inward:

I. *Molecular (or Plexiform) Layer:* The molecular layer contains the terminations of dendrites from neurons that lie deeper within the cortex, horizontal cells, and a few cells having short axons (Golgi type II).

II. *External Granular Layer:* The external granular layer is composed of many small granule (or satellite) and pyramidal cells. The dendrites of neurons that lie within the deeper layers pass through the rather dense external granular

A.

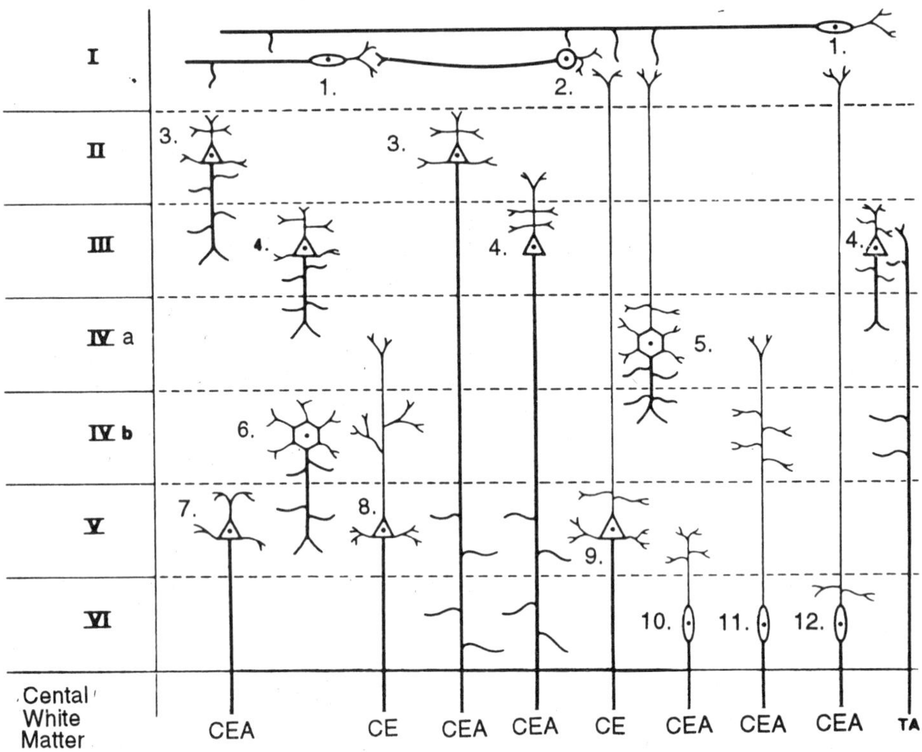

Fig. 2.44. A. Layers of the cerebral cortex (sensory area) presented in highly diagrammatic form. Heavy lines on individual cells represent axons, light lines represent dendrites. The six cortical layers (Roman numerals) are: I, Molecular (plexiform) layer. II, External granular layer. III, Pyramidal layer. IV, Internal granular layer. V, Ganglionic layer. VI, Polymorphic layer. The specific cortical cells found in these layers are: 1. Horizontal cell. 2. Golgi type II cell. 3. Small pyramidal cell. 4. Medium pyramidal cell of layer III. 5. Star pyramidal cell. 6. Stellate cell. 7. Short pyramidal cell. 8. Medium pyramidal cell of layer V. 9. Large pyramidal cell. 10. Short spindle cell. 11. Medium spindle cell. 12. Long spindle cell. Axons found in the central white matter are as follows. CEA = cortical efferent (association) fibers; CE = cortical efferent (projection) fibers; TA = thalamic afferent fibers.

B.

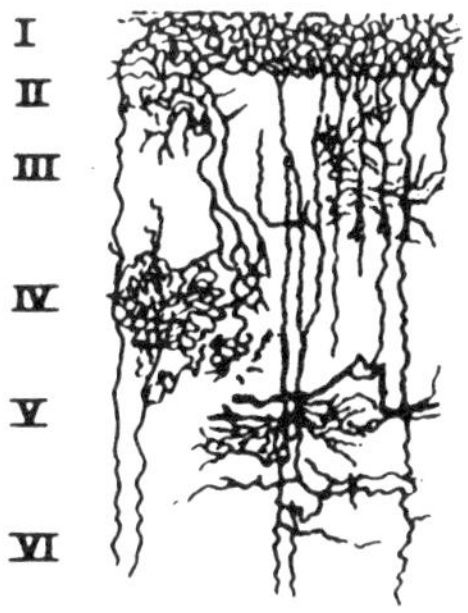

C

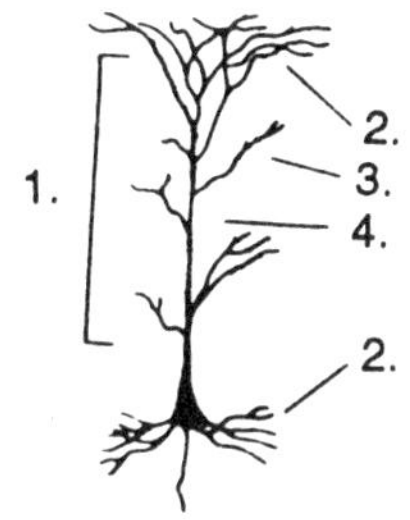

Fig. 2.44. B. Neural interconnections within the cerebral cortex. On the left side are two thalamic afferent fibers, nonspecific and specific respectively. Note particularly the density of the dendritic processes in the different cortical layers.

Fig. 2.44. C. Pyramidal cell of the cortex illustrating the sites of presynaptic terminals as follows: 1. Nonspecific afferent fibers of the reticular formation and thalamus. 2. Recurrent collaterals from pyramidal cell axons. 3. Commissural fibers from contralateral hemisphere (mirrior image loci). 4. Afferent fibers from specific thalamic sensory projection nuclei.

layer, whereas some of the dendrites of cells in the pyramidal layer (layer three) terminate here.

III. *Pyramidal Layer:* The pyramidal layer consists of an outer region that contains mostly medium-sized pyramidal cells and an inner region that is composed principally of larger pyramidal cells. A number of afferent thalamic fibers terminate upon the dendrites of the pyramidal cells located in the inner zone of the pyramidal layer.

IV. *Internal Granular Layer:* The internal granular layer contains an abundance of small pyramidal cells in addition to small satellite cells. Characteristically, this layer has many dense plexuses of fibrils. In the parietal area of the cortex, the plexuses of the internal granular area are composed of afferent fibers that arise within the thalamus, whereas in the temporal and occipital areas the plexuses are formed by afferent fibers that arise from neurons located within the medial and lateral geniculate bodies.

V. *Ganglionic Layer:* The ganglionic layer consists of large, medium, and short pyramidal cells. These pyramidal cells are somewhat more sparse, but in general are large, than those found in layer III. The long dendrites of the large pyramidal cells extend to the molecular layer (I), while their collateral branches and basal dendrites terminate entirely within the ganglionic layer itself.

Dendrites of the medium-sized pyramidal cells of layer V terminate in the internal granular layer (IV); thus an abundance of synaptic connections is present between these neurons and thalamic as well as geniculate afferent fibers. Dendrites of the short pyramidal cells terminate entirely within layer V.

VI. *Polymorphic Layer:* The polymorphic layer contains long, medium, and short fusiform (or spindle) cells. Dendrites of the long spindle cells emit collaterals in layer VI, then ascend without yielding additional collaterals to terminate in the molecular layer (I). Dendrites of the medium fusiform cells terminate in the internal granular layer (IV) on the thalamic afferent fibers, whereas the dendrites of the short fusiform cells terminate in the ganglionic layer (V).

In certain areas of the cerebral cortex the presence of myelinated layers of nerve fibers between the cortical layers is responsible for the presence of macroscopically visible white lines. In the striate area of the occipital lobe, the line of Gennari is present on the outer zone of the internal granular layer (IV). Elsewhere in the cortex, a similarly located but thinner line is found, and this is called the external line of Baillarger. At the inner zone of the ganglionic layer (V) is found the internal line of Baillarger.

The cytoarchitecture in various regions of the cerebral cortex has been studied intensively by many investigators in order to attempt a correlation between structure and function in different areas of the brain. One such classification is that developed by Brodmann, who labeled particular areas of the cortex with numbers depending upon the individual cytoarchitectural characteristics of each area. This classification is useful as it gives reference points for the localization of physiologic as well as pathologic processes in the cerebral cortex.

Many cortical functions have been related experimentally to specific brain areas by means of electric and chemical stimulation in addition to ablation of particular cortical areas. Much of this experimental work has been carried out on the brains of higher primates (i.e., monkeys and chimpanzees), as well as on human subjects during as well as following neurosurgical procedures. In addition, clinical and postmortem data have added considerably to out knowledge of localized functions in various areas of the brain.

Functional Correlates. The general physiologic properties of the four major cortical regions will be summarized briefly, and this information will be followed by a more complete discussion of the functions carried out by particular cortical areas.

Area 4 of the frontal lobe is the primary motor area of the cerebral cortex, whereas area 6 forms a part of the extrapyramidal system. Eye movements and changes in pupillary diameter are related to area 8. The frontal association areas are located in areas 9, 10, 11, and 12.

Areas 1, 2, and 3 of the parietal lobe are the primary cortical sensory areas. Sensory association areas are found in areas 5 and 7.

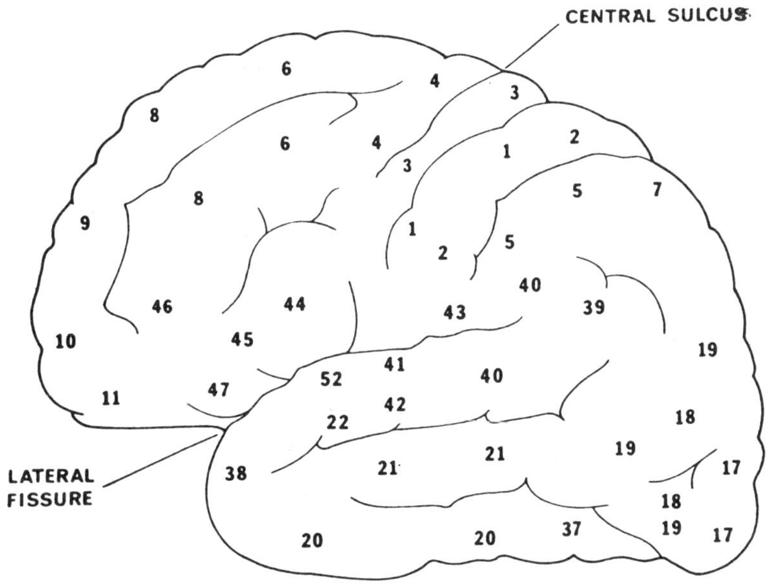

Fig. 2.45. Lateral aspect of the left cerebral hemisphere showing the cortical areas according to Brodmann. Area 8 = frontal eye movement, pupillary change area. Area 6 = premotor area (portion of extrapyramidal system). Area 4 (precentral gyrus) is the primary motor area. Area 3, 2, 1 (postcentral gyrus) are the primary sensory areas. Areas 5, 6, 7 = secondary sensory association areas. Areas 39, 40 = association areas. Areas 18, 19 = visual association areas. Areas 17 = primary visual cortex. Area 41 = primary auditory cortex. Area 42 = associative auditory cortex. Area 44 = motor speech area of Broca.

Within the temporal lobe, the primary auditory cortex is located in area 41, whereas the secondary (or associative) auditory area is found in area 42. Areas 20, 21, 22, 38 and 40 are association areas.

Area 17 of the occipital lobe is the primary visual cortex, whereas the visual association areas are found in areas 18 and 19.

The Primary Sensory Projection Cortex. The primary sensory cortex for the receipt of general sensory information which is transmitted from receptors located throughout the body is found in areas 1, 2, and 3. This region, called the somesthetic area, is located in the postcentral gyrus immediately dorsal to the central sulcus.

The somesthetic area receives afferent impulses that arise within skin, muscle, joint, and tendon receptors and are transmitted via thalamic radiations to the cortex from the contralateral side of the body.

It has been determined experimentally that a relatively large area of the frontal lobe also can receive sensory impulses (areas 4 and 6), whereas certain motor responses can

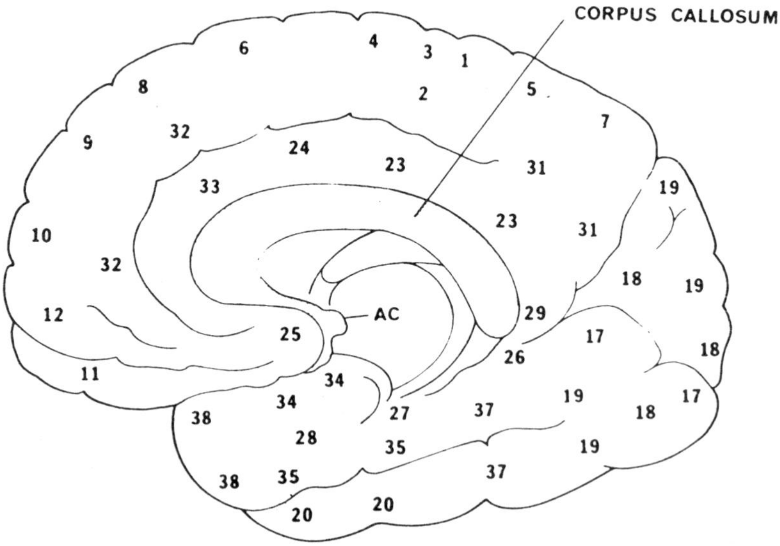

Fig. 2.46. Medial aspect of the left cerebral hemisphere showing the cortical areas according to Brodmann.

be elicited by stimulation of areas 1, 2, and 3. Therefore the primary sensorimotor area of the cortex is considered able to subserve both motor as well as sensory functions. However, the region dorsal to the central sulcus (of Rolando) is considered to have principally sensory functions, whereas the region ventral to this sulcus has principally motor functions.

The cortical localization of sensory information received from various parts of the body. The high degree of topographic specificity that is present between the various peripheral regions and the cortical pattern for the expression of these regions.

The Primary Motor Projection Cortex. The primary motor cortex is found on the anterior wall of the central sulcus as well as in the precentral gyrus immediately adjacent to this sulcus (area 4). This motor area correlates well with the distribution of the giant pyramidal cells of Betz; and as noted earlier, these cells control the voluntary contractions of skeletal muscles on the contralateral side of the body. Efferent impulses generated within the Betz cells are transmitted over their axons via the corticobulbar and corticospinal tracts to the nuclei of particular cerebrospinal nerves.

It has been determined experimentally that the topographic organization of the primary sensory areas of the postcentral gyrus bear a mirror-image relationship to those of the primary motor areas of the adjacent precentral gyrus.

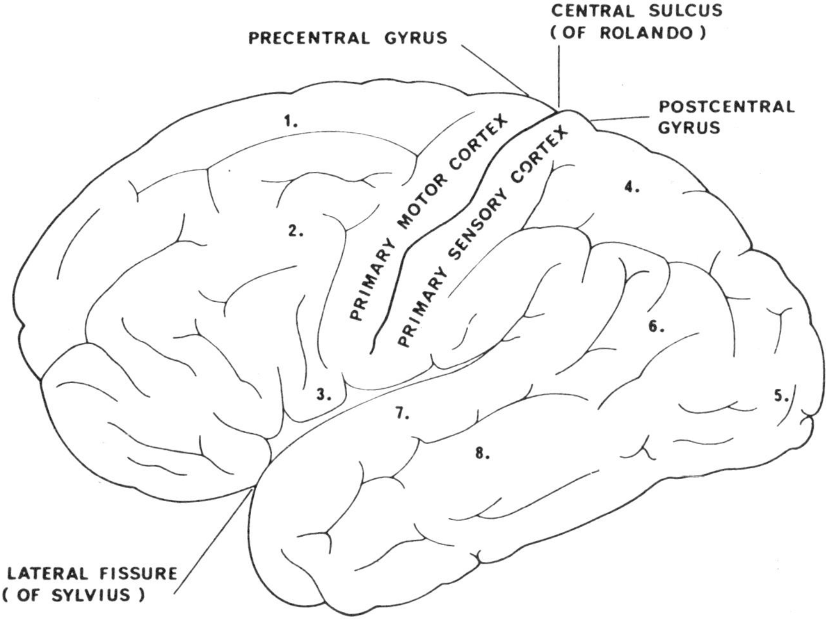

Fig. 2.47. Some effects obtained by electric stimulation of particular areas of the cerebral cortex. Note: The numbers in this figure merely indicate areas stimulated, and are not Brodmann areas. Stimuli applied to the primary motor cortex and areas 1., 2., and 3. elicited as follows: 1. Head, eyes, and trunk turn toward the opposite side. Complex synergistic movements of the contralateral arm and leg can be produced. 2. Eyes turn toward contralateral side; no visual aura experienced. 3. Chewing, licking, swallowing movements. 4. Sensory aura in contralateral leg followed by complex synergistic movements. Also, poorly localized and vague but disagreeable sensations. 5. Complex optical hallucinations, including stars, lights, flames, colors. 6. Eyes turn to opposite side of body. 7. Auditory hallucinations, e.g., roaring, buzzing. 8. Head, eyes, and trunk rotate to contralateral side coupled to complex synergistic movements of contralateral extremities. The specific sensations and movements evoked by simulations of the primary sensory and motor cortices are highly localized insofar as regions of the body are concerned.

Area 4 is the most sensitive region of the cerebral cortex, insofar as motor stimulation is concerned, and it appears that the ganglionic layer (V), which contains the giant pyramidal cells, is responsible for modulating the excitability of the neurons located within this area. Thus facilitation and suppression are phenomena that may be evoked in response to appropriate stimulation of the cortex. Facilitation (or temporal summation) refers to the ability of a neuron to respond by firing an all-or-none impulse in response to a rapidly applied series of subthreshold stimuli. Suppression; on the other hand, is an inhibition of the contraction of skeletal muscle following prolonged cortical or subcortical stimulation. Both of these effects, of course, could modify profoundly the contractile state of the somatic musculature in vivo.

Stimulation of area 6, sometimes referred to as the premotor area, evokes contractions of skeletal muscles similar to those elicited by stimulation of area 4. If one extirpates area

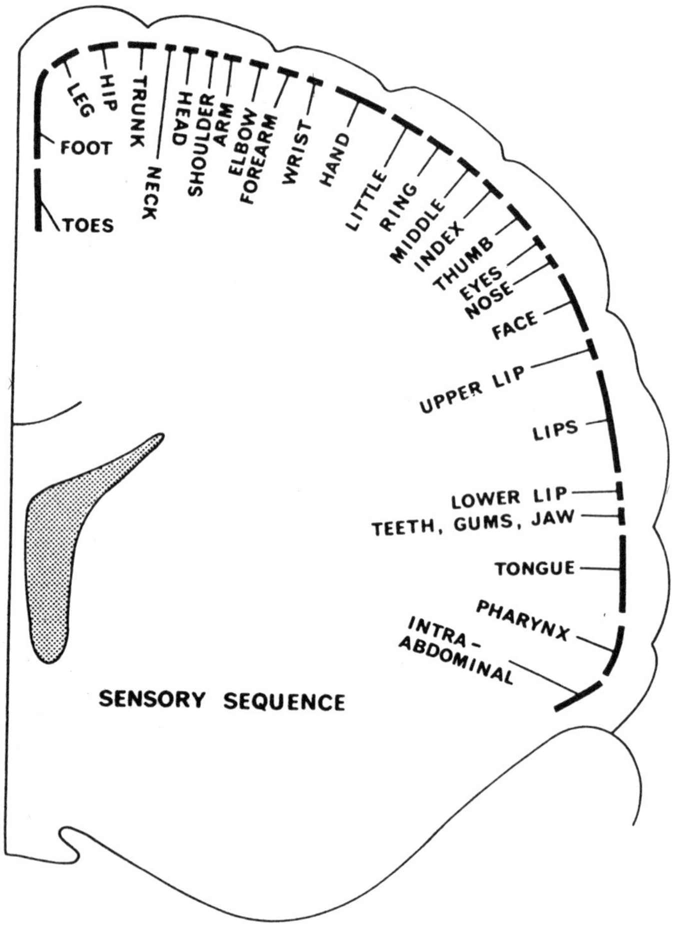

Fig. 2.48. Cross section through the postcentral gyrus of the left cerebral hemisphere (i.e., the primary sensory cortex) illustrating the sequence in which sensory phenomena are localized. The sensory sequence in the right hemisphere is an exact mirror image of that shown in this figure. The length of the heavy black bars for each area indicates the approximate brain area that subserves each function in this and the following figure.

4, or sections the nerve fibers that connect areas 4 and 6, however, stimulation of these regions now produces stereotyped motor responses, including twisting of the body and rotation of the head.

The Primary Visual Cortex. The primary cortical area for the reception of visual impulses is found in the occipital lobe (area 17; the calcarine fissure and nearby parts of the cuneus and lingual gyri). Thus stimulation of this region can produce visual hallucinations including bursts of light, rainbows, or bright stars.

The dorsal most region of the occipital lobe in primates (including man) is concerned principally with macular vision. The more ventral portions of the calcarine fissure, on the other hand, are related to peripheral vision.

The association of visual impulses takes place in areas 18 and 19. Area 18 receives impulses principally from the primary visual cortex (area 17), whereas area 19 is able to receive impulses from the entire cerebral cortex.

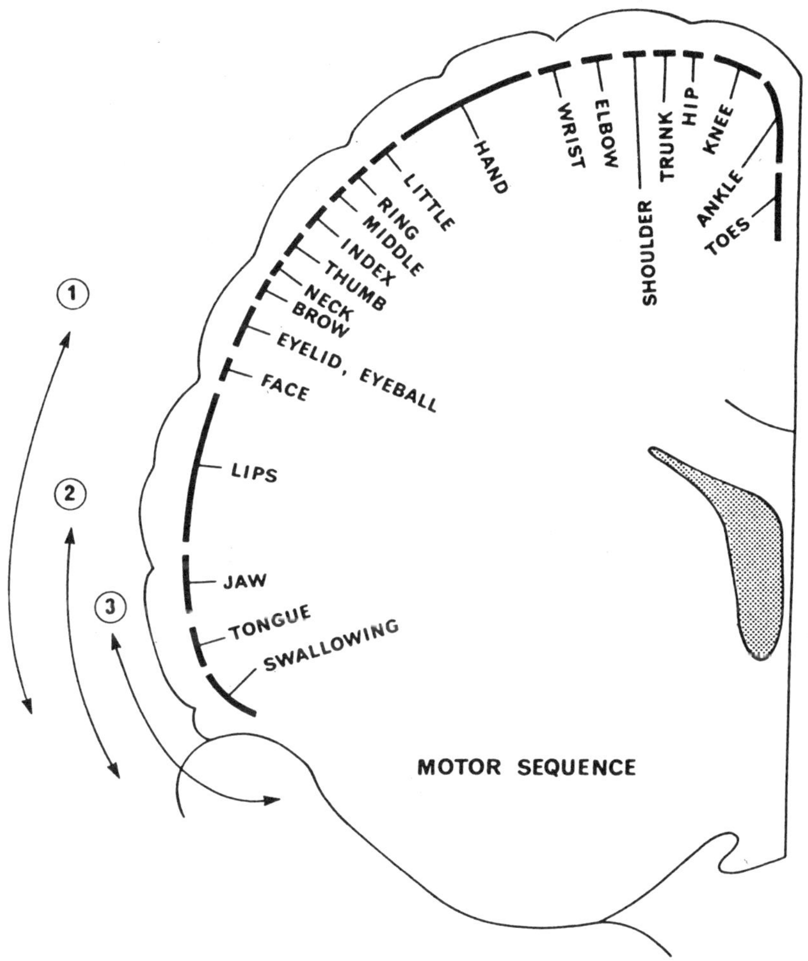

Fig. 2.49. Cross section through the precentral gyrus of the right cerebral hemisphere (i.e., the primary motor cortex) illustrating the sequence in which motor phenomena are localized. The motor sequence in the left hemisphere is an exact mirror image of that shown in this figure. The numbers signify the approximate cortical areas given to complex motor functions as follows. 1. Vocalization. 2. Salivation. 3. Mastication.

The Primary Auditory Area. The primary cortical area for the receipt of auditory impulses is found in the transverse temporal gynus (area 41; Heschl's gyrus). This convlution is located within the floor of the lateral cerebral ventricle, and it receives auditory fibers which radiate from the medial geniculate body; the sensory end organ for hearing, in turn, is the cochlea.

Unilateral lesions of the primary auditory area produce only mild deafness, as the perception of auditory impulses from one ear is represented bilaterally on each primary auditory area. This fact is in marked contrast to the unilateral neuroanatomic arrangement of nerve fibers that is found in all other sensory pathways in the brain.

The Olfactory Area. The olfactory area for receipt of impulses from the olfactory tract is located within the uncus as well as the nearby regions of the hippocampal gyrus of the temporal lobe.

Primary Association Areas of the Cerebral Cortex. The association areas of the sensory and motor regions of the cerebral cortex are connected by a number of tracts within the white matter which contain association fibers. The association areas are of major importance for the maintenance of the higher mental processes in man, and these will be considered in more detail in relation to specific topics that fall under this heading.

Briefly, however, the frontal lobe anterior to area 4 is concerned with higher intellectual and psychic functions, e.g., thought processes. This orbitofrontal area, which includes areas 9, 10, 11, and 12, receives afferent nerves from the dorsomedial thalamic nuclei which in turn receive hypothalamic connections.

When stimulated electrically, the posterior region of the orbital surface as well as the anterior region of the insula evoke profound autonomic responses, as well as alteration of blood pressure and respiratory inhibition. When the anterior cingulate area is stimulated inhibition of skeletal muscle tone as well as autonomic responses are elicited. Furthermore, extirpation of this area in lower primates (male monkeys) reduces their aggressive behavior somewhat so that the animals become more tractable and less fearful.

The primary association areas located within the parietal lobe (areas 5 and 7) are necessary for the integration of cutaneous sensations with other perceptual cues. Thus a subject can recognize various common objects placed in his hand when his eyes are closed. This function is called the sterognostic sense. The parietal lobe also contains secondary sensory and motor association areas that are broadly connected to the primary motor and sensory areas.

Complex memory patterns are retained within the temporal lobes of the cortex.

The aphasias further illustrate the importance of the cortical association areas to the higher mental processes. An aphasia can be defined as a defect or loss of the power of expression, whether by speech, writing, or signs (i.e., the use of symbols or language). The term aphasia also denotes a loss of comprehension of spoken or written language. Various clinically recognized aphasias can result from lesions in the association areas of the brain. In right-handed individuals, aphasias are produced by lesions in the contralateral (or the dominant) hemisphere, whereas the opposite situation obtains for

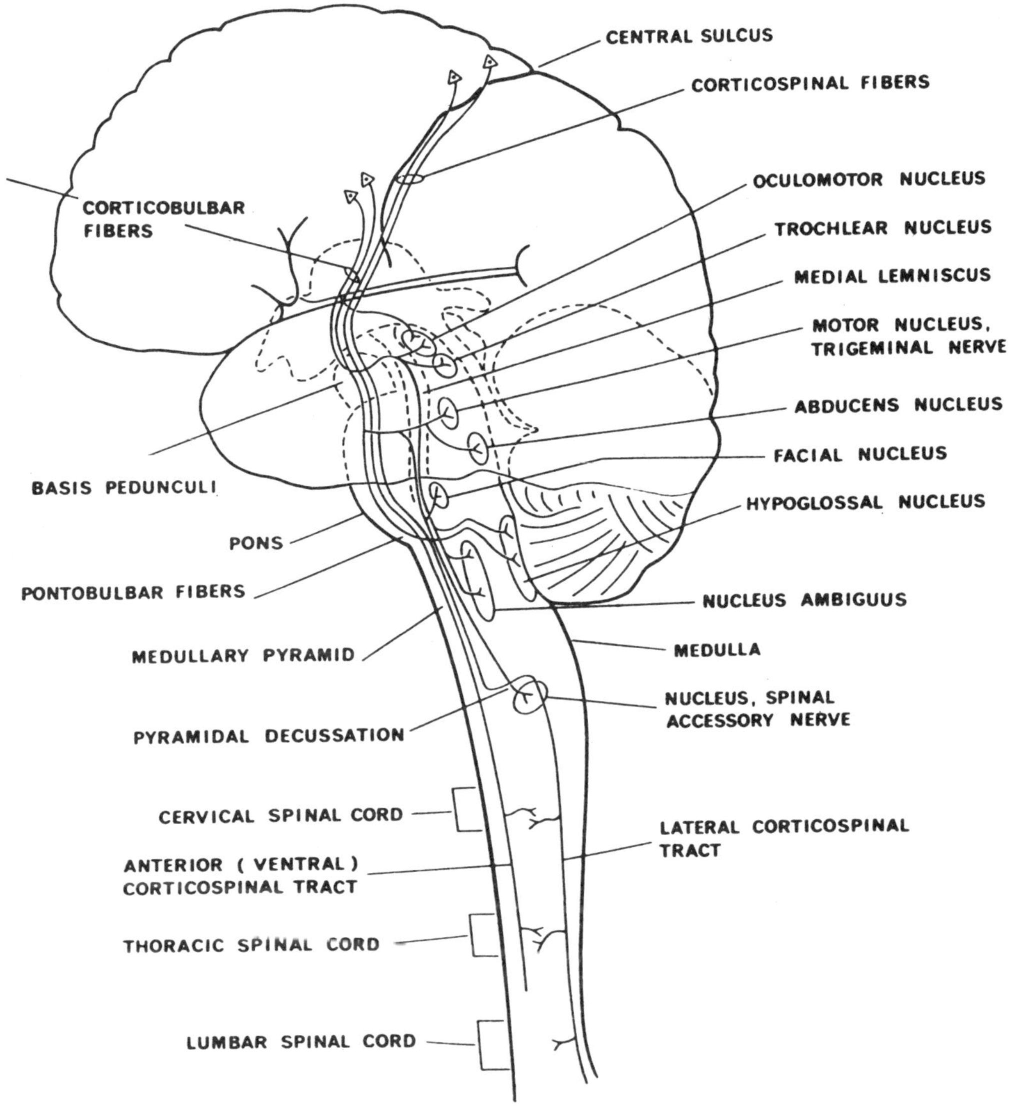

Fig. 2.50. The origin and distribution of the corticospinal (pyramidal) and corticomedullary fibers.

left-handed individuals. For example, motor aphasia results from damage to the motor speech area of Broca (area 44). The patient can move both tongue and lips but is incapable of producing the coordinated movements necessary for coherent speech. Agraphia, or the inability to write words, often accompanies motor aphasia. Lesions within the posterior region of the superior temporal gyrus cause sensory aphasia (area 39). The victim cannot understand the meaning of spoken words, although hearing may be unimpaired. Damage

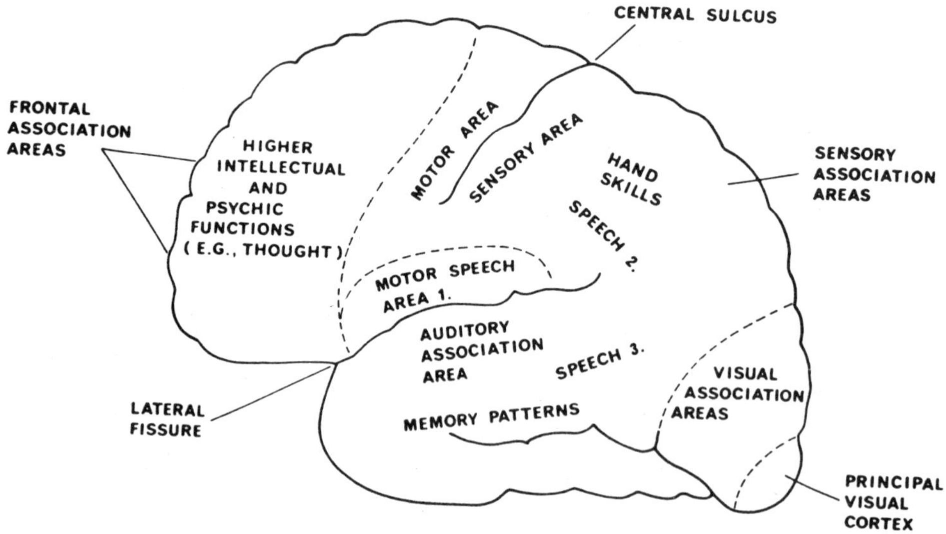

Fig. 2.51. Some general functional areas of the left cerebral cortex. The crude localizations shown here are those as would be found primarily in the categorical hemisphere of a right-handed person as discussed in the text.

to the angular gyrus (areas 39 and 40) may result in word blindness; that is, the patient is unable to understand the meaning of written words although vision is unimpaired.

In conclusion, it must be emphasized that the association areas and their functions are closely integrated, and that many of the higher sensorimotor functions of the brain do not take place in circumscribed regions. Rather, higher mental processes such as thought or memory involve the participation of large cortical association areas that function in a cooperative fashion and are connected by association fibers. It is, of course, impossible to localize anatomically any particular mental process.

The Limbic System (Rhinencephalon). The term rhinencephalon was applied earlier in this text to designate those phylogenetically ancient structures of the cerebral hemisphere that are concerned with the perception of olfactory stimuli. However, since the rhinencephalic portion of the brain has been demonstrated unequivocally to possess a number of important functional roles in a variety of physiologic processes in addition to olfaction, the term limbic system generally is employed preferentially to denote the rhinencephalic structures of the cerebral hemisphere. In fact, the terms rhinencephalon, limbic lobe, and limbic system often are used interchangeably. Henceforth the term limbic system will be used in this text to denote collectively the following structurally

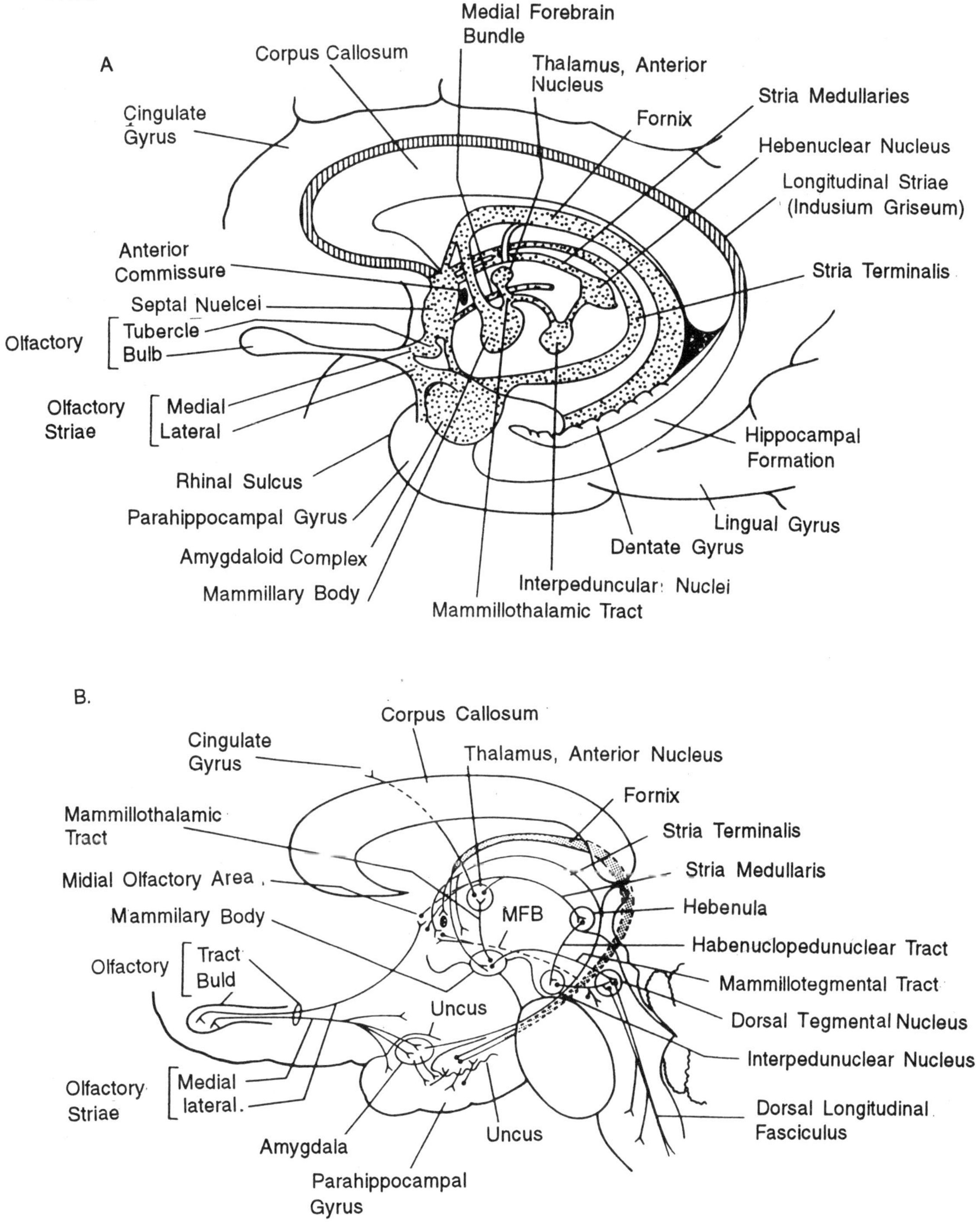

Fig. 2.52. A. The relationships among the component structure of the limbic system (rhinencephalon) as found in a medial section of the right cerebral hemisphere. **B.** Similar view of the limbic system illustrating the interconnections among the component structures. MFB = medial forebrain bundle.

and functionally interconnected neural elements; the limbic lobe and hippocampus together with their related subcortical neural connections; the amygdala; the septal nuclei; the hypothalamus; the anterior thalamic nuclei; portions of the basal ganglia. The epithalamus sometimes is considered part of the limbic system.

Each cortical lobe of the limbic system is composed of a band of primitive (allocortical) tissue that surrounds the hilum of the cerebral hemisphere. Histologically, this allocortical tissue does not have the characteristic six-layered cytoarchitectural pattern found in the neocortex.

The fornix connects the hippocampus to the mamillary bodies, and these structures in turn are connected to the anterior thalamic nuclei via the mamillothalamic tract (of Vicq d'Azyr). The anterior nuclei of the thalamus then project fibers to the cingulate gyrus, and from this cortical area neural connections pass to the hippocampus, thereby completing a closed neural circuit or loop, sometimes referred to as the Papez circuit after the worker who described it originally.

One peculiarity of the limbic system is that it has only a few connections with the neocortex. A small number of nerve fibers pass from the frontal lobe to the nearby limbic structures, and possibly some indirect functional are present via the thalamus.

The functions of the limbic system now may be summarized briefly, and this information has been gained out only from stimulation and ablation experiments performed on animals, but from clinical studies as well.

In man, the role of the limbic system in olfaction is relatively minor. In general, the limbic system is concerned with a wide variety of autonomic somatosensory and somatomotor responses. Specifically, the activity of the limbic system is concerned initimately with such complex phenomena as emotions of rage and fear as well as their genesis; the control of various biologic rhythms sexual behavior; motivation; and together with the hypothalamus, drinking and feeding behavior. These manifestations of limbic function will be dealt with more fully in later sections of this chapter.

Electric stimulation of various components of the limbic system can evoke a wide variety of responses, including the inhibition of respiratory movements, shivering, and swallowing, as well as voluntary movements that are initiated by discharge of impulses from the premotor area of the cerebral cortex. Alternatively, such stimulation can elicit chewing, swallowing, facial-vocal movements, licking, tonic movements of the extremities and trunk, changes in pupillary diameter, piloerection, and salivation, as well as reflex micturition and defecation. The inherent electric activity of practically the entire cerebral cortex also can be modified by stimulation of various limbic structures.

Certain components of the limbic system, such as the anterior limbic region as well as the posterior orbital surface, appear to exert an inhibitory role upon those mechanisms in the brain stem that are related to the expression of emotions such as fear and anger. Lesions in these structures produce hyperactivity.

Physiologically, the activity of the neocortex can modify emotional behavior and the opposite also is true, despite the lack of abundant neural pathways between the

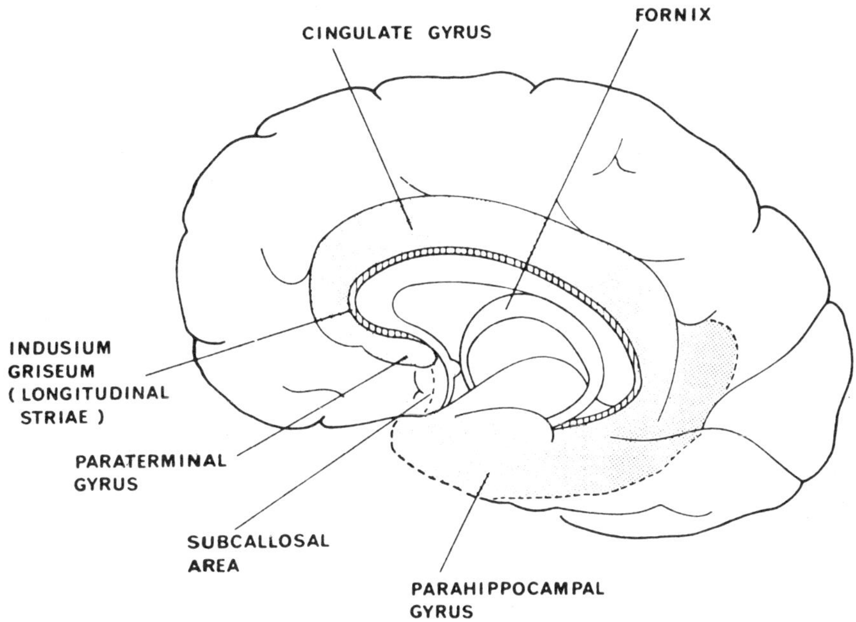

Fig. 2.53. Medial surface of right cerebral hemisphere showing the limbic cortex (shaded area).

limbic system and other cortical areas. Nevertheless, one of the basic characteristics of emotional behavior is that it cannot be evoked or terminated voluntarily. In this regard, it is of interest that limbic circuits once stimulated exhibit a prolonged after-discharge. Consequently this fact may explain (at least partially) the fact that emotional responses generally are of long, rather than of transient, duration. Hence such responses tend to persist for a much longer interval than do the stimuli that elicit them.

Memory for recent events may be lost following bilateral lesions of the hippocampus in humans, indicating that the limbic system is involved in some way in the process of information retention.

It has been demonstrated that the limbic system has major relationships with the reticular formation of the brain stem, and thus presumably has a role in the alerting or arousal process.

Lastly, the limbic system has been implicated in the hypothalamic regulation of pituitary activity, and possibly this limbic control is manifest via the hypothalamic neurosecretory cells.

Since the functions of the limbic system are related so intimately to the control of a broad variety of autonomic and other functions, the term "visceral brain" sometimes is

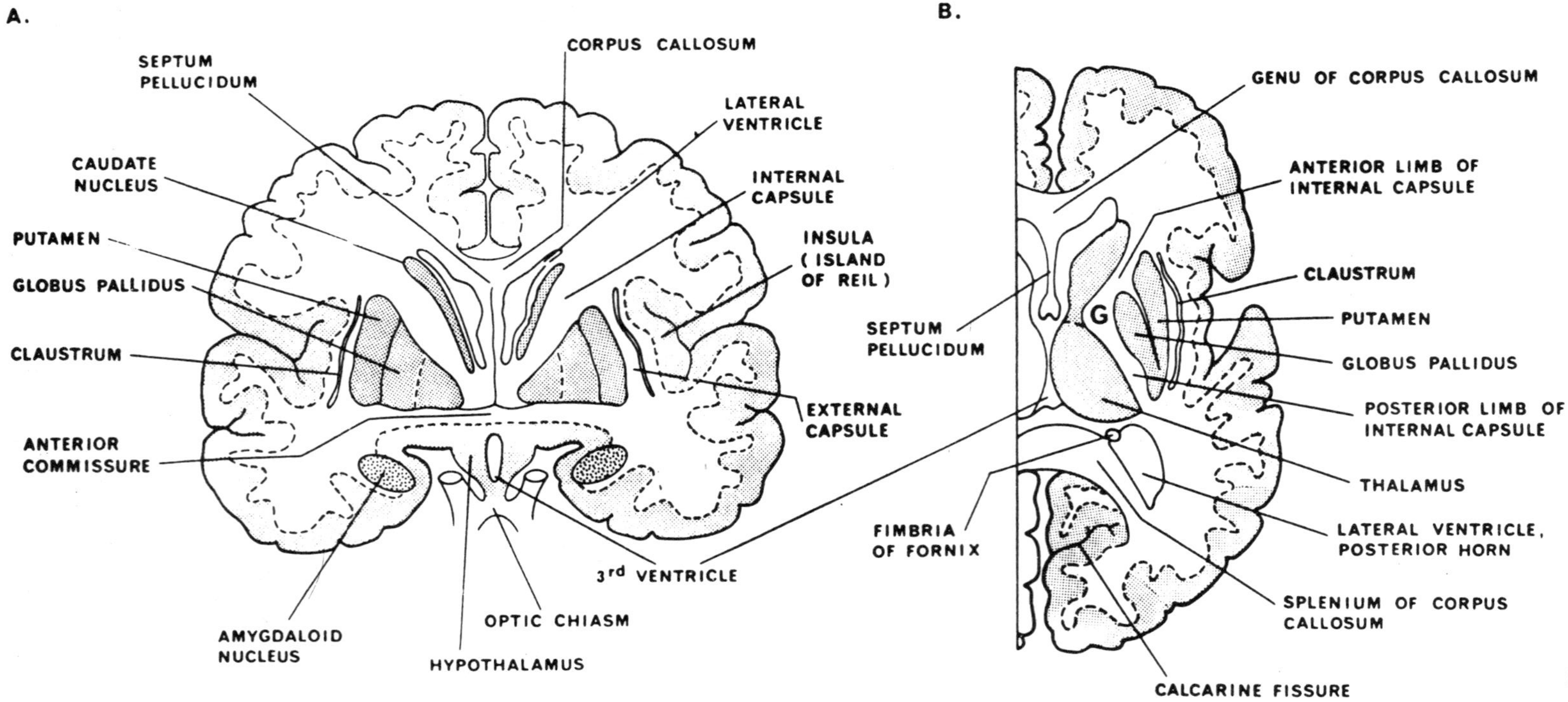

Fig. 2.54. A. Transverse section through the cerebral hemispheres at the level of the anterior commissure. **B.** Horizontal section through the right cerebral hemisphere showing the relationships among the anterior limb, genu (or flexure, G), and the posterior limb of the internal capsule.

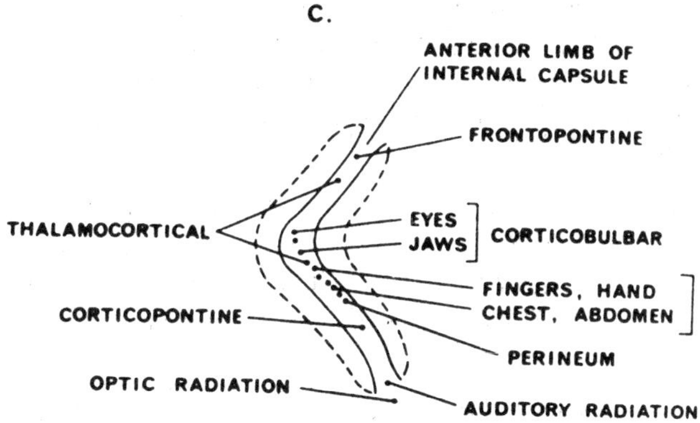

Fig. 2.54. C. Detail of the internal capsule illustrating the general spatial orientation of certain ascending and descending tracts.

used to denote the limbic structures. In conclusion, it is unclear at present which structural components of the limbic system should be assigned particular functional roles, a fact which can be appreciated readily when one considers the anatomic complexity of this system as well as its intimate relationships to, and interconnections with, other parts of the brain.

The Basal Ganglia and the Internal Capsule. The basal ganglia are large masses of gray matter that are located deep within each cerebral hemisphere. The term "basal ganglia" usually is applied to those nuclear masses called the caudate nucleus, the putamen, and the globus pallidus. The term *corpus striatum* (or *striatum*) denotes the caudate nucleus plus the putamen, because of the striped appearance of the bundles of white matter that are located between these two nuclear structures. Hence this region of the brain sometimes is referred to as the striatal level. The term *lenticular (or lentiform)* nucleus denotes the putamen plus the globus pallidus.

Some authors also include the claustrum, amygdaloid nucleus, red nucleus, red and substantia nigra as components of the system of basal ganglia because of the elaborate interconnections between these structures and the striatum as well as the lenticular nucleus. However, for the purposes of this text the basal ganglia are considered to be only the caudate nucleus, putamen, and globus pallidus.

Many afferent nerve fibers pass from the caudate nucleus to the putamen; thence short fibers course to the globus pallidus. The putamen as well as the globus pallidus receives afferent fibers from the substantia nigra, whereas fibers pass from the thalamus to the caudate nucleus.

Efferent fibers that arise within the corpus striatum leave this nucleus by way of the globus pallidus. Some of these efferents run through the internal capsule and form a bundle, called the fasciculus lenticularis, on the medial side of the capsule. Additional fibers course to the medial region of the internal capsule and form a loop called the ansa enticularis. Both the fasciculus lenticularis and the ansa lenticularis yield terminals to the subthalamic nucleus (of Luys), whereas other fibers pass to the thalamus by way of the fasciculus thalamicus.

The internal capsule is continuous with the cerebral peduncle, and this structure is composed of a wide band of white matter that separates the lenticular nucleus from the medially located caudate nucleus and thalamus. When the brain is sectioned horizontally, the internal capsule appears as a widely expanded V, whose apex (the genu) is directed medially.

The anterior limb of the internal capsule separates the caudate nucleus from the lenticular nucleus, and this region contains thalamocortical as well as corticothalamic fibers which interconnect the lateral thalamic nucleus with the frontal lobe of the cerebral cortex. The anterior limb of the internal capsule also contains frontopontine (or frontopontile) tracts that descend from the frontal lobe to nuclei within the pons, as well as fibers that run from the caudate nucleus to the putamen.

The posterior limb of the internal capsule is located between the thalamus and the lenticular nucleus. This region sometimes is divided into lenticulothalamic, retrolenticular, and sublenticular regions. The anterior portion of the lenticulothalamic region contains the corticobulbar and corticospinal tracts which provide motor innervation to the arm and leg. Corticorubral fibers from the frontal lobe of the cortex course together with the fibers of the corticospinal tract, to terminate within the red nucleus. The retrolenticular portion of the internal capsule contains fibers from the lateral thalamic nucleus to the postcentral gyrus of the cortex. The sublenticular region of the internal capsule lies beneath the lenticular nucleus and contains parietotemporopontine fibers from the temporal and parietal lobes of the cerebral cortex that pass to pontine nuclei. In addition, the sublenticular region contains auditory radiations from the medial geniculate body that pass to the transverse temporal gyrus (Heschl's gyrus), as well as optic fibers that course from the lateral geniculate body to the calcarine cortex.

It should be reiterated here that all of the afferent pathways to the cerebral cortex (excepting the olfactory pathway) have synaptic junctions (or relay stations) within the various thalamic nuclei, and that in every instance the axon of the final sensory neuron passes to the cortex via the internal capsule, which in turn is continuous with the cerebral peduncle.

The exact functions of the basal ganglia are a mystery, although experimental as well as clinical data support the contention that these nuclei have an important role in the control of bodily movements.

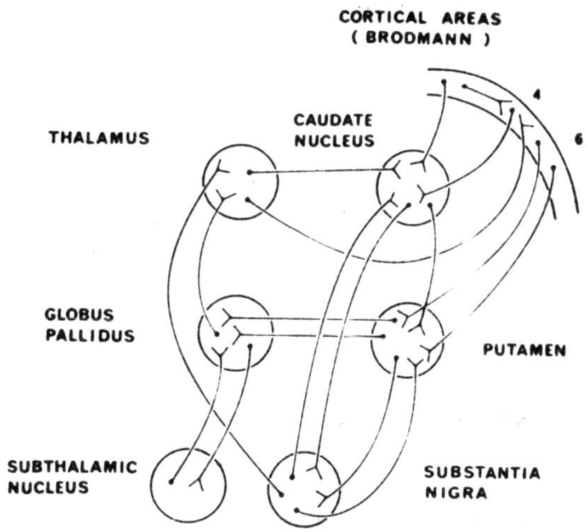

Fig. 2.55. Highly schematic diagram illustrating the interconnections among the basal ganglia and the cerebral cortex.

The caudate and lenticular nuclei, in combination with the fibers of the internal capsule which lie between these structures, comprise an important structural unit of the extrapyramidal system, the corpus striatum (qv, next section). From the corpus striatum efferent fibers course to the globus pallidus, and this unit also receives afferent fibers from the frontal lobe (areas 4 and 6) as well as the thalamus and hypothalamus.

An important efferent route from the globus pallidus passes to the cerebral and brain-stem nuclei by way of the ansa lenticularis.

When the basal ganglia are stimulated electrically, skeletal muscle tone may be inhibited, and movements that originate within the cortex either may be evoked or inhibited, although such results usually are negative.

The globus pallidus and the lateral thalamic nuclear groups apparently are regions of the brain within which many efferent (motor) pathways converge. Consequently these nuclei would seem to act as regulatory as well as integrating centers for motor activities, in addition to functioning as relay centers for afferent impulses to the cerebral cortex.

It has been demonstrated experimentally that certain neurons within the basal ganglia discharge impulses only during slow and smooth eye movements, whereas they do not fire during rapid and jerky (or saccadic) eye movements such as are found when one reads a printed page. These facts tend to corroborate the hypothesis that the basal ganglia are involved in some way with the control of movement. Furthermore certain clinical states involving the basal ganglia also tend to support this idea (see Clinical Correlates).

The Comparative Anatomy of the Brain

The essential features of the comparative anatomy of the vertebrate brain may be passed in review by an examination of diagrams of the brain of various vertebrate types which may be compared also with the diagram of a vertebrate brain principally upon that of a cyclostome.

(a) *Cyclostomes.*— The brain of the lamprey eel, *Petromyzon*, is without marked flexures and quite primitive in plan. Connected with the relatively large medulla

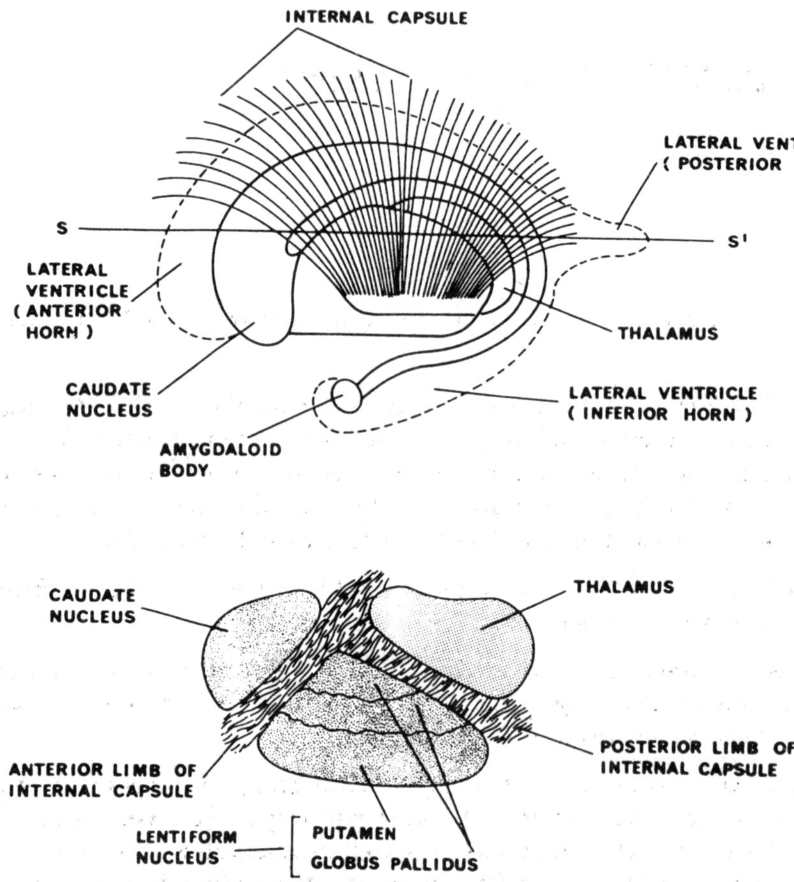

Fig. 2.56. The basal ganglia are adjacent structures as seen in a lateral view. A horizontal cross section of the basal ganglia through the plane S—S′ is shown at the bottom of the figure.

are six pairs of cranial nerves (V-X, inclusive), there being only ten pairs in these animals, as in fishes and amphibians. The roof of the fourth ventricle has an extensive vascular network.

The metencephalon of *Petromyzon* includes a rudimentary lip-like *cerebellum* but no *pons*, while both are lacking in *Myxine*. The roof of the mesencephalon has but one pair of swellings, the *optic lobes*. As the wall of this region remains relatively thin there are large *optic ventricles* which are not separated from the aqueduct.

The *infundibular* region and the *thalamus* proper are small. The epithalamus includes a pair of *habenular ganglia* connected by a *commissure* as in all vertebrates. There are two outgrowths from the habenular region: a well developed *epiphysis* (*pineal organ*), anterior to which is a smaller parietal body. These two organs, arising from a common origin, were probably originally paired, since the pineal body is in intimate relation with the right habenular ganglion and the parietal body with the left.

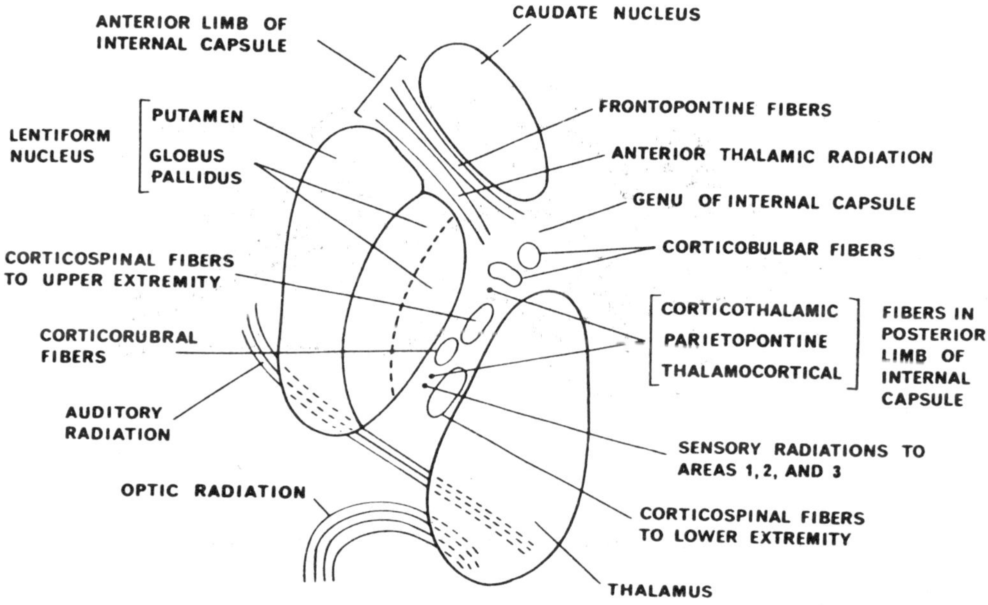

Fig. 2.57. Horizontal section illustrating the regions of the internal capsule and its fiber systems in relation to adjacent structures.

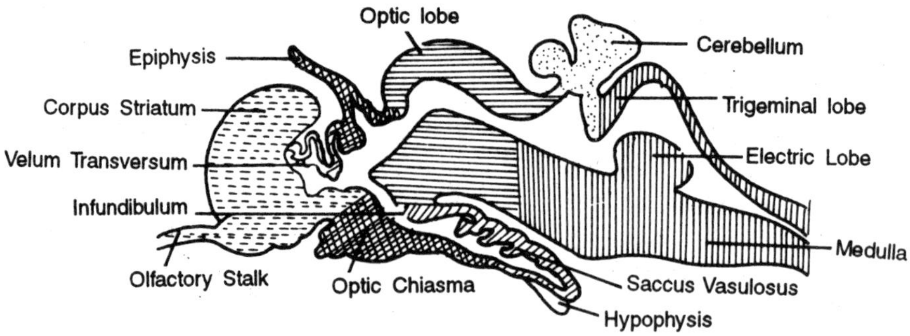

Fig. 2.58. Sagittal section diagram of the brain of the electric ray, Torpedo.

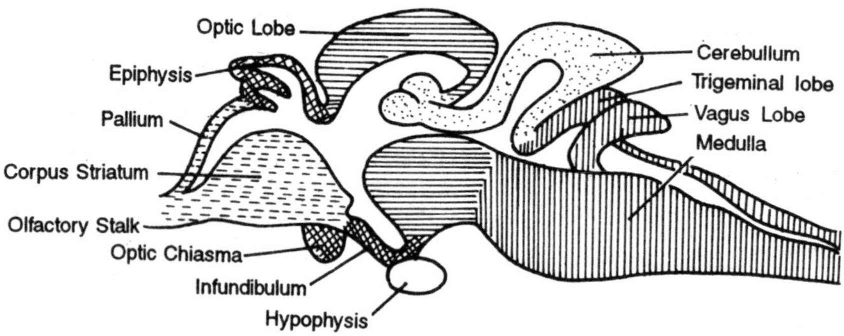

Fig. 2.59. Sagittal section diagram of the brain of a teleost.

The presence in certain fossil fishes, for example *Titanichthys*, of a pair of foramina located side by side in the skull directly above this region in the brain, also seems to point to the originally paired relation of these organs. Apparently the tandem-like position of the pineal and parietal bodies in cyclostomes is the result of a secondary displacement of the former side-by-side arrangement.

The histological structure of the epiphysis, or pineal body, as well as its access to light through a foramen in the dorsal region of the skull, seems to indicate that it is, in

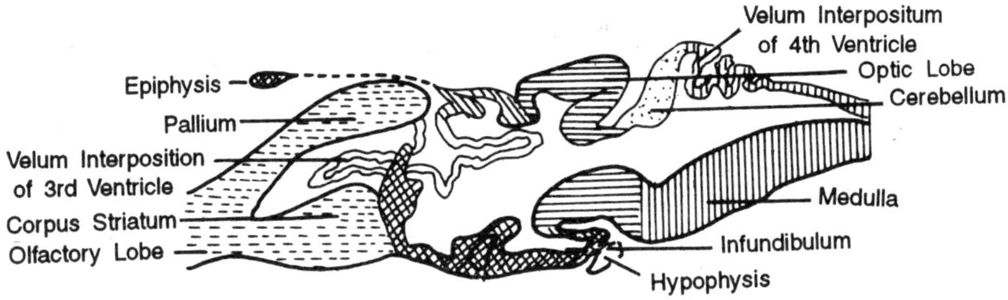

Fig. 2.60. Sagittal section diagram of the brain of an amphibian.

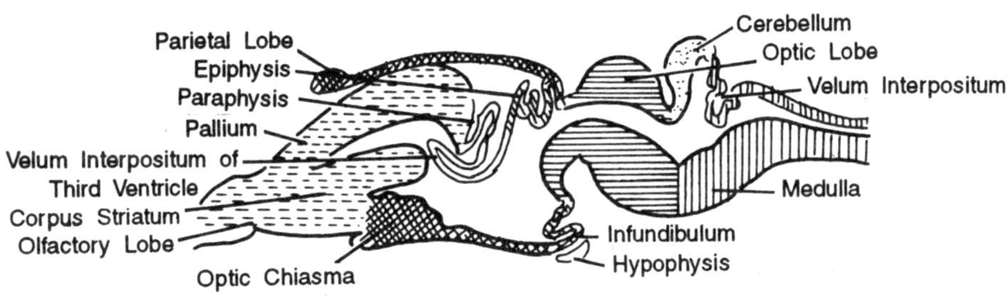

Fig. 2.61. Sagittal section diagram of the brain of a reptile.

cyclostomes at least, a photoreceptive organ by means of which light and darkness are distinguished.

The rather small telencephalon, olfactory in function, includes paired *olfactory bulbs*, *olfactory lobes*, and weakly differentiated *corpora striata. An anterior commissure*, found in all vertebrates, connects the two sides of the brain in the region of the *lamina terminalis*.

(b) *Elasmobranchs.*— In elasmobranchs the bulging *corpora striata*, which even grow into the lamina terminalis, and the dominant *olfactory lobes* constitute the bulk of the telencephalon. From each olfactory lobe there extends forward a conspicuous *olfactory stalk*, terminating in an *olfactory bulb* which may be quite large. The *velum interpositum*, the thin roof of the third ventricle, develops an invaginated transverse fold, or *velum transversum*, which marks the posterior limit of the dorsal part of the telencephalon.

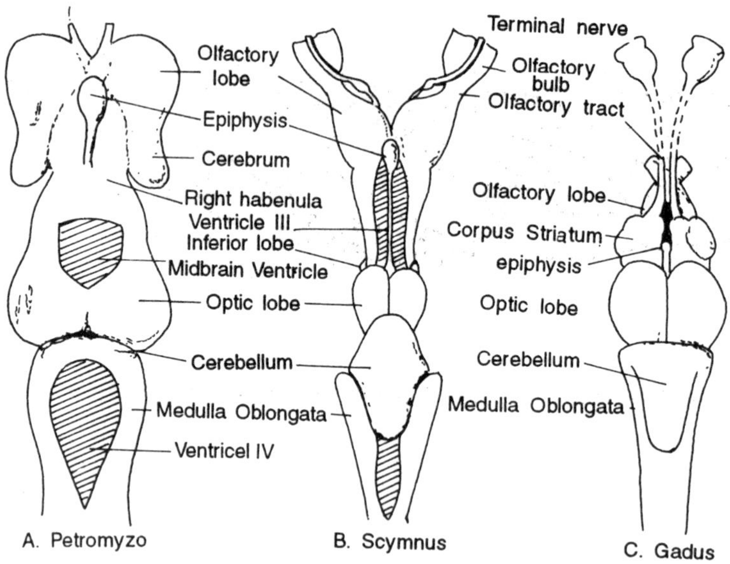

Fig. 2.62. Dorsal views of the brain of A, a lamprey; B, a shark; C, a teleost (codfish). Hatched areas are those in which a choroid plexus has been removed, exposing the underlying ventricle.

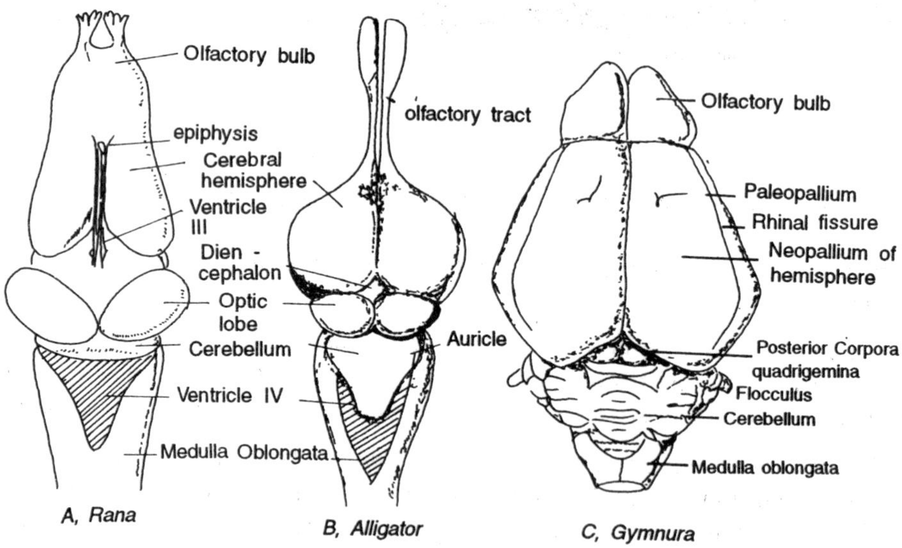

Fig. 2.63. Dorsal views of the brain of A, a frog; B, an alligator; C, a tree shrew. Hatched areas are those in which a choroid plexus has been removed, exposing the underlying ventricle. (After Gaupp, Crosby, Wettstein, Clark.)

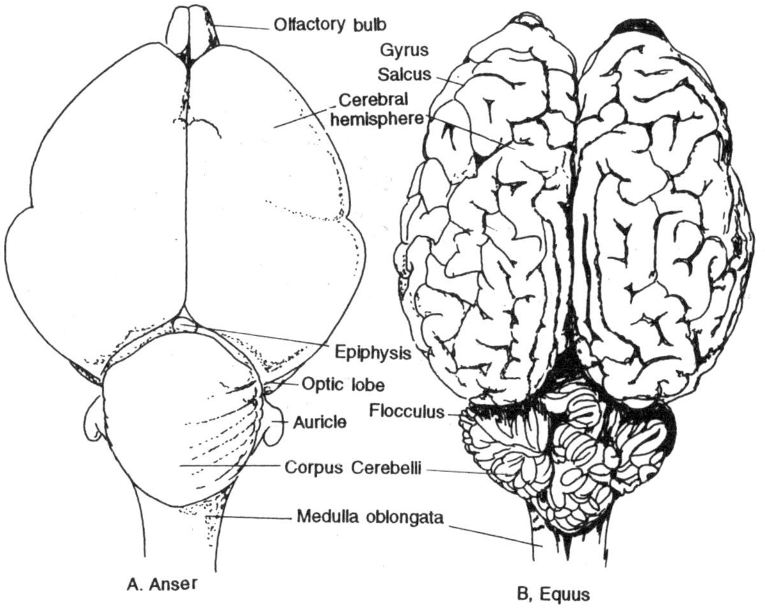

Fig. 2.64. Dorsal views of the brain of A, a goose; B, a horse. (After Butschli, Kuenzi, Sisson.)

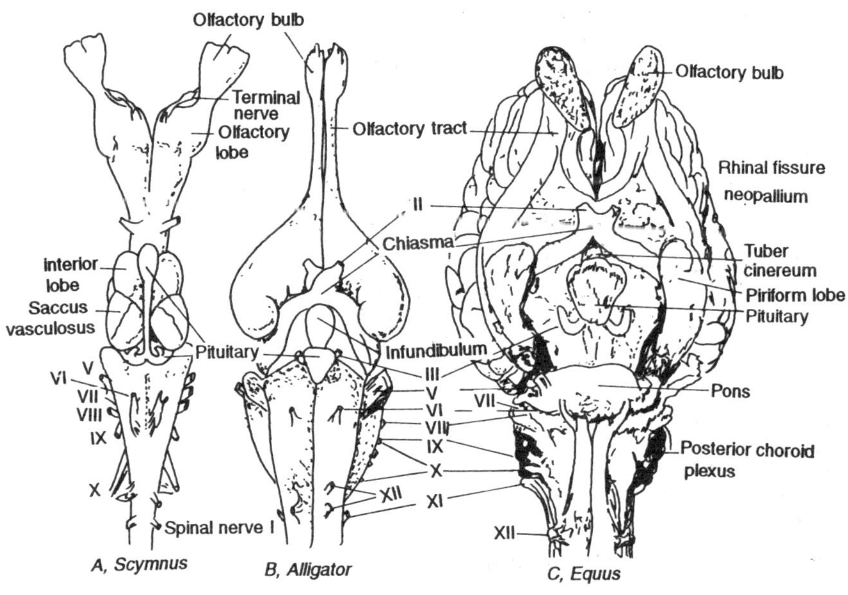

Fig. 2.65. Ventral views of the brain of A, a shark; B, an alligator; C, a horse. Roman numerals indicate cranial nerves. (After Butschli, Wettstein, Sisson.)

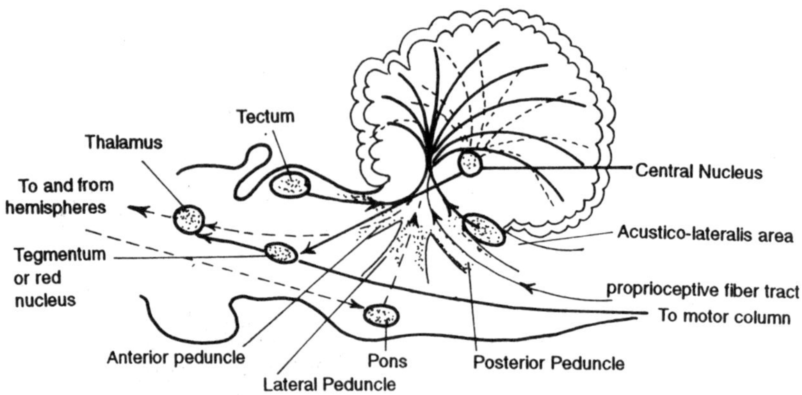

Fig. 2.66. Diagram to show the main connections of the cerebellum. The connections with the cerebral cortex, peculiar to mammals, are shown in broken lines.

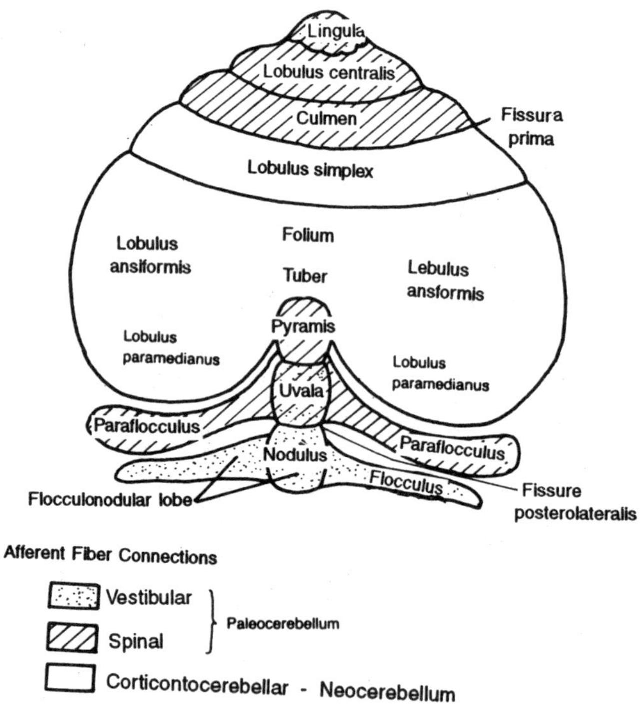

Fig. 2.67. Diagram of a surface view of a mammalian cerebellum (showing details not discussed in the text). The stippled and hatched portions, associated with equilibrium (vestibular) and with muscle sensations (spinal), are the phylogenetically oldest parts of the cerebellum; the white area is a mammalian addition associated with the cortex of the cerebral hemispheres.

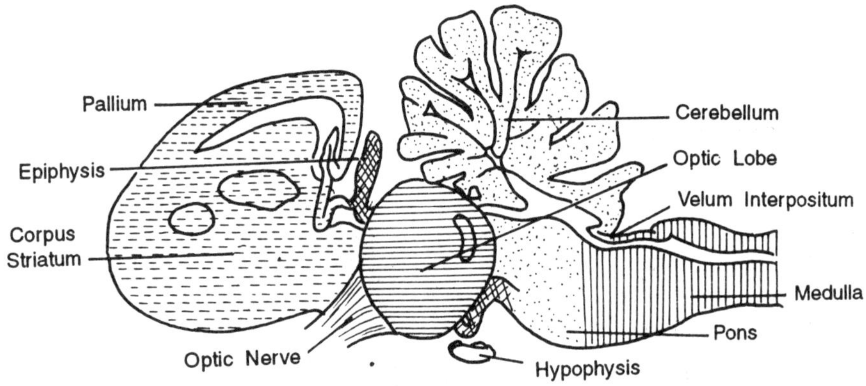

Fig. 2.68. Sagittal section diagram of the brain of a bird. (After Edinger.)

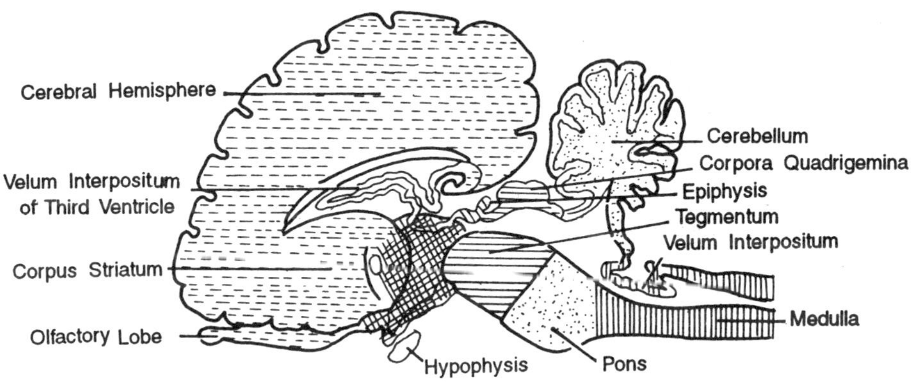

Fig. 2.69. Sagittal section diagram of the brain of a mammal. (After Edinger.)

In the diencephalon the epiphysis is stalked, reaching as far as the cartilaginous roof of the cranium in many cases. The parietal organ disappears after temporary appearance during embryonic development. The *infundibulum* develops a pair of elongate swellings, the *inferior lobes*, between which the hypophysis is attached. Posterior to the inferior lobes and dorsal to the neuro-hypophysis proper, is a thin-walled *vascular sac*, or *saccus vasculosus*, lined with a sensory epithelium of problematical significance. This sac is not found in cyclostomes or tetrapods.

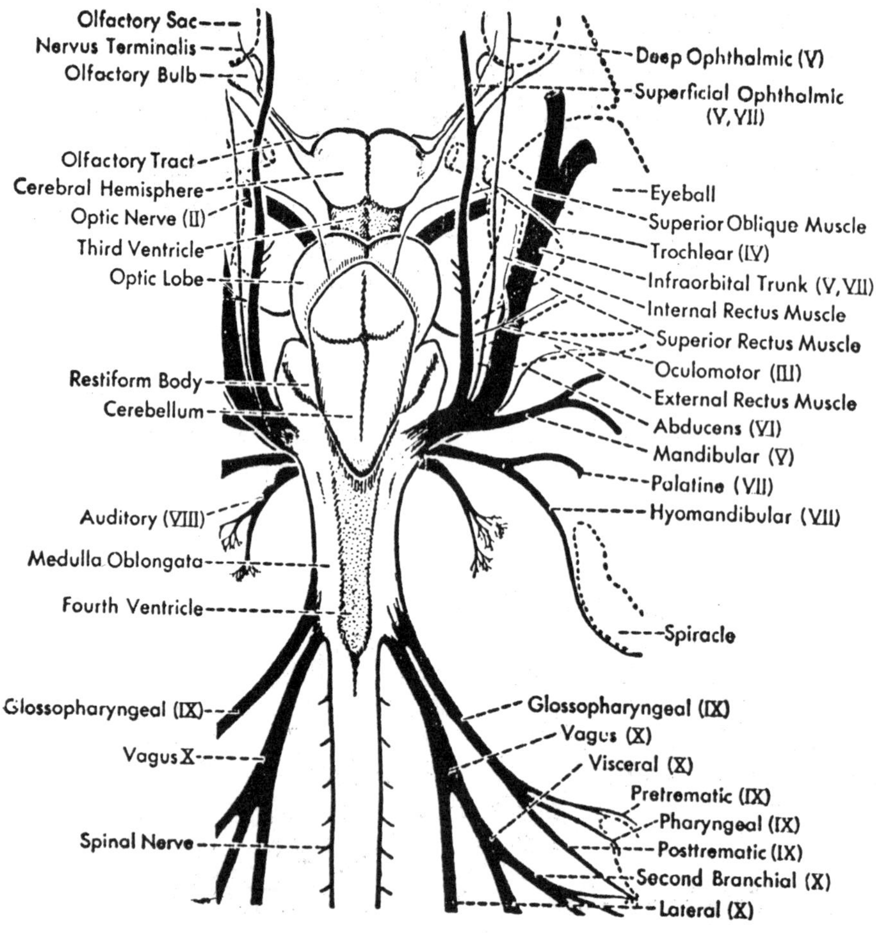

Fig. 2.70. Dorsal view of the brain of an elasmobranch, *Squalus.*

The well developed *optic lobes* may be partially covered by a large cerebellum. As would be expected, the cerebellum is much larger in the active dogfishes and sharks than in the sluggish skates and rays.

In the antero-lateral part of the medulla, connecting it with the cerebellum, are prominent *restiform bodies* which stand out like a pair of ears on either side of the cerebellum. In elasmobranchs, as in embryonic stages of higher vertebrates, the differentiation of the medulla into four longitudinal areas is clearly visible. These four columns represent the same four nervous components described for the cord. On either side of the thin ependymal velum which forms the roof of the fourth ventricle are the *somatic sensory columns* ventral to which are the *visceral sensory columns*, then the *visceral*

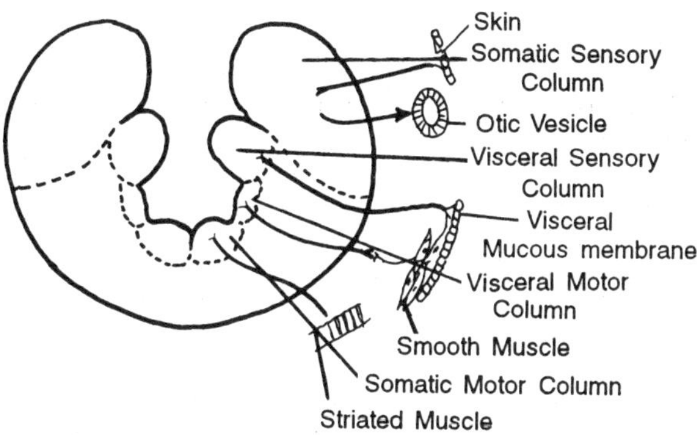

Fig. 2.71. Diagrammatic cross section through the medulla of an elasmobranch to show the four areas and the parts they supply. (After Johnston.)

motor columns, and finally the *somatic motor columns* which lie on either side of the median plane in the floor of the ventricle.

The electric *Torpedo* has two *electric lobes* that project into the fourth ventricle. These structures are hypertrophied nuclei of the vagus (X) nerve which supplies the electric organ of these animals.

(c) *Other Fishes* — In bony fishes the brains are small and show great variations. The roof of the telencephalon is thin and non-nervous. Convex corpora striata occupy the floor of this region. The shortened epiphysis is on the downward road of degeneration. The optic lobes are large, especially in teleosts. The cerebellum, small in dipnoans and ganoids, is large in most teleosts, especially the most active ones.

(d) *Amphibians.*— In amphibians, the large elongated *olfactory lobes*, which are continuous with the distinctly separated *cerebral lobes*, lie closely side by side and are joined medially together.

The *corpora striata* project upward from the telencephalic floor only slightly, allowing for fairly large *lateral ventricles* and invaginated anterior choroid plexuses inside the cerebral lobes. The latter are without an external layer of gray matter, although scattered neurons begin to appear in the thickening pallial wall.

The diencephalon is uncrowded, and visible from above, without inferior lobes or saccus vasculosus. In adult anurans the epiphysis is represented by a small median vesicle, the pineal gland, close under the dorsal wall of the cranium, which by its development is shown to be the bulbous tip of the vanished stalk of the epiphysis. Skulls of stegocephals have a dorsal foramen, which shows the presence in those primitive amphibians of either a pineal or a parietal eye in this region. The parietal body is absent in modern amphibians.

The optic lobes have been so spread apart as to occupy a more lateral position, and the cerebellum, reduced to a transverse lip in most forms, is quite rudimentary in the caecilians as well as in some urodeles.

(e) *Reptiles.*— The reptilian brain shows an advance in the telencephalic region, since a gray cortex, although not pronounced, is definitely laid down, and the commissures between the cerebral lobes are somewhat more developed than in the amphibian brain.

The corpora striata are so large that only small lateral ventricles remain. In most reptiles the olfactory lobes are hardly distinguishable from the neopallial part of the telencephalon, but in those lizards and alligators with prominent projecting snouts the olfactory lobes are extended into salks and bulbs, as in elasmobranchs.

The diencephalic region of the brain of reptiles is of particular interest. The thalami are large, while the hypophysis attached to the infundibulum is definitely differentiated into an anterior and a posterior part, the former enveloping the latter. On the thin dorsal wall of the third ventricle there are, at least embryonically, not only pineal and parietal outgrowths, but also a third evagination, the paraphysis, which is so far anterior in position that it actually belongs to the telencephalon. The paraphysis usually undergoes degeneration in adult life and its function is still unknown.

Except in crocodiles and alligators, the epiphysis is always present as a glandular pineal structure. The parietal organ is also always present in close association with the same habenular centers as those of the pineal body. Reaching its highest development in *Sphenodon,* in which it extends as far as a transparent window on the roof of the skull, it is unmistakably a third median eye, equipped with a retina and a lens.

In snakes distinct corpora quadrigemina occur in the dorsal part of the mesencephalon. It has been shown however, that other reptiles and possibly amphibians have small auditory centers, corresponding to posterior colliculi. These auditory centers do not show as a pair of elevations until the optic centers become reduced to anterior colliculi occupying only the anterior part of the roof of the mesencephalon. The thickening of the mesencephalic wall reduces the cavity of this region to a slender canal, the aqueduct.

The cerebellum of reptiles is usually small, although fairly well developed in swimming forms. Eight pairs of cranial nerves connect with the medulla as in birds and mammals, whereas only six pairs occur here in anamniotes.

(f) *Birds.*— The brain of birds is more of an "eye brain" than a "nose brain", thus showing an advance over its forerunners. The cerebral cortex, however, is less well developed than in reptiles, with the corpora striata more in evidence. The lateral ventricles, due to the increased thickness of the corpora striata, are reduced to very restricted spaces.

The olfactory lobes were fairly prominent in the tooth-bearing cretaceous birds, but are small and degenerate in their modern representatives. No trace of a parietal organ appears in birds, and since the degenerate pineal body is buried between the encroaching cerebrum and cerebellum, the entire brain gives the impression of compact crowding and centralization, characteristic of the bird's structure generally. This is due not only to the fact that the greatly enlarged optic lobes are crowded over laterally in position, but also to a considerable backward growth of the cerebrum which tends to bury the diencephalon and the mesencephalon from dorsal view.

The cerebellum, consisting of a well-defined median *vermis* as well as two *lateral lobes*, is very large, as might be expected in these extremely active animals.

(g) *Mammals.*— Tertiary mammals, as methods of exploring the cranial cavity of fossil skulls reveal, had a reptilian type of brain. In modern mammals also, the brain is more like that of reptiles than that of birds, since the outstanding size of the cerebrum is due to the development of the cortex rather than to an enlargement of the corpora striata, as is the case among birds.

The commissural systems between the cerebral lobes are better developed than in other vertebrates, particularly by the elaboration of the large corpus callosum, although this is small in the monotremes and marsupials.

While still prominent in the monotremes, marsupials, and other lower mammals, the archipallial olfactory part of the brain becomes reduced among the higher mammals, until in man it is very small, and in seals and whales almost entirely lacking.

In the diencephalon the thalami are large. The epiphysis, now connected with endocrine activity and having lost its eyelike structure, is reduced to an organ degenerate in size, although indispensable in function. It is usually covered over by the hemispheres and is relatively large in ungulates and rodents but missing in armadillos and other edentates.

The two optic lobes of lower forms become changed in mammals into four corpora quadrigemina, which are relatively smaller than is this region of the mesencephalon in any other vertebrate. The corpora quadrigemina are quite covered by the overgrowth of the massive cerebrum and the cerebellum which have so enlarged that they meet dorsally.

In addition to enlarged vermis and lateral lobes, *flocculi* of considerable size are present. Thus the correlation tissue of the cerebellum is notably increased.

A further characteristic of the mammalian brain is a definite band of fibers encircling the brain stem, known as the *pons*, in the metencephalic region. The medulla of mammals is comparatively short, and appears to be drawn under the prominent cerebellum.

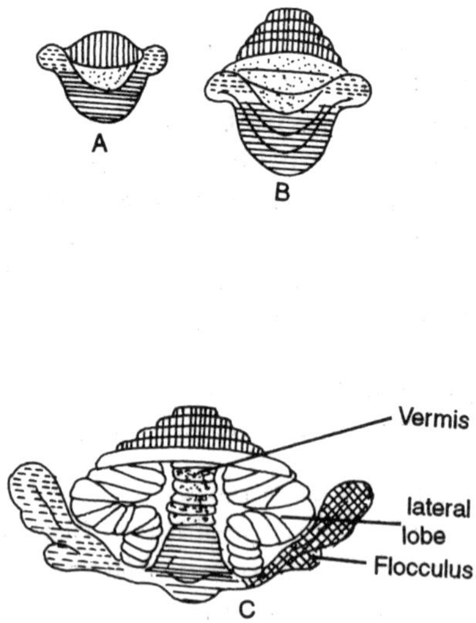

Fig. 2.72. Evolution of the cerebellum. A, crocodile; B, bird; C, mammal. Anterior lobe, vertical lines; median lobe, dots; posterior lobe, horizontal lines.

Comparison of Brain and Cord

The central nervous system of amphioxus is all cord and no brain. The true rise of the vertebrate brain begins in fishes, where the cord still cutweighs the brain. Among amphibians the brain overtakes the cord in bulk and weight, while in modern reptiles it gets the lead, which ever afterwards in the vertebrate series is maintained.

In mammals there is an ascending dominance of the brain over the cord. A cat and a macaque monkey, for example, with cords of the same weight (7.5 grams), have been found to have brains weighing 29 and 62 grams respectively, or ratios of 1:4 and 1:8. The ratio in man is nearer 1:50, an average measurement being 26 grams for the cord as compared with 1350 grams for the brain.

The absolute weight of the brain, it should be noted, is not in itself a reliable criterion of intelligence, since various factors, such as age, sex, form of skull, and weight of body, as well as the comparative size of different parts of the brain, must be taken into account. It is quality rather than quantity that counts.

The average human male has a brain of about 1350 grams in weight, while that of the average human female, not to start an argument but to state a fact, is something like 100 grams less. Sometimes the size of a brain is determined more by the non-nervous neuroglia cells than by the neurons.

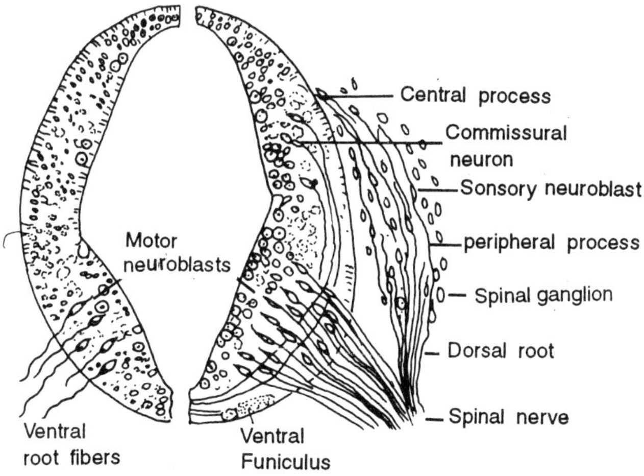

Fig. 2.74. Sections of the spinal cord of early mammalian embryos. Left, axons are growing outward from motor nerve cells. Right, association commissural neurons are developing within the cord and sensory neurons are developing externally from neural crest cells (fig. 77). These sensory neuroblasts are at this stage bipolar, i.e., with separate proximal and distal processes; later the two processes fuse proximally in higher vertebrates to give a unipolar condition to the mature ganglion cell (but one with a T-shaped process).

Some notable deviations from the average weight of human brains are recorded as follows: Thackeray, the novelist, 1644; Cuvier, the comparative anatomist, 1830; Turgenieff, the historian, 2012; Haeckel, the biologist, 1575; Agassiz, the zoologist, 1495; Schumann, the musician, 1475; Gambetta, the statesman, 1294; Whitman, the poet, 1282; Dollinger, the anatomist, 1207; and Anatole France, the writer, 1017. It is not the size of your wrist watch that is of importance, but how good time it keeps.

The weight of the brain of a dog, gorilla, and man, having approximately the same weight of body, has been found to be 135, 430, and 1350 grams respectively.

The actual mass of the human brain is exceeded among animals only by that of the gigantic elephants and whales, the size of whose body is many times that of man. An examination of the cranial cavities of the great reptiles of the Mesozoic age reveals the fact that they had significant brains in proportion to the enormous bulk of their bodies. Indeed it is a source of astonishment that these monsters of the past were able to get about with brains relatively so small, but it must be remembered that eventually, after an evolutionary experiment of several million years, they did succumb. It is doubtless

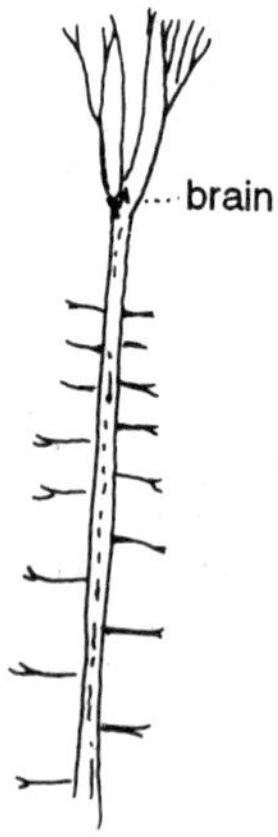

Fig. 2.74. Central nervous system of amphioxus, showing the alternation of the spinal nerves. Photoreceptor cells, represented by dots, are embedded in the nerve cord.

more than a coincidence that the twilight of the dinosaurs and their reptilian contemporaries fell at about the same time as the dawn of the mammals who were at first comparatively insignificant in size, but who had a new and revolutionary ratio established between weight of brain and weight of body.

3

The Spinal Cord

The portion of the neural tube which forms the spinal cord undergoes considerably less modification than that forming the brain. It generally assumes the shape of a more or less cylindrical, but slightly flattened, tube. It widens at the anterior end, where it is continuous with the medulla oblongata. The posterior end usually tapers down to a fine thread, the *filum terminale*.

In cyclostomes and fishes, the spinal cord is of fairly uniform diameter throughout its length, but in most tetrapods two conspicuous swellings, or enlargements, occur at points where the nerves going to the limbs arise. Since, with the development of limbs, the nerve supply to these structures is increased, the enlargements are actually places in which greater numbers of nerve-cell bodies are situated than are present at other levels

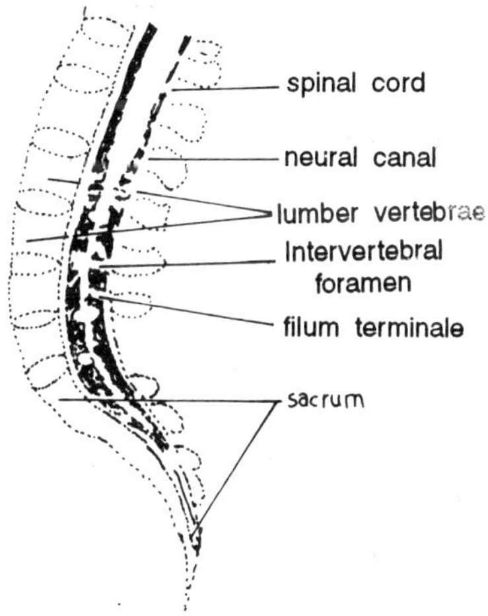

Fig. 3.1. Diagram of sagittal section of lower end of vertebral column of man, showing its relation to spinal cord and filum terminale.

of the cord. The *cervical enlargement* is the more anterior of the two. Here the white matter also shows an increase. It is the region where the large nerves supplying the forelimbs arise. The *lumbar enlargement,* near the posterior end of the spinal cord, marks the point of origin of nerves supplying the hind limbs. The difference in degree of development of forelimbs and hind limbs in various tetrapods accounts for the fact that in some forms the cervical enlargement exceeds the lumbar enlargement in size, whereas in others, the reverse condition obtains. In such limbless forms as snakes, neither enlargement is present. It is probable that in certain extinct dinosaurs, which possessed enormous limbs but had relatively little cranial capacity, the nervous tissue composing the cervical and lumbar enlargements exceeded that of the brain itself in size. Casts of the neural canal of the dinosaur *Stegosaurus* indicate that the lumbar enlargement may have been twelve times as large as the brain.

The spinal cord in higher forms has a conspicuous *ventral fissure* on its undersurface. A slight median depression, or sulcus, may be present on the dorsal side. From the sulcus a *dorsal septum* extends toward the interior of the cord. The dorsal septum and ventral fissure incompletely divide the spinal cord into symmetrical halves, connected across the middle by commissures of nervous tissue. The central canal lined with a single layer of ependymal cells is very small and lies in the center of the nervous mass connecting the two halves of the cord.

Length of Cord. At first, during embryonic development, the spinal cord and vertebral column are of approximately the same length. During subsequent development in many vertebrates, the growth of the spinal cord fails to keep pace with that of the vertebral column. As a result, the spinal cord of the adult may be considerably shorter than the backbone. In man it averages slightly less than 18 in. in length and reaches down only to the upper border of the second lumbar vertebra. The filum terminate, however, continues on to the first segment of the coccyx. In other vertebrates, the spinal cord may be relatively much longer than in man, but within the entire group there is a very definite tendency toward a reduction in length.

Gray and White Matter of Cord. In cross section the spinal cord is seen to be composed of gray and white matter, the former being almost completely surrounded by the latter. The gray matter in amniotes is arranged somewhat in the form of a butterfly, or in the shape of the letter H. The portions corresponding to the upper of the H extend dorsally and are known as *dorsal columns.* The lower bars are the *ventral columns,* and the connecting bar, in which the central canal lies, forms the *dorsal* and *ventral gray commissures,* above and below the central canal, respectively. Considerable variation exists in the arrangement of the gray matter within the spinal cords of different vertebrates, the H-shaped distribution being more typical of higher forms. The small nerve-cell bodies in the dorsal columns are, for the most part, those of *association neurons,* or *interneurons.* Their dendrites form synapses with the axons of sensory, or afferent, nerve fibers which enter the spinal cord via the dorsal roots of spinal nerves. The axons of the association neurons, which are of variable length, course up or down the spinal cord, cross to the opposite side, or pass ventrally on the same side, to form synapses with the dendrites of motor, or efferent, neurons, the very large cell bodies of which are located in the ventral columns. The

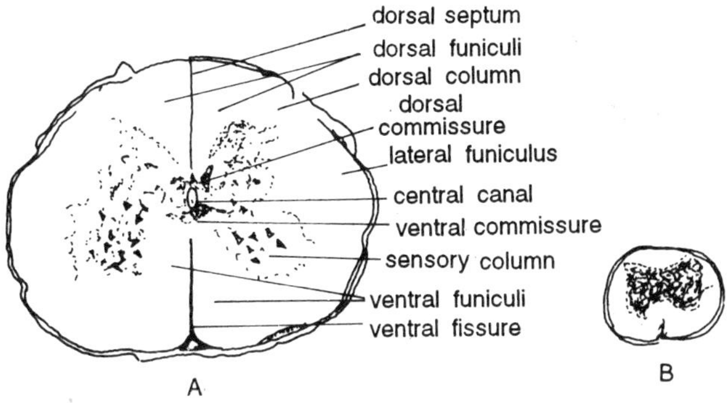

Fig. 3.2. Cross sections of spinal cords of A, cat, and B frog, shown at same magnification. Gray matter is heavily stippled; white matter is lightly stippled.

axons of the motor neurons in higher forms typically emerge via the ventral roots of the spinal nerves, but in lower forms some may emerge through the dorsal roots as well. It is the cell bodies of these efferent motor neurons, which are frequently destroyed in the disease known as infantile paralysis (anterior poliomyelitis). In such cases these results a paralysis of the muscles which would normally be supplied by the axons of these cells.

Neurologists have discovered that the cells in the dorsal and ventral columns show a rather definite arrangement into areas, each of which is associated with a certain type of function. All functions carried on by the body can be resolved into two main categories, *somatic* and *visceral*. Somatic functions are those carried on by the skin and its derivatives, the voluntary musculature and skeletal structures. Visceral functions are those performed by the other organ systems of the body, i.e., digestive, respiratory, excretory, reproductive, endocrine, and circulatory systems. Somatic sensory fibers carry impulses from the somatic tissues to the central nervous system. They form synapses with cells in the *upper portion* of the dorsal columns. Visceral sensory fibers are those carrying impulses from the visceral organs. They form synapses with cells in the *lower portion* of the dorsal columns. The motor neurons, the cell bodies of which are located in the ventral columns, are likewise of two types, somatic and visceral. The cell bodies of somatic motor neurons are located primarily in the lower portions of the ventral columns, whereas visceral motor neurons have their origin in the *upper* and *lateral* portions of the ventral columns. There are thus four areas in the gray matter on each side of the spinal cord, arranged in a dorsoventral sequence as follows: somatic sensory, visceral sensory, visceral motor, somatic motor. The visceral areas are, in general, smaller than the somatic areas. A similar arrangement is present in the gray matter of the medulla oblongata.

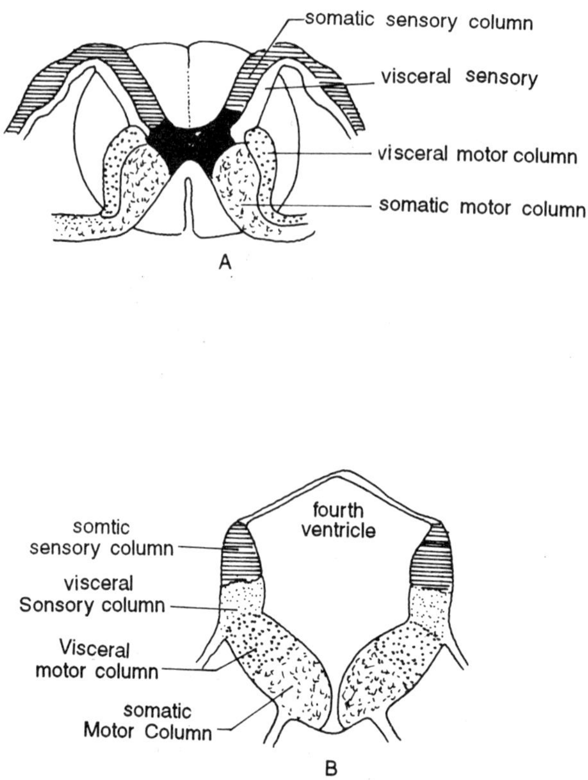

Fig. 3.3. Diagrams indicating the relative positions of the four columns of gray matter on each side of A, the spinal cord, and B, the medulla oblongata.

The white matter of the cord is arranged in longitudinal columns called *funiculi* which lie outside the gray matter. The funiculi are in turn divided into *fasciculi*, or *fiber tracts*, composed of medullated fibers that carry impulses up and down the cord and to and from the brain. A *lateral funiculus* is present on each side between dorsal and ventral columns. A *dorsal funiculus* lies between the dorsal septum and the dorsal column on each side, and a ventral funiculus is located between the ventral fissure and the ventral column of gray matter. The two ventral funiculi are in communication through the *white commissure* which lies just below the ventral *gray commissure*. This serves as a bridge between the white matter of the two sides.

It is beyond the scope of this book to discuss the detailed arrangement of fiber tracts in which nerve fibers ascend and descend the spinal cord. Suffice it to say that those in the dorsal funiculi, for the most part, carry sensory nerve impulses *up* the cord and *to* the brain. Those in the ventral funiculi are primarily motor, carrying impulses *down* the cord and *from* the brain. The lateral funiculi carry both ascending (sensory) and descending (motor) fibers. In general, the lower vertebrates do not show so elaborate an organization or arrangement of the columns, funiculi and fasciculi in the spinal cord as do higher forms.

Comparative Anatomy of the Spinal Cord. AMPHIOXUS. The spinal cord of amphioxus is of uniform diameter throughout except for a gradual tapering toward the end of the tail. It appears to be somewhat triangular in shape when viewed in cross section. The central canal is slit-shaped. There is no clear-cut distinction between gray matter and white matter, since in amphioxus medullated fibers have not as yet made their appearance. Only in a very general way does a cross section of the spinal cord of amphioxus bear a resemblance to that of the typical vertebrate. Nerve-cell bodies, some of exceptional size, lie in the central region in the vicinity of the central canal. The canal is not lined with a continuous layer of ependymal cells. Some of the giant cells even cross the slitlike central canal.

Cyclostomes. A truly tubular spinal cord first appears in cyclostomes. The cord is considerably flattened and is ribbon-shaped. The dorsal side is more or less convex, and the ventral side concave. Of fairly uniform diameter, the cord tapers gradually toward the posterior end. Gray and white matter are not sharply differentiated, the gray matter being in the form of a broad, longitudinal band surrounded on all sides by white matter, except where the roots of spinal nerves emerge. Dorsal septum and ventral fissure are lacking. In the lamprey a mass of tough, pigmented, fibrous tissue lies above the spinal cord, filling in the spaces between the incomplete neural processes and completing the enclosure of the neural canal dorsally and laterally. No other special function has been demonstrated for this peculiar fibrous tissue of the neural canal.

Fishes. A dorsal fissure is present in the spinal cords of most fishes, but a ventral fissure is absent. Gray matter is arranged in the form of a triangle, the apex of which points dorsally. Paired ventral columns of gray matter are present for the first time. In most fishes the cord tapers gradually to the end of the tail, but in certain teleosts there is a marked shortening and the spinal cord terminates at some distance from the end of the vertebral column. Thus the position of the posterior end is considerably anterior to the parts of the body which it supplies with nerves. The spinal cord of the marine sunfish. *Orthagoriscus,* has been reduced to almost ridiculous proportions. In this large fish, which may reach a length of 8 ft and weigh a ton or more, the spinal cord is less than ¾ in. long and is even shorter than the brain.

Amphibians. In salamanders the spinal cord extends to the posterior end of the vertebral column, but in frogs and toads it has been considerably shortened. The filum terminale in these forms extends into the urostyle. Cervical and lumbar enlargements appear for the first time since these are the first forms in which the appendages have been modified into true limbs. A dorsal sulcus may be present, and a ventral fissure appears for the first time. Gray matter may appear in the form of an oval in cross section, but dorsal and ventral columns are usually present and the beginning of the typical H-shaped arrangement found in higher forms is apparent. Fasciculi, or fiber tracts, in the white matter are more clearly indicated than in lower forms.

Reptiles. The reptilian spinal cord extends the entire length of the vertebral column. Cervical and lumbar enlargements are absent in the snakes and limbless lizards but are present in other forms. They seem to be unduly conspicuous in turtles, however. The trunk muscles in turtles have been reduced, and their nerve supply is correspondingly less. Therefore, the portion of the spinal cord between the two enlargements is more slender than usual. The H-shaped arrangement of gray matter is typical of the condition found in other amniotes.

Birds. The spinal cord of birds extends the full length of the vertebral column, and a filum terminale is absent. The most conspicuous feature which distinguishes the spinal cord of birds from that of other vertebrates is the separation of the two halves of the cord on the dorsal side of the lumbar enlargement. An elliptical space, the *sinus rhomboidalis*, is present, filled with neuroglia cells of a gelatinous character. These make up the so-called *glycogen body*. The relative sizes of cervical and lumbar enlargements depend upon the degree of development of wings and legs. The ostrich is notable for the large size of its lumbar enlargement.

Mammals. In the duckbill platypus and a few rodents, the spinal cord extends to the sacral region of the vertebral column, but in other mammals it has been shortened. Even in mammals with well-developed tails, the cord fails to extend into the caudal region. Such tails are moved primarily by means of longitudinal muscles and ligaments which are innervated by nerves at their bases. In addition to the median dorsal sulcus, dorsolateral and ventrolateral sulci are frequently present. The ventral fissure is conspicuous. A marked discrepancy exists in the size of cervical and lumbar enlargements in bats, which have an unusually large cervical enlargement associated with the large wing muscles used in flight.

Extent of the Cord

In a typical human adult the nervous part of the cord from the level of the foramen magnum of the skull to the beginning of the non-nervous filum terminale, reaches only about eighteen inches, or to near the level the first lumbar vertebra. Thus the entire axial central nervous system including the brain and the functional part of the cord, extends only from the region of the forehead to the "small of the back". Embryologically as well as phylogenetically the cord is originally practically as long as the backbone itself.

In Orni throghynchus and a few rodents it reaches as far as the sacrum, but there is a pronounced evolutionary tendency of it to shorten.

Among insects the process of Cephalization, on, or shrinkage in the length of the cord, is very striking. The lower insects have a primitive nerve chain extending along the entire floor of the body, whereas "higher forms present a condensed cord, composed of ganglia that have telescoped together into compact masses. During the metamorphosis of an insect, such as a honey bee for example, a ganglionic chain streches the whole length of the long larval body, but in the adult worker bee, which eventually emerges from the larva, the nerve chain is represented by ganglionic masses that are drain much more closely together.

In primates the degree of shortening marks the relative position in animal aristrocracy which each form occupies, as the following table shows:

Lemur cord ends at the 7th lumbar vertebrates.

Marmoset (Hapale) ends at the 6th lumbar vertebrates.

Monkey (Macacus) ends at the 4th lumbar vertebrates.

Man ends at the 1st lumbar vertebrates.

It is interesting to speculate as to the possible fate of the shrinking nerve cord in the far distant future. Probably the time will nerve come when the cord will be entirely dispensed with, since there must always remain a structure of sufficient length to furnish a point of departure for the nerves supplying the body.

Spinal Nerves

In man there are typically 31 pairs of spinal nerves, as follows Cervical 8, Thoracic 12, Lumbar 5, Sacral 5, and Caudal, 1. The total number of spinal nerves in vertebrates other than man in naturally subject to wide variation.

Each pair of spinal nerves, with the exception of the cervical ones, takes its name from the vertebrate just anterior to its exit. The reason for a reversal of designation in the cervical nerves is that the first pair emerges between the skull and the first cervical vertebra, or atlas, and so having no vertebra infront of it takes its name from the vertebra immediately behind it. This method of nomenclature is followed throughout the cervical series, leaving the eighth pair of nerves without any cervical, vertebral godfather standing behind it, and accordingly it is called the eighth pair, although mammals have only seven neck vertebrae.

The next pair of nerves plainly belongs to the trunk, and so begins a new series as the first thoracic pair, taking its name from the vertebra behind which it emerges.

The size of the spinal nerves is dependent upon the relative area of the body which they supply, the largest in man being the first sacral pair that goes to the legs. The general distribution of every spinal nerve in connection with the region which it supplies is indicated.

The relation between the spinal nerves and the metameric embryonic muscles is very regular and constant, but the rearrangement and migration of these muscles in the adult organism brings about apparent irregularities. A nerve once associated with a muscle, however, remains faithfully to it throughout all its subsequent transformations. Since metameric muscles in mammals do not extend to a tail, as in fishes and urodeles, decides differences in the abundance of post and spinal nerves appear in the higher vertebrates.

In man particularly, the nerve cord is shortened as already described, so that it does not extend through the entire length of the vertebral column. Nevertheless the emerging spinal nerves maintain their people intervertebral exits. This necessities the continuation the posterior pairs of spinal nerves within the neural canal of the vertebral column for increasingly lengthened distances before they finally emerge, with the result that a brush of spinal nerves, the cauda equina, or the horse tail is formed at the end of the cord. Moreover, while the anterior spinal nerves leave the cord at practically right angles, the angle of departure for posters or pairs becomes more and more acute until it may be said of the sacrad nerves that for some distance they run almost or quite parallel to the filum terminale, that is, to the non nervous continuation of the cord itself.

Roots. The connection between the peripheral nervous apparatus and the central nervous system is effected on either side through the dorsal and ventral roots of the nervous which differ not only in structure and function, but also in their origin and manner of development.

Dorsal roots are composed primarily of neurons whose polarity is afferent or centripetal, that is, toward the central nervous system. Ventral roots on the contrary, are efferent or centrifugal carrying massages outward to glandular or muscular effectors. Since these effectors, which are mostly muscular bring about motion, the ventral roots are commonly designated as motor roots.

For the most part dorsal roots are made up of fibers from neurons apparently unipolar, although in reality bipolar, located in the dorsal ganglia, whose origin from the neural crests has already been described. Neurites in the ventral roots, on the other hand, which have no ganglia, take their origin from cell bodies grouped together in a gray matter of the ventral area of the cord.

Among lower vertebrates, dorsal roots in some instances are not always purely sensory but may also contain efferent fibers going to the autonomic system. A few recurrent sensory fibers also may find their way from the dorsal to the ventral root, thus modifying the character of the motor roots.

The spinal nerves of amphioxus show several primitive features. The dorsal root is mixed, including visceral (autonomic) motor as well as the usual complement of sensory fibers. No dorsal ganglion is present, the sensory neurons having their cell bodies in the dorsal part of the cord. Further the dorsal and ventral roots, alternating in their attachment to the cord, do not unite into a spinal nerve.

In cyclostomes the dorsal roots are also mixed and alternate with the ventral roots, but, in contrast with amphioxus, the cell bodies of their sensory fibers are located in dorsal ganglia, as in all other vertebrates. In the myxinoid the two roots join to form a united spinal nerve as in all gnathostomes. The combined spinal nerve, therefore, probably represent a secondary evolutionary adaptation.

The dorsal and ventral roots in elasmobranch fishes also emerge from the cord alternately. The dorsal root makes an inter-vertebral exit, through the inter-calary plate, while the ventral root comes out vertebrally through a foramen which penetrates the neural plate. They then join to form a spinal nerve. In higher vertebrates both roots of a spinal nerve emerge intervertably in the same transverse plane.

In fishes the dorsal ganglia and the point of union of the roots of the spinal nerves are usually located out side the vertebral column, but in other vertebrates the junction of the roots is affected closer and closer to the cord itself so that it comes to lie within the neural arch.

Branches. Near the junction of the two roots the spinal nerve divides into four branches, or rami, namely (1) a thinner, shorter dorsal branch, supplying epaxial sense organs, musculature, and glands (2) a thicker, longer ventral branch, to similar hepaxial branch (3) a small meningeal branch, going back into the neural canal to supply the blood vessels of the cord and its membrane and (4) an autonomic branch, communicating with the autonomic nervous system.

The important generalization that the branches of spinal nerves are mixed, while their roots are not independently established over a century ago by the French man Magendie and by Sircharles Bell, an Englishman, who has been characterized by professor Keinth as "an autonomical detective of the highest rank."

Plexuses. In the regions of the appendages, the ventral rami of certain spinal nerves are drawn out into the appendages. In such cases a more or less complicated network, or *plexus,* may be present, formed by the connection of branches of certain nerves with those of others. In lower forms an anterior *cervicobrachial plexus* is present for each pectoral appendage and a posterior *lumbosacral plexus* for each hind limb. In higher vertebrates a further differentiation takes place, so that separate cervical brachial, lumbar, and sacral plexuses may be present. In mammals such large nerves as the *ulnar* and *median nerves* of the forelimbs and the *femoral and sciatic nerves* of the hind legs represent convergences of portions of the above-names plexuses.

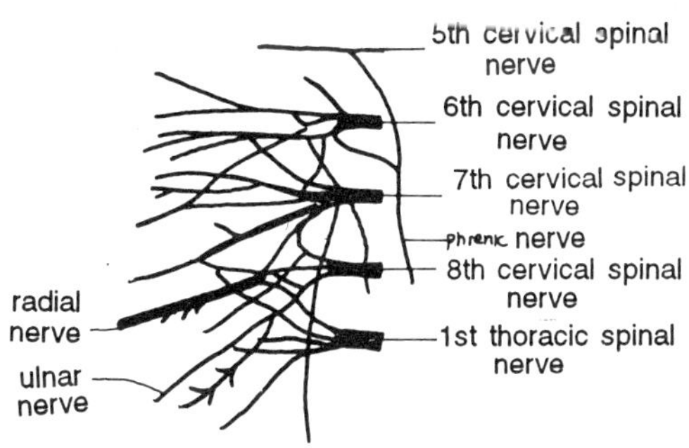

Fig. 3.4. Diagram of right brachial plexus of cat, ventral view.

Cauda Equina. Since the spinal cord lies in the canal formed by the neural arches of vertebrae, the spinal nerve must pass out of the vertebral column in order to reach their destination. Dorsal and ventral roots, except in certain lower forms, lie within the neural canal. Openings, known as *intervertebral foramina*, are present between adjacent vertebrae, providing for the passage of spinal nerves. At first, during embryonic development, each spinal nerve passes through intervertebral foramen located at the spinal level as the part of the cord from which the nerve arises. Later, however, growth of the cord fails to keep pace with that of the vertebral column. As a result, the spinal nerves, particularly those toward the posterior end, are drawn posteriorly so that they emerge through foramina which may be a considerable distance posterior to the point at which the spinal nerve leaves the cord. These nerves, therefore, must course for some distance through the neural canal, running obliquely or else parallel to the spinal cord, before they finally emerge. The more posterior the spinal nerve are greater distance must it travel before reaching the foramen through which it passes. Because of the brushlike appearance of the posterior spinal nerves of higher forms and their fancied resemblance to a horse tail, early anatomists gave to these nerves the name *cauda equina*.

Comparative Anatomy of Spinal Nerves. Amphioxus. The roots of the spinal nerves of amphioxus do not arise from the spinal cord in symmetrical pairs as do those of higher forms. Instead, those of one side alternate with those of the other in a manner similar to that of the myotomes, or muscle segments. Dorsal and ventral roots do not immune. Furthermore, they do not arise from the same level, the dorsal roots emerging opposite the myocommata and the ventral roots opposite the myotomes. The dorsal roots are composed of compactly arranged fibers, and dorsal root ganglia are lacking. The cell bodies of the sensory neurons in the dorsal roots lie within the spinal cord itself. The ventral roots are less compact, each missing from the cord by a number of loosely arranged bundles. The dorsal roots of the animal nerves in amphioxus carry somatic sensory, visceral sensory, and visceral motor fibers, the ventral roots being composed of somatic motor fibers alone. Each dorsal root branches into dorsal and ventral rami soon after leaving the cord. The ventral ramus gives off a visceral branch.

Cyclostomes. As in amphioxus, the dorsal and ventral roots of the spinal nerves of cyclostomes alternate with each other as they arise from the cord, the dorsal root coming off somewhat posterior to the ventral root. In lampreys the roots do not join each other, but in hagfishes such a union is usual except in the caudal region. In either case each dorsal root bears a ganglion.

In the gill region of lampreys fibers from adjacent dorsal roots unite as do fibers from adjacent ventral roots so as to form two nerves, one sensory and the other motor. These together form the *hypobranchial nerve*, which supplies the ventral part of the gill region. The motor components of this nerve presage the appearance of the hypoglossal nerve of amniotes.

Since paired appendages are lacking in cyclostomes, no spinal nerve plexuses are present.

Fishes. Dorsal and ventral roots unite in fishes, but the union occurs outside the vertebral column. In elasmobranchs the components form a looser union than is commonly

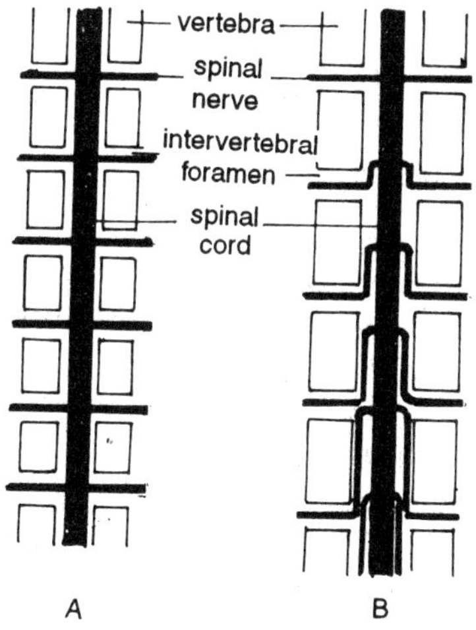

Fig. 3.5. Diagram illustrating the formation of cauda equina: A, the spinal nerves emerge through the vertebral column at right angles to the spinal cord, B, because of the disproportionate growth of vertebrae and spinal cord, the nerves emerge at some distance posterior to their point of origin.

the case. Also in elasmobranchs the roots do not arise from the cord in the same transverse plane, the dorsal roots coming off a short distance posterior to the ventral roots. A separate foramen is present for each root, that for the dorsal root being located in the intercalary plate and that for the ventral root in the neural arch proper.

In some of the anterior spinal nerves, the dorsal roots have disappeared and only the ventral, motor roots of the original spinal nerves persist. They are called *spino-occipital nerves*. Fibers from these nerves contribute to the formation of a hypobranchial nerve similar to that described for cyclostomes except that it is composed of efferent fibers alone.

There is much variation in the complexity of the cervicobrachial and lumbosacral plexuses in fishes. The most complicated conditions is found in skates, with their highly developed pectoral fins. As many as 25 spinal nerves may contribute to the formation of the cervicobrachial plexus in these fishes.

Amphibians. In amphibians, as in previous forms, the dorsal roots of the spinal nerves arise somewhat posterior to the level at which the ventral roots come off. The two roots unite as they pass through the inter-vertebral foramen. A swelling, the dorsal root ganglion, is located at the point of junction just outside the foramen. It is protected anteriorly by the transverse process of the vertebra and dorsally by the articular processes. From the spinal ganglion arise a dorsal ramus, in the form of a number of twigs, and a large ventral ramus. The visceral ramus comes off the ventral ramus.

In anurans, chalky masses known as *calcareous bodies*, apparently of lymphatic origin, surround the spinal ganglia. They are believed to serve as reserve supplies of calcium. In urodeles there are no calcareous bodies but the ganglia are surrounded by spongy, fatty tissue.

Between the occipital condyles and the first, or atlas, vertebra, the ventral root of a small *suboccipital nerve* emerges on each side. Some authorities consider it to be the first spinal nerve, but there is disagreement on this point. Usually the nerve emerging between the first and second vertebrae is called the first spinal nerve, at least in the anamniota. It also consists only of a ventral root, the dorsal root and ganglion having disappeared at the time of metamorphosis. The nerve is purely motor and may represent the hypoglossal cranial nerve of higher forms. The remaining spinal nerves are typical. In urodeles the number varies with the number of segments in the body. At the time of metamorphosis in anurans, there is a reduction in number of spinal nerves, so that in most cases only 10 or 11 remain. Cervico-brachial and lumbosacral plexuses are present, the latter being more complex in anurans in accordance with the greater degree of development of the hind limbs. A conspicuous cauda equina is present in frogs and toads.

Reptiles. In the amniota there are 12 pairs of cranial nerves, in contrast to the condition in lower forms in which there are but 10. It is generally believed that the eleventh cranial nerve (spinal accessory) represents a separation of a visceral motor component of cranial nerve X (vagus) together with certain fibers contributed by spino-occipital nerves. The twelfth cranial nerve (hypoglossal) represents a union of two or three spino-occipital nerves which have been incorporated within the skull and, therefore, arise from the medulla oblongata. The hypoglossal is a motor nerve which lacks a dorsal root, as is the case with the spino-occipital nerves which contain only efferent fibers. The probable homology of the hypoglossal nerve with the hypobranchial nerve of lower forms has already been alluded to. With the appearance of the hypoglossal nerve in amniotes, spino-occipital nerves are no longer present.

The spinal nerves of reptiles show no peculiarities. As in other amniotes, dorsal roots contain only sensory fibers. Both visceral motor and somatic motor fibers are confined to the ventral roots. It is of interest that in certain snakes and limbless lizards a distinct although poorly developed, lumbosacral plexus is present, indicating that these limbless forms those in evolution from ancestors with limbs.

Birds. The arrangement of spinal nerves in birds is typical. In certain long-necked forms, the nerves making up the cervico-brachial plexus arise from the cord much farther posteriorly than is usually the case. The lumbosacral plexus may be composed of two or three distinct components, in which case the names *lumbar, sacral,* and *pudendal plexuses* are applied. The lumbar plexus supplies the thigh. The nerves of the sacral plexus unite to form the sciatic nerve passing through the thigh to the lower leg. The pudendal plexus sends branches to the cloacal and tail regions.

Mammals. The spinal nerves of mammals are named according to their relation to the vertebral column. There are, therefore, cervical, thoracic, lumbar, sacral, and caudal or coccygeal spinal nerves. Each is numbered according to the number of the vertebra which lies anterior to it except in the case of the cervical spinal nerves, the first of which emerges between the occipital bone and the atlas. In man there are 31 pairs of spinal nerves: 8 cervical, 12 thoracic, 5 lumbar, 5 sacral, and 1 caudal. The number varies a great deal in different mammals. The horse, for example, has the following numbers: 8 cervical, 18 thoracic, 6 lumbar, 5 sacral, and 5 caudal.

As a general rule, the somatic motor fibers of each spinal nerve supply a single myotome, or muscle segment. In each case the myotome supplied is the one adjacent to the spinal nerve during ėarly embryonic development. No matter how the muscles derived from a certain myotome change or shift in position later on, the original nerve is maintained. This is the basis for determining muscle homologies which otherwise might be quite obscure. There are few exceptions to this.

The limb plexuses of mammals may be very complicated. They are commonly divided into cervical, brachial, lumbar, and sacral divisions. The *phrenic nerve* which supplies the diaphragm, arises from the cervical plexus, indicating that at least some of the musculature of the diaphragm has been derived from myotomes in the cervical region. In the rat the phrenic nerve on each side arises from the fourth and fifth cervical nerves: in the cat cervical nerve 5 and 6 are involved: in man the phrenic nerve arises mainly from the fourth cervical nerve but also receives some branches from the third and fifth.

Development of the Spinal Cord

With the formation of the medullary tube there are established around the central canal above and below, roof and floor plates, respectively, which do not increase notably in thickness, and two sides that enlarge enormously until they overshadow both roof and floor.

In early stages there are two types of cells in the wall of the medullary tube, namely, germinal cells, near the central canal, and spongioblasts, extending from the canal to the outer surface of the cord. Soon several additional types appear, namely, non-nervous ependymal cells, non-nervous neuroglass cells and neuroblasts, destined to become the important neurons. Germinal cells may give rise to any of these five types with the possible exception of ependymal elements, while spongioblasts defferentiate into neuroglia and ependymal cells.

Three zones may now be recognized in the wall of the medullary tube, especially in its thick lateral regions namely (1) an inner ependymal layer, bordering directly on the central canal (2) a middle mantle layer, containing many nuclei and (3) an outer marginal layer, practically devoid of nuclei.

The spongioblasts, with the ependymal cells, form a supporting framework which extends through all three layers. Although the ependymal cells are concentrated in the inner layer, they send long slender processes to the outer surface of the cord. The spider web like neuroglia cells form a supporting meshwork in the middle and outer layers.

Germinal cells are especially abundant within the staining neuroglial network of the mantle layer where they divide repeatedly to produce larger numbers of neuroblasts. The thickening of the mantle layer, due to this rapid cell poliferation, is most marked in two regions on each side of the cord, one dorso-lateral forming the dorsal horn, the other ventro-lateral, the ventral horn.

Many neuroblasts when they begin to sprout, send their nerve fibers into the marginal layer. At first these fibers are naked but gradually myelin sheaths are added, probably through the activity of certain neuroglia cells which become temporarily associated with the fibers but do not remain to form a neurolemma. This massing of myelinated fibers in the marginal layer converts it into white matter in contrast with the middle layer, composed chiefly of neuroblasts, cell bodies of neurons and neuroglia, which remains gray matter. Eventually the inner zone becomes reduced to a thin ependymal layer lining the central canal.

Neurons of the ventral gray matter also send out neurites which establish the ventral roots of the spinal nerves and continue into the several branches. Along with the fibers go non-nervous cells which give rise to the two sheaths, myelin and neurolemma. At the same time neurons in the dorsal ganglia are sprouting. Their dendrites, accompanied by sheath cells, grow out through the several branches of the spinal nerves to the surface of the body or to the internal organs. Their neurites complete the dorsal roots and extend into the cord where many of them grow forward to the brain by way of the dorsal part of the white matter. These myelinated neurites also have a neurolemmal sheath up to the point where they enter the cord.

Thus the alae plate, the dorsal part of the lateral walls of the cord is given over to cells and fibers of afferent, or sensory, neurons, concerned with bringing in impression from without while the ventral part, or basal plate, becomes headquarters for efferent or motor neurons that convey messages outward to various effector mechanisms.

As the sensory fibers enter the cord those from the outer surface of the body, somatic sensory component, are more medial than these from the internal organs, visceral sensory component, which supplies the voluntary muscles, are in the more medial ventral horn while those of the visceral motor component running chiefly to the autonomic nervous systems, are in the lateral columns, the more lateral part of the gray matter of the basal plate. Thus the gray matter includes four kinds of neurons, or component, in sequence from dorsal to ventral as follows—somatic sensory, visceral sensory, visceral motor, somatic motor.

In cross section the nerve cord at first has an oval outline while the central canal appears like a dorso-ventral slit. With the formation and enlargement of the ventral horns, together with the addition of the surrounding white matter, the cord bulges ventrally on either side of the thin floor plate leaving a median longitudinal groove, the ventral fissure. The formation of less extensive dorsal bulges results in a shallou dorsal fissure. Further the two sides of the dorsal part of the central canal grow together, giving rise to a dorsal medium septum, composed of ependymal cells, which extends from the bottom of the dorsal fissure nearly to the central canal. The septum is separated from the canal by a thin sheet of non myelinated nerve fibers which grow across between the gray matter regions of the two sides, forming the dorsal commissure. A somewhat similar cross connection between the two sides of the cord is found ventral to the canal, but this ventral comunussure courists of a white portion, next to the ventral fissure, in addition to the gray part near the canal.

Thus the nervous elements of the two sides of the cord are almost completely separated from one another, dorsally by a fissure and septum, ventrally by a fissure only the commissure act as nervous bridges between the two sides.

Internal Architecture of the Adult Cord

In a crossection of a fully formed cord, the gray matter somewhat resemble a butterfly, or a capital letter H with a hole through a centre of cross bar. On each side of the projecting horn of the gray matter, the upper and lower parts of one upright of the letter H, seperate the white matter into three large masses, the dorsal lateral and ventral funiculi. These funiculi are further differentiated into parallel tracts or fasiculi, each of which is a group of fibers of common function and with their cell bodies in the same general location. These fibers arise from cell bodies located (1) in the dorsal ganglia (2) in the cord itself and (3) in the brain. Together they constitute pathways of communication between more or less distant parts of the entire body.

The determination of the facts now known concerning these tracts has been a difficult though fasicinating work, engaging many different investigators over a long period of time nevertheless our knowledge in these matters is all too limited. In tracing the course of the pathways over which the countless message of communication go, workers have employed four outstanding methods, namely, Wallerian degeneration, study of pathological changes observation of the order of myelimation, and electrical stimulation.

As long ago as 1852 Waller found out that when a fiber is at the part of the individual fiber seperated from the nucleus degenerate. This serves to indicate in which direction the nucleus of a nerve cell is situated. Animals whose nerve fibers have been allowed to degenerate following a particular type of cut are observed for motor paralysis, loss of sensation or both in any region of the body. These experiments reveal the nature of the fibers involved, the location of their cell bodies and the region or regions of the body which they supply. This type of research is aided by methods of differential staining which render fibers and sheaths visible.

Pathological conditions, especially in man, furnish similar information cadavers of individuals who have suffered the loss of sensation or motor paralysis during life may, upon autopsy, reveal what group of cell bodies or fibers was concerned with the symptoms.

Another method of determining the course and direction of fiber groups is dependent upon the fact that the nerve fibers, which are at first naked, do not all require their medullary sheaths at the same time. Because most of the fibers belonging to any one tract tend to myelinize concurrently, it is possible to recognize different pathways by this means.

The fourth method, employed considerably in recent years, involves the use of electrical stimulation. Minute electrodes are used to stimulate limited group of nerve cells in anesthetized animals. After tabulation of the effects produced in numerous experiments of essentially on type, it is possible to determine at least some of the connections of the stimulated areas. By this means it has been possible to obtain detailed information concerning many complicated pathways, especially those in which only a few or scattered fibers are involved and therefore other methods do not suceed.

Thus the details of the invisible individual highways of the nervous system have been pieced together accumulatively, until now quite a complete picture of the whole complicated system of nervous traffic lanes is available. As would be expected, the various paths in the great white way studied in higher groups than in lower vertebras. Representative tracts, as found in man, may be grouped as—

I Ascending (sensory) tracts.

(1) Dorsal columns

Fasciculus gracilis (Tract of Goll)

Fasciculus cuneatus (Tract of Burdach)

(2) Spinocerebrallar system

Dorsal spinocerebellar tract

Ventral spinocerebellar tract

(3) Spino thalamic system

Lateral spinothalamic tract

Ventral spinothalamic tract

II Descending (Motor) Tracts

Fasciculus corticospinalis lateralis (crossed pyramidal tract)

Fasciculus corticospinalis ventralis (Direct pyramidal tract)

III Association Tracts

Fasciculus proprius dorsalis

(Dorsal ground bundle)

Fasciculus proprius lateralis

(Lateral ground bundle)

Fasciculus proprius ventralis

(Ventral ground bundle)

Ascending Sensory tract. The fiber which give rise to the so-called dorsal columns are neurites coming from cell bodies located in the dorsal ganglia of the spinal nerves, outside the cord. As they come into the cord by way of the dorsal root of the spinal nerve, they branch & go both anteriorly and posteriorly, with the longer branch toward the head, and the shorter branch away from the head. Both the longer ascending craniad fibers and the shorter descending cauded fibers send off collaterals that enter the gray matter, where they form synapses with either intermediate neurons or motor neurons. Many of the cranially directed fibers reach without relay as far as the brain itself.

Thus a neurite entering the cord through a dorsal root makes numerous central connections many of which are through its large number of collaterals. Some collaterals terminate in the ventral gray matter where they synapse with motor neurons which run out through the ventral roots to muscles or to the autonomic nervous system. Others collateral, ending in the dorsal gray matter, synapse there with intermediate neurons, the cell bodies of which are in this part of the gray matter. The neurites of these intermediate neurons usually run into the white matter where they may enter one of several tracts, either ascending or association. Still other collaterals run through the dorsal commissure to end in the dorsal gray matter of the opposite side of the cord.

The fasciculus gracilis and fasciculus cuneatus, which make up most of the dorsal fasiculus are composed mainly of ascending branches of the neurites of sensory neurons. Fibers from sacral, lumbar and lower thoracic spinal ganglia from the fasciculus gracilis, while those from anterior thoracic and cervical ganglia constitute the cuneatus. In the cervical regions these two tracts are seperated from one another by the dorsal intermediate septum. The courses which these and other tracts take upon entering the brain will be considered later. Although some of the short descending branches of the sensory neurons may also run in these two tracts, most of them take other pathways.

Some of the intermediate neurons with which the collaterals synapse, as mentioned above, run into the spino cerebellar tracts, located chiefly near the surface of the cord in the lateral funiculus. The dorsal spinocerebellar tract arise from cell bodies located in the dorso-median gray matter (nucleus dorsalis, sometimes known as Clarke's column) of the same side of the corrd. The cell bodies of the fibers making up the ventral spinocerebellar tract are found in the dorsal and intermediate gray matter, of the opposite side of the cord as well as the same side.

Other intermediate neurons, with which collaterals join in the dorsal gray matter, run through the ventral white commissure to enter the spinothalamic tracts, which are therefore crossed tracts, being composed of fibers which have their cell bodies on the side opposite that in which they run. The ventral spinothalamic tract is at the surface in the ventral funiculus while the lateral spinothalamic tract lies just medial to the ventral spinocerebellar tract.

The primary sensory neurons associated with the lateral spinothalamic tract differ in two important respects from those connected with the other tracts. First of all, they are entirely unmyelinated. In addition they do not send branches up and down the cord but, instead, enter the gray matter almost at once to synapse with neurons of the second order whose fibers then run into the white matter where they enter the lateral spinothalamic tract.

We may further observe that of these six ascending tracts the fasiculi gracilis and cuneaties have their cell bodies in spinal ganglia, while the other four have theirs in dorsal gray matter. Also, the spinothalamic tracts and some fibers of the ventral spinocerebellar are crossed while the other three have their cell bodies on the same side as that in which they run.

These tracts also differ in function. Impulses from muscular sense organs in muscles, joints and tendons and those from sense organs of touch in the skin are carried by sensory fibers which run at least a short distance in the fasciculi gracilis and cuneatus. These impulses are carried to the brain through three different paths, namely, (1) the original fibers of these two fasiculi (2) the spinocerebellar tracts and (3) the ventral spinothalamic tract. In the case of muscular sense, most of the impulse going to conscious levels are carried to the brain in the original fibers while those going to the sub-conscious areas of the cerebellum are transferred to the spinocerebellar tracts. Tactile impulses may also be carried along distances in the original fibers, but most of them are transferred to ventral spinothalamic tract before reaching the brain. The pathways for sensations of pain, and cold go at once into the gray matter, then across to the opposite side and forward in the lateral spinothalamic tract.

Descending Motor Tract. The cortical spinal system, on the other hand, runs from the brain to the cord, constituting a motor transmission highway that reaches its highest expression in mammals. Arising from cell bodies in the cortex of the cerebrum in the anterior part of the brain, it grows down by means of neurites into the cord, eventually reaching the ventral horn of the gray area to synapse with the neurons these whose fibers extend outward through the ventral roots of the spinal nerves to the effector mechanism.

Not all the cortico spinal fibers follow the same course most of them, upon reaching the posterior part of the brain, cross over from the side of their cortical origin to enter the cord on the opposite side, forming the crossed pyramydial tracts, which are broadered on the outside by the spinocerebellar bundles of the lateral funiculi. These tracts together form a great motor stand which bring the spinal motor apparatus under the control of the wall. Other fibers, fervee in number continues from cortex to cord on the same side of their origin, forming the direct pyramidial tract, that come to lie on either side in the ventral funiculus close to the ventral fissure. These latter tracts are found only in a few mammals including the anthropoid apes and man. Just before the fibers composing them terminate, they also cross over, through the white commissure of the cord, and synapse with motor neurons of the cortico-spinal system make connections with effector neurons on the side of the body opposite to that occupied by the cell bodies from which they originate in the brain.

Other lesser descending bundles run from different parts of the brain to the cord where they synapse with motor neurons. These tracts aid in the complicated regulation of the effectors of the body.

Association Bundle Fibers

Earlier we described simple intro-segmental reflex arcs, limited to one segment and involving one sensory, one motor, and usually one association neuron we have also shown inter-segmental reflex arcs, may extend over segments in addition to the one through which the sensory neuron entered. In the latter type neuritis of the sensory neurons ran in the dorsal columns giving off collaterals of various levels. These collaterals in turn went into the gray matter to carry impulses to motor neurons either directly or through an association neuron.

Another type of intersegmental reflex arc is that in which impulses are transmitted from one sensory neuron to motor neuron in a number of segments through an intermediate neuron. A collateral form a sensory neuron enters the gray matter where it synapses with the short dendrite of an intermediate cell. The neurite of this cell runs into one of the white ground bundle lying immediately around the gray area. These bundles or, fasciculi propril, are found in all the gray matter. A neurite entering one of these bundles splits into ascending and descending branches each of which runs for only a few segments. Along their courses these fibers give off collaterals which return to the gray matter where they synapse with motor neurons. In this manner reflex responses are spread over several segments through association neurons.

As in the case of intersegmental reflex arcs and intersegmental type in which the different levels are reached through sensory neuritis, this type involving proper fasciculi is not limited to one side of the cord. Some of the intermediate fibers cross in the ventral white commissures to send impulses out through motor neurons of the side of the body opposite that to which the sensory neuron belonged. In these various ways the two sides of the body and the various segments are inter-connected so that a response is by no means limited to a localized area. Under ordinary circumstances, however, the response will not be diffuse as in the case of nerve net transmission. Instead the impulses pass along appropriate pathways as determined by synoptic connections within the cord.

It is evident from the above description that motor neurons may synapse with fibers coming from a variety of places. In fact a single motor neuron with its much branched set of dendrites may have impulses funneled to it through several primary sensory neurons as well as by fibers from fasciculi propril, corticospinal tracts, and other tracts which space has prevented us from discussing. As sherrington has no aptly said, a motor neuron is "the final common path" of many reflex arcs.

Also it is evident that the cell bodies of the fibers which make up the single tracts of the spinal cord have three different locations (1) spinal ganglia, giving rise to the fasiculus gracilis and fasciculus cuaeatus, as well as many collateral, which enter the gray matter of the cord (2) gray matter of the cord, giving rise to the three fasciculi propril the dorsal and ventral spinocerebellar tracts and the lateral and ventral spinothalamic tracts and (3) the brain, giving rise to the crossed and direct pyramidial tracts.

The pattern of gray and white matter, as well as the actual size of the whole cord, varies greatly at different levels in any individual. Since the white is the transmission highway between the cord and the brain, it naturally becomes cumulatively larger the nearer it approaches to the brain itself relative increase in the white matter at different levels within the cord of mammals is explained as machinery that makes possible more reliance on the brain in regulating the behaviour of the animal.

The relative amount in sq. mm of the white and gray matter throughout the human cord is shown by the curves plotted.

4

Craniospinal Nervous Pathways

Of the different bundles of fibers connecting brain and spinal cord, four groups were mentioned in the discussion of the cord. Three of these were the dorsal columns (fasciculi gracilis and cuneatus), the spinothalamic tracts, and the spinocerebellar tracts, all of which are made up of ascending fibers; the fourth was the descending corticospinal group. We are now in a position to consider some of the cranial portions of these pathways.

(a) *Fasciculi gracilis and cuneatus.*— As mentioned during the discussion of the spinal cord, sensory neurons with their bodies in the dorsal ganglia send their neurites into the dorsal funiculus. Many of these neurites continue forward as the *fasciculus gracilis,* in the case of sensory neurons from posterior parts of the body, or the *fasciculus cuneatus,* for anterior sensory neurons. These bundles extend into the medulla as the *funiculi gracilis* and *cuneatus,* respectively. Here the neurites terminate, synapsing with the short dendrites of relaying neurons, or *sensory neurons of the second order,* which carry the impulses to more anterior parts of the brain.

The neurons of the second order for the fasciculus gracilis have their cell bodies in the *nucleus gracilis* which lies near the region where the roof plate is broadening to form the thin velum. The *nucleus cuneatus,* for the relaying neurons of the cuneate tract, is just lateral to the gracile nucleus. Most of the neurites of these relaying neurons swing in an arc ventrally to decussate (cross to the other side of the medulla), beneath the central canal and posterior part of the fourth ventricle, thus forming what is known as the *sensory decussation.* As soon as they cross the mid-line they turn sharply to run anteriorly, as the *median lemniscus* which lies near the mid-line.

In the thalamus the fibers of the second order terminate and synapse with *sensory neurons of the third order* which have their cell bodies in one of the thalamic nuclei. The neurites of these third neurons go to the *somatesthetic area* of the cerebral cortex.

These tracts form pathways for sensations of touch and pressure as well as for proprioceptive impulses from the muscles, joints, and tendons.

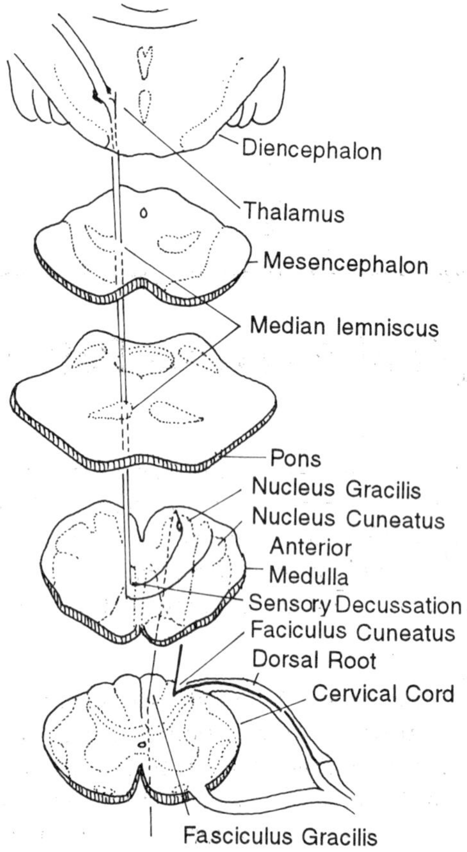

Fig. 4.1. Sensory pathways through the dorsal columns.

(b) *Spinothalamic Tracts.*— In the case of the spinothalamic tracts the sensory neurons (neurons I) synapse with neurons II within the dorsal gray matter of the cord. The neurites of these neurons of the second order cross, through the *ventral commissure*, into the spinothalamic tracts of the other side of the cord. The fibers of each of these tracts reach the thalamus, where they synapse with the neurons of the third order which have their cell bodies in one of the *thalamic nuclei*. From this nucleus, the neurites extend to the *somatesthetic area* of the cerebral cortex.

It will be recalled that physiologically the two tracts of this group are not the same. The *ventral spinothalamic* tract is a pathway for sensations of touch and pressure, the *lateral spinothalamic* for pain and temperature. Also the neurites of the primary sensory neurons associated with each of these tracts take somewhat different courses. The neurites carrying touch and pressure impulses run in the dorsal columns before sending collaterals into the dorsal gray horn. The neurites carrying pain and temperature impulses go directly into the gray matter at the level of entrance into the cord.

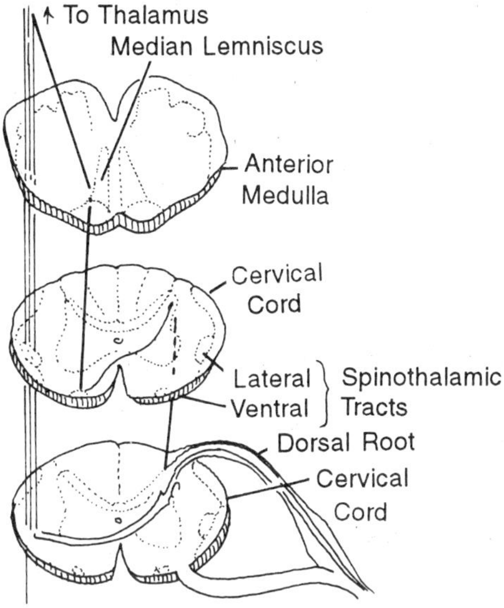

Fig. 4.2. Sensory pathways through the spinothalamic tracts.

(c) *Spinocerebellar Tracts.*— The spinocerebellar tracts are important proprioceptive pathways to the cerebellum, the chief center of correlation of these impulses as well as of coordination of muscular activity. In both of these tracts the primary sensory neurons are similar to those described for the fasciculi gracilis and cuneatus. Collaterals, leaving these neurons along their course, enter the dorsal gray matter to synapse with the neurons of the second order.

The cell bodies of the dorsal *spinocerebellar tract* are located in the *nucleus dorsalis* (Clarke's column) from which neurites run into the dorsal tract of the same side of the cord. These fibers run forward through the medulla and enter the cerebellum by way of the *restiform body*.

The *ventral spinocerebellar* tracts are composed of neurites whose cell bodies are in the *dorsal horns* and adjacent portions of the gray matter. Some fibers enter the nearby tract of the same side of the cord; other cross over, through the *ventral commissure*, to run forward through the ventral tract of the opposite side. Each ventral spinocerebellar tract passes through the *medulla* and deeper part of the *pons to enter the anterior cerebellar peduncle*, through which it swings back into the anterior part of the cerebellum.

(d) *Corticospinal Tracts.*— Numerous motor pathways eventually leave the spinal cord through the primary motor neurons or "final common path," as mentioned previously. Many groups of fibers exert involuntary control over the muscles, while several which descend from the cerebral cortex place the skeletal muscles under voluntary control. The most important voluntary tracts entering the spinal cord are the corticospinals which originate in giantpyramidal cells of the motor cortex, immediately anterior to the central sulcus.

The neurites of these pyramidal cells pass successively through the white matter of the cerebral hemisphere, the *crura cerebri* and the *deeper part of the pons* to enter the

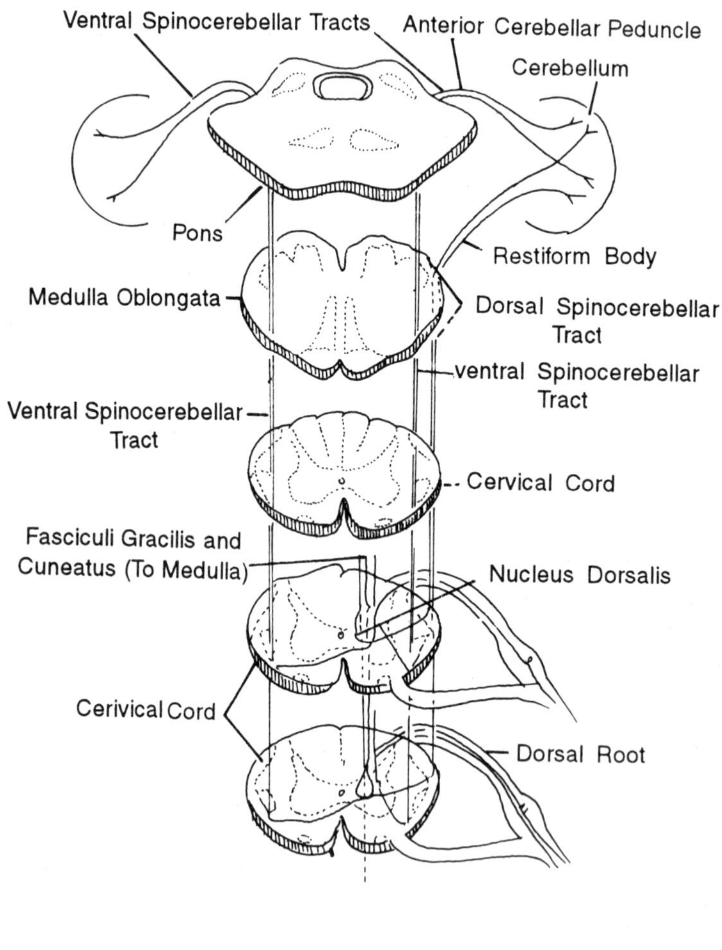

Fig. 4.3. Sensory pathways through the spinocerebellar tracts.

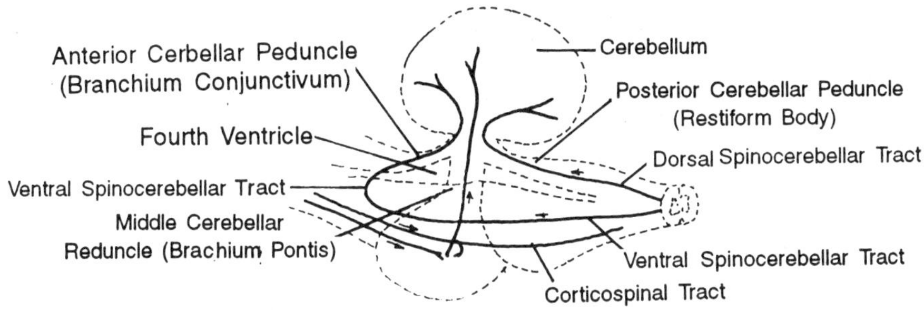

Fig. 4.4. The three cerebellar peduncles.

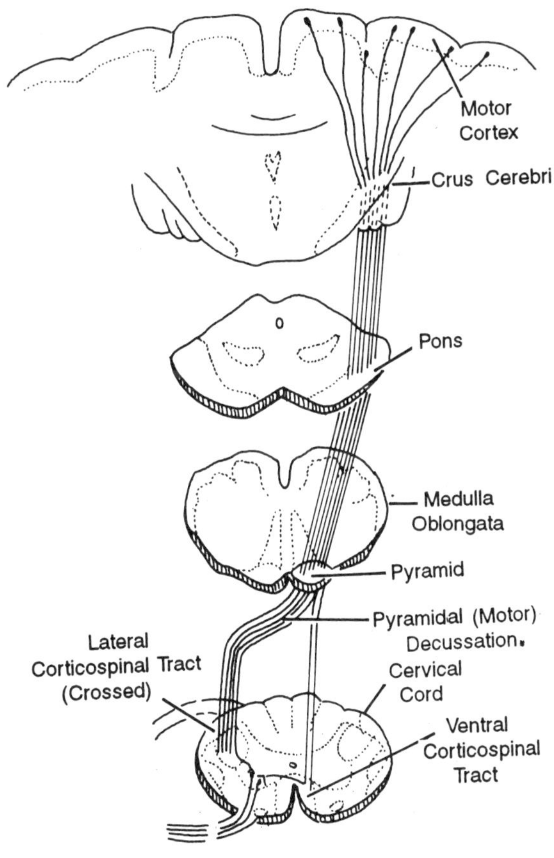

Fig. 4.5. The corticospinal (motor) pathways.

pyramids of the medulla oblongata (Fig. 4.5). In the *pyramidal decussation*, at the posterior end of the medulla, most of these fibers cross over to become the *lateral pyramidal*, or *lateral corticospinal, tract* which continues the entire length of the cord. At every segment some of these fibers enter the ventral horn of the gray matter to synapse with primary motor neurons. In man, about one-fourth of the fibers do not decussate but continue posteriorly as the *ventral pyramidal tract*, which ordinarily does not extend below the mid-thoracic region. When these direct fibers leave the tract, a few at a time, they cross to the other side of the cord and enter the ventral gray horn where they synapse with the primary motor neurons. Thus while in one case the fibers cross in the medulla, in the other they cross near their termination in the cord; but all of them cross. Consequently all of the skeletal muscles of one side of the body are under the voluntary control of the motor cortex to the opposite side of the brain.

Sensory Pathways to the Brain

Signals entering the spinal cord through nerve fibers from sensory receptors not only produce spinal reflexes but must also travel to the brain, where, among other things, they can produce conscious appreciation of the various stimuli which the body receives. The route by which sensory information travels from the spinal cord to the brain depends upon the degree of discrimination and the urgency with which information must reach the brain. Thus, information about joint position, for example, is transmitted rapidly to the brain by the dorsal column system. On the other hand, temperature sensation, which is less urgent and not precisely localised, is conveyed to the brain via the spinothalamic system.

Sensory-nerve fibers forming the dorsal column system enter the spinal cord in the dorsal roots and branch in the dorsal horn. Some branches are short and form synapses locally while the longest branch travels up the spinal cord to the medulla in the dorsal columns. On each side of the medulla there are two sensory nuclei, the dorsal column nuclei (the gracile and cuneate nuclei). The gracile nuclei receive sensory fibers from the hindlimbs and lower body, while the cuneate nuclei receive sensory fibers from the forelimbs and upper body. Within these nuclei sensory fibers of the dorsal column system form synaptic connections with second-order sensory neurons (those neurones which are second in the chain joining sensory receptors to the brain). The axons of the second-order neurones then cross the midline to the opposite side of the medulla and travel up to synapse in the thalamus. These fibers then pass to the somatic sensory area of the cerebral cortex. The actual part of the somatic sensory cortex to which nerve fibers travel depends upon the part of the body those fibers represent. Thus, signals from the leg arrive in that part of the somatic sensory cortex near the midline. In this way there is a spatial representation of the body across the somatic sensory cortex. The size of the cortical area devoted to each part of the body, however, is not proportional to the physical size of that part, but is related to the density of sensory receptors therefore the fingers and lips, which have a high degree of discrimination for tactile stimuli, have a large area of cortical representation in comparison with the trunk, which has relatively poor discrimination.

Sensory-nerve fibers carrying less precise information to the somatic sensory cortex via the spinothalamic system enter the spinal cord through the dorsal roots, then travel up or down the spinal cord for several segments before forming synaptic connections with second-order neurones. Fibers of the pathway then cross the midline and travel up the spinal cord, through the medulla, finally terminating in the thalamus. Here they synapse with neurones which convey the signals to the somatic sensory cortex. Fibers of the spinothalamic system are generally smaller in diameter and hence have a lower conduction velocity than those of the dorsal column system. Each system does, however, consist of a chain of neurones which carries signals from sensory receptors to the somatic sensory cortex.

In the above description of the sensory pathways to the brain each successive synapse was considered merely as a relay by which sensory information is passed from one neurone to another; each synapse in the pathways does, however, modify the sensory signals in some way, so that the pattern of signals arriving at the somatic sensory cortex is not an exact replica of that in the sensory-nerve fibers entering the spinal cord. An example of the way in which signals may be processed by successive neurones in a sensory pathway is given with reference to the visual system.

Control of Movement

Although motor acts are often classified as conscious or unconscious, the distinction between the two is often blurred. Thus, when learning a new skill, such as riding a bicycle, we must attempt to concentrate simultaneously on many different aspects of our often unsuccessful attempts to maintain equilibrium. In the light of painful mistakes we are able to voluntarily focus on the most faulty aspects of our performance. Once the skill has been learned we are able to keep balance without the need to concentrate on the details of the task and are able to devote our thoughts to other matters as we cycle along. In this way a given series of motor commands have passed from the conscious to the automatic domain of control.

At present we do not know exactly how the brain comes to a decision to perform a particular action, or where this decision is made; instead we are limited to descriptions of those pathways by which movements are controlled once they have been initiated. It has been known for some time that localised muscular contractions can be produced by electrical stimulation of that area of the cerebral cortex known as the precentral gyrus. This lies just in front of the somatic sensory area and is known as the motor cortex. Different muscles can be activated by electrically stimulating different parts of the motor cortex. In this way it is possible to construct a map of the muscles controlled by each part of the motor cortex. As with the somatic sensory cortex, the cortical area representing a given part of the body is not directly related to its physical size. Instead muscles capable to delicate movements have a relatively large representation on the motor cortex, while muscles under comparatively poor nervous control have a small area of cortical representation.

There are two major systems by which signals are transmitted from the brain to the spinal cord to produce movement. These are known as the pyramidal (corticospinal) system and the extrapyramidal (extra-corticospinal) system. Both systems send nerve fibers down the spinal cord where they activate directly, or indirectly, α- or γ-motor neurones. Neurones of the pyramidal tract have their cell bodies in the cerebral cortex. Their nerve fibers pass down into the white matter of the cerebrum where they all converge to pass through a narrow gap (the internal capsule) between brain centres. From the internal capsule, the nerve fibers travel on down through the brainstem, where most fibers cross to the opposite side of the midline at the caudal end of the medulla. The fibers then continue down the spinal cord and terminate in the spinal segment containing the motor neurons they are to control. Thus, signals descending in the pyramidal tract are transmitted from the cerebral cortex to their destination in the spinal cord without intervening synapses.

The extrapyramidal system can be defined as any system other than the pyramidal system by which the brain sends motor commands to the spinal cord. The extrapyramidal system is anatomically more complex than the pyramidal system for two main reasons: first because of its heterogeneity and, second, because there are a number of synaptic relays in the system. The extrapyramidal system consists of the basal ganglia (a group of nerve centres deep within the cerebrum), several brainstem nuclei and the brainstem reticular formation (an area containing a complex network of small cells). Motor signals from the cerebral cortex are received and modified by this system, then sent down the spinal cord. The extrapyramidal system also receives information concerning such things as balance, body position and the visual work from sources other than the cerebral cortex. All this information is integrated and contributes to the final motor commands sent to the spinal cord by the extrapyramidal system.

Although, so far, the pyramidal and extrapyramidal systems have been considered separately, they are functionally interdependent. Thus signals travel back from parts of the extrapyramidal system to the motor cortex, where they influenced the activity of neurones in the pyramid tract.

Because the extrapyramidal system receives sensory information from a number of sources and uses this to modify motor signals in the pyramidal system, it is extremely important for the maintenance posture and balance and also for the production of smooth slow movements. In view of this, it is perhaps not surprising that malfunction of the basal ganglia results in a number of motor disturbances such as a resting tremor which can often be observed in patients suffering from Parkinson's disease.

The cerebellum has a large modifying influence on motor signals from the brain to the spinal cord via both the pyramidal and extra pyramidal systems. The functions of the cerebellum are in some times complementary to those of some components of the extrapyramidal system. Thus, the extrapyramidal system predominates in the production of smooth, slow movements, while the cerebellum is of primary importance in the generation of coordinated rapid movements.

Like the extrapyramidal system, the cerebellum receives signals related to body position and movement from a variety of sources. Thus, information about head movement (from the vestibular apparatus) and limb movement (mainly from muscle

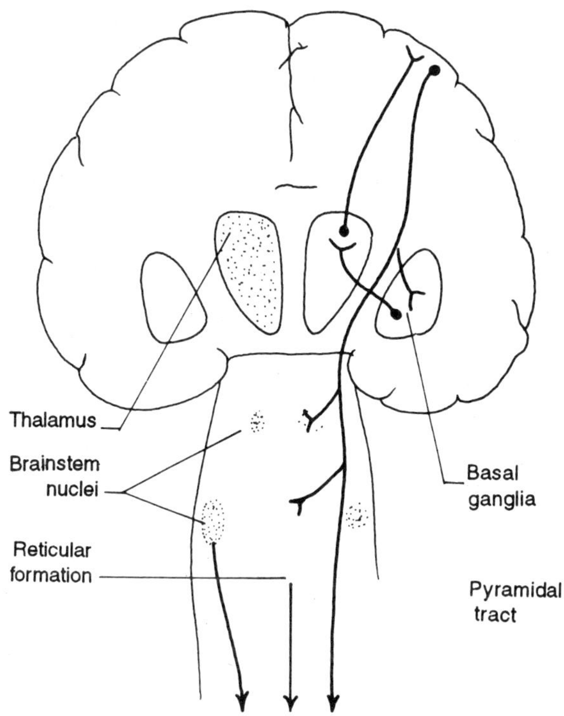

Fig. 4.6. Extrapyramidal system. This system is more heterogeneous than the pyramidal system; it carries signals from a number of different brain areas to spinal motor centres. These brain areas include the basal ganglia, brainstem nuclei and the brainstem reticular formation, all of which are influenced directly or indirectly by motor signals from the cerebral cortex.

spindles and Golgi tendon organs) and signals from the visual and auditory systems converge upon the same region of the cerebellar cortex, so that, like the somatic sensory cortex, a map can be made to show where each part of the body is represented on it. Although the cerebellum receives such a wide range of information, it plays no part in the conscious perception of sensory stimuli. The cerebellum is itself also unable to initiate movements. For these reasons electrical stimulation of the cerebellum leads neither to sensations nor to movements; instead, the cerebellum uses incoming sensory information to compute the position in space of different parts of the body. In addition to sensory signals the cerebellum also receives signals from the motor cortex and from elements of the extrapyramidal system reflecting their output to spinal motor centres. By combining sensory and motor signals the cerebellum can predict the movements and positions of different parts of the body which will result from motor commands leaving the brain via the pyramidal and extrapyramidal systems. In this way the cerebellum can compare an intended movement with that which is actually being produced. The cerebellum also has connections with both the motor cortex and parts of the extrapyramidal system through which it can modify their subsequent output. Thus, if for example the cerebellum computes that a limb is moving too fast for a particular action, it will send messages to the relevant motor systems, inhibiting the overactive muscles and causing excitation of antagonists. In this way the limb movement stops at the right moment without appreciable overshoot.

It appears, in fact, that the motor systems normally send commands to the spinal motor centres which would, in themselves, produce exaggerated movements; the moderating influence of the cerebellum, however, allows the production of smooth, accurate movements. Thus, impairment of cerebellar function results in movements which are jerky, less precise and which often overshoot the desired final position; this overshoot can lead to pendular limb movements, which result from successive unsuccessful attempts to bring a limb to rest at a given final position. Cerebellar damage can also be associated with 'intention tremor', in which muscular tremor develops when movement is attempted, but is absent at rest. Like other movement disorders which result from cerebellar malfunction, 'intention tremor' might be expected if commands from the motor systems are not modulated by the cerebellum. 'Intention tremor' contrasts markedly with that seen after damage to the basal ganglia in which tremor occurs at rest and is reduced during muscular activity. Loss of cerebellar corrective functions can also result in an inability to coordinate movements involving several different joints. Instead, movements of each joint are produced separately. This is perhaps not surprising if the patient has difficulty even executing and terminating movements about a single joint.

One of the major sources of sensory input to the cerebellum is the vestibular apparatus, which provides information about the orientation and movement of the head in space. This information alone cannot be used by the cerebellum to compute the position of the whole body; the cerebellum also receives signals from joint receptors in the neck, which indicate the angle of the neck. By analysing the signals from both the vestibular apparatus and the neck-joint receptors the cerebellum is able to compute the position of the whole body in space. In the light of this it is not surprising to find that cerebellar damage can be associated with a loss of balance.

We have already seen that the cerebellum receives a wide range of sensory information. Under normal circumstances the information from all the different sources should correspond, and all will contribute to the signals sent from cerebellum to the motor centres. As conditions change, however, the relative importance of the sensory signals from different sources can vary. Thus, in the dark the cerebellum receives no visual information. The cerebellum of an astronaut in a space capsule, on the other hand, receives no information about head position from the vestibular apparatus, since there is no gravitational force to act upon the macular hair cells. Instead the cerebellum of the astronaut has to rely heavily on visual information.

In summary, movements are controlled by the two major motor systems which have their origins in the brain. The activity of both systems can strongly be influenced by the inflow of sensory information from a number of sources, some of which can act directly through the extrapyramidal system and some of which acts via the cerebellum

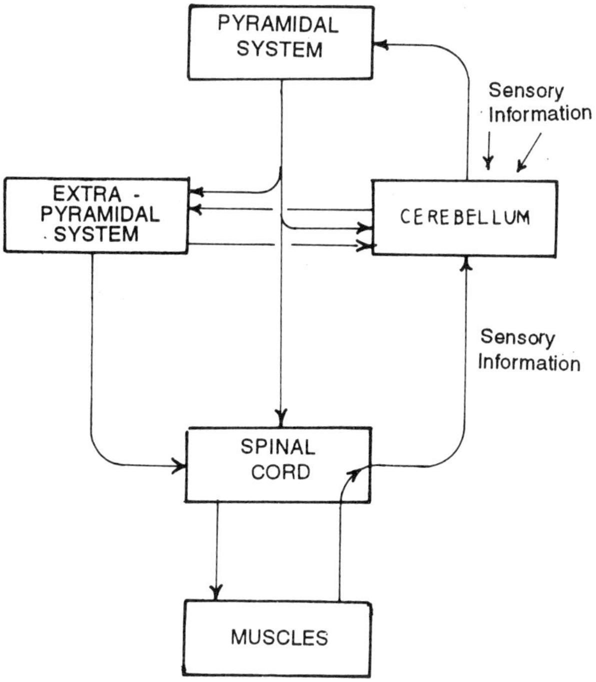

Fig. 4.7. Interactions of the cerebellum with the two motor systems. The cerebellum receives information about the motor commands travelling to the spinal cord via both the pyramidal and extrapyramidal systems; it also receives sensory information from a number of different sources, including muscles. In the light of all this information the cerebellum sends corrective signals back to the motor systems to modulate their subsequent output.

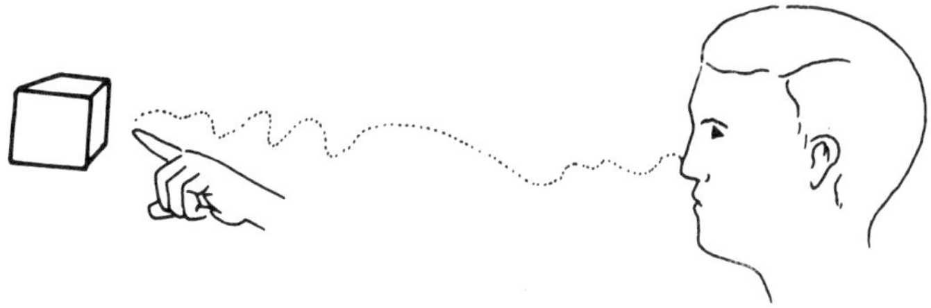

Fig. 4.8. Effect of cerebellar malfunction on movement. Damage to the cerebellum can disturb its corrective influence on motor commands; as a result movements become poorly controlled. Thus, when such a patient attempts to move his finger from his nose to a particular object the movement is irregular and becomes progressively more jerky as the object is approached.

to maintain balance and to produce coordinated, smooth and precise movements. At the present time, though, we have little insight into the way in which the 'decision' to produce movements is made in the brain.

The Reticular Formation

So far we have discussed the routes by which relatively specific information is transmitted from one part of nervous system to another. We are all aware that the overall level of activity in the nervous system can alter under different conditions; thus, at some times we may be very alert and excited and could not sleep even if we wished, while at others it is hard to remain awake. These alterations in the degree of arousal are a result of variations in the level of activity in the area of the brainstem core known as the reticular formation. This consists of an extremely complex network of small interconnected neurones; it is not homogeneous but contains a number of nuclei with quite specific functions in addition to more diffuse areas. Thus, the reticular formation has a number of discrete functions in addition to that of setting the level of consciousness. We have already seen that some nuclei embedded in the reticular formation form part of the extrapyramidal system and are concerned with the maintenance of posture and balance. In addition, other areas of the reticular formation are responsible for, among other functions, the regulation of respiration, heart rate and blood pressure.

The reticular formation has widespread inputs, including the cerebrum, cerebellum, spinal cord and other regions of the brainstem; it has widespread outputs and is able to influence the activity of many areas from which it receives signals. In this way the reticular formation samples much of the activity in the CNS and can use this information to modulate overall nervous activity.

Reticular Activating System

Stimulation of one particular area of the reticular formation can cause an individual to become aroused or alert. This part of the reticular formation is known as the reticular activating system. The reticular activating system projects diffusely to most of the cerebral cortex, largely via the thalamus. In this way activation of the reticular activating system in turn alerts the cerebral cortex and makes it more receptive to incoming signals.

Although the reticular activating system is directly responsible for the production of the alert state, it is itself under the influence of two other regions of the reticular formation, both of which lower the overall level of arousal. Both these centres act together to produce sleep, although the role of each is different. (See below for a discussion of sleep.)

Electroencephalogram

Electrodes placed on the scalp can be used to record electrical activity of the brain. Such a recording is known as an electroencephalogram (EEG). The EEG does not reveal the electrical activity of single nerve cells, but shows electrical changes which result from the activity of large populations of nerve cells in the cerebral cortex. The nature of the activity recorded depends upon the level of consciousness of the individual. Figure

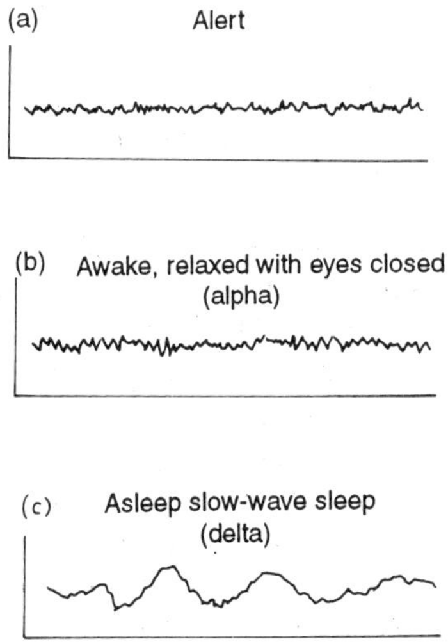

Fig. 4.9. Electroencephalogram (EEG) Electrical activity of the brain can be recorded by electrodes placed on the scalp; such recordings reflect activity in large numbers of cortical nerve cells and are known as electroencephalograms. (a) Recordings made from an alert subject show irregular low-amplitude electrical activity. (b) If the subject relaxes with his eyes closed, regular waves appear with a frequency of 8-12 Hz. This type of electrical activity is known as the α-rhythm. (c) When a subject first falls asleep the α-rhythm is replaced by larger, slower δ-waves.

4.9 shows some of the types of wave which can be observed. If a subject is awake but relaxed with his eyes closed his EEG pattern shows regular waves with a frequency of 8-12 Hz; this is known as the α-rhythm and apparently results from synchronised activity of many cortical neurones. If the subject opens his eyes and becomes alert, the α-rhythm is replaced by irregular low amplitude activity which results from desynchronisation of neuronal activity. The actual changes which take place at the cellular level to produce the different types of EEG pattern are unclear. The EEG can be used clinically, however, to determine the position of localised brain abnormalities. Normally the shape and timing of the EEG patterns recorded from corresponding points on each cerebral hemisphere are similar. A tumor or other localised lesion on one hemisphere would upset this bilateral symmetry in the EEG allowing its position to be determined. The EEG can also be used in the diagnosis of the various forms of epilepsy. Epilepsy results from excessive activity of whole or part of the CNS and can be divided into partial and generalised forms. Partial epilepsy usually results from local brain damage. The damaged area causes very rapid discharge of neighbouring neurones. During an epileptic attack this abnormal discharge may remain localised or may spread to other brain areas. Generalised epilepsy involves larger areas of the brain and can be subdivided into grand mal and petit mal epilepsy. Grand mal is associated with convulsions which may last from several seconds to several minutes. Petit mal epilepsy is closely related to grand mal, and may similarly be associated with convulsions; these are, however, much shorter in duration. During both grand mal and petit mal episodes the EEG has a characteristic form.

Sleep

Although we spend a considerable proportion of our lives asleep, at present the physiological reason why we need sleep is not understood. It is, however, clear that the brain does not switch off during sleep.

Sleep can be divided into two types: slow-wave sleep and paradoxical sleep. Initially, on falling asleep, the α-rhythm is replaced by slower, larger (delta) waves (Fig. 4.9) and the person is said to be in slow-wave sleep. At intervals slow-wave sleep is interrupted by periods of paradoxical sleep, in which the EEG pattern resembles that of an alert individual. In spite of this, a subject is less easily aroused during paradoxical sleep than during slow-wave sleep; paradoxical sleep is associated with a reduction in the tone of limb and body muscles, but can be accompanied by rapid movements of the eyes. For this reason paradoxical sleep is also known as 'rapid eye movement sleep' (REM sleep). Dreaming usually takes place during REM sleep. Periods of REM sleep normally last about 20 minutes and constitute approximately 20% of the total time spent asleep.

We have already said that the level of consciousness depends upon the interplay between three regions of the reticular formation. It is thought that slow-wave sleep is produced by a centre in the reticular formation of the medulla. It does this by depressing the activity of the reticular activating system (RAS). This depression apparently results from the inhibitory action on the reticular activating system of 5-hydroxytryptamine produced by cells of the sleep centre in the medulla. While the centre in the medulla inhibits the RAS it simultaneously activates the second sleep centre, which is located in the pons. This pontine sleep centre is responsible for the generation of paradoxical sleep. Sleep cycles probably result from fluctuations in the levels of 5-hydroxytryptamine in the reticular formation.

Emotion—the limbic system

Both emotion and motivation are entities which can be only poorly defined neurophysiologically: it seems that both are controlled by a part of the brain previously known as the rhinencephalon (=nose brain). Originally this part of the brain was thought to be primarily concerned with the sense of smell; it is now known to have several other important functions. For this reason the term 'rhinencephalon' has been replaced by 'limbic system' to describe these structures. The limbic system is heterogeneous and consists of a ring of primitive cortical tissue on each side of the midline encircling a number of subcortical structures, including parts of the hypothalamus and thalamus, the amygdaloid nuclei, the septal nuclei and the hippocampus. These components of the limbic system have relatively complex interconnections. Much of the output of the limbic system is channelled through the hypothalamus, which, therefore, has a central role in limbic function.

The limbic system is important in a number of different brain functions. These include analysis of olfactory signals, generation of some feeding behaviour, and the control of several biological rhythms, the emotions of fear and rage and the motivational state of the animal. For this reason these activities may become enhanced or depressed by damage to different parts of the limbic system.

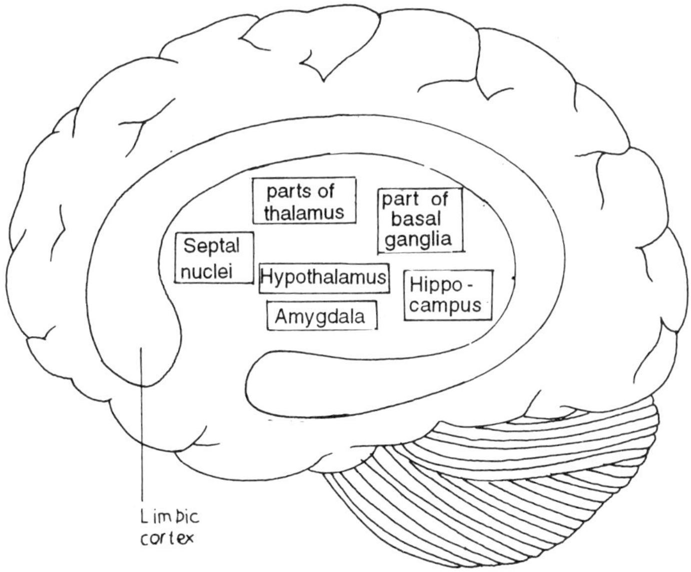

Fig. 4.10. Limbic system. This system is concerned with a number of functions including the perception of smell, production of feeding behaviour and the control of some biological rhythms, fear and rage and motivation. It consists of a ring of cortical tissue encircling a number of underlying structures all of which interact by means of a complex series of interconnections.

Normally there is a balance between rage and placidity, so that an animal will only become enraged if severely provoked; lesions in certain parts of the limbic system, however, can turn a previously placid animal into one which will show rage with minimal provocation. A similar transformation in behaviour can also be produced by electrical stimulation of other regions of the limbic system. Enragement produced in this way not only results in the behavioural changes directly associated with rage, but also the characteristic effects of changes in activity of the autonomic nervous system, such as an increase in heart rate, blood pressure and respiration. Thus, artificially produced rage is indistinguishable from rage observed in normal animals. Fear and rage are related emotions, and so it is perhaps not surprising that experimental manipulations of limbic function can enhance or suppress fear as they can rage.

Experiments have been performed to discover whether electrical stimulation of particular brain areas has a rewarding or punishing effect. To do this electrodes are chronically implanted into a selected brain area of an animal. The electrode is then wired-up so that, by pressing a lever, the animal can deliver stimulating pulses to its own brain. If the effect of stimulation is unpleasant, the animal will learn to avoid pressing the bar; if the effect of electrical stimulation is rewarding, the animal will press the bar repetitively. In fact, animals find stimulation of some brain areas so rewarding that they will ignore food to continue bar pressing and will only stop when completely

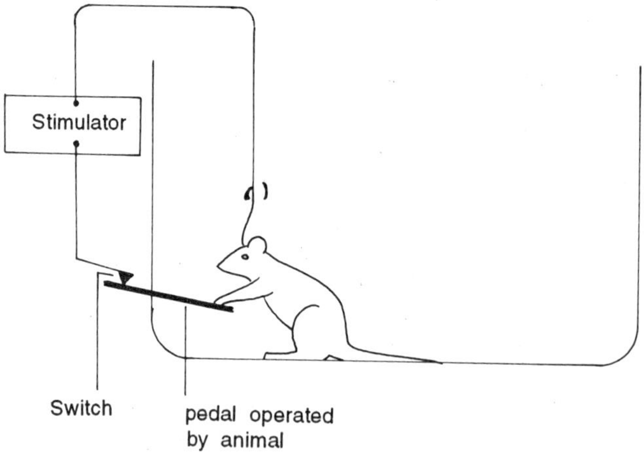

Fig. 4.11. Apparatus used to study reward and punishment. An electrode chronically implanted in the brain of the experimental animal is connected via a pedal switch to a stimulating device. The animal is able to operate the pedal and so stimulate its own brain; if stimulation has a rewarding effect, the animal will repeatedly press the pedal.

exhausted. Among the areas producing the highest rates of bar pressing are the hypothalamic centres controlling thirst, food intake and sexual behaviour. The effectiveness of some areas as centres for reward are dependent on the motivational state of the animal. For example, with certain electrode placements, bar pressing may be more frequent when the animal is hungry.

Cerebral Cortex

So far we have discussed those areas of the cerebral cortex which are involved in somatic sensations, motor control and those cortical regions which constitute part of the limbic system. The cortical areas concerned with the analysis of visual and auditory information. In addition to these areas there are three 'association' areas. One occupies part of the frontal lobe, a second occupies part of the temporal lobe, while the third occupies part of both the parietal and the occipital lobes.

One of the most remarkable characteristics of the human brain is its ability to deal with complex language. The ability to comprehend and produce language is located in parts of the cerebral cortex; disorders known as aphasias have provided a great insight into the way in which the brain deals with language. Aphasias are language deficits which result not from deafness or blindness nor, on the motor side, from paralysis of respiratory or oral muscles, but instead from an inability directly related to language. Aphasias may be classified as sensory or motor. In sensory aphasias there is a deficit in the ability to understand language. This deficiency may be limited to comprehension of written or of spoken language. The cortical areas responsible for comprehension of

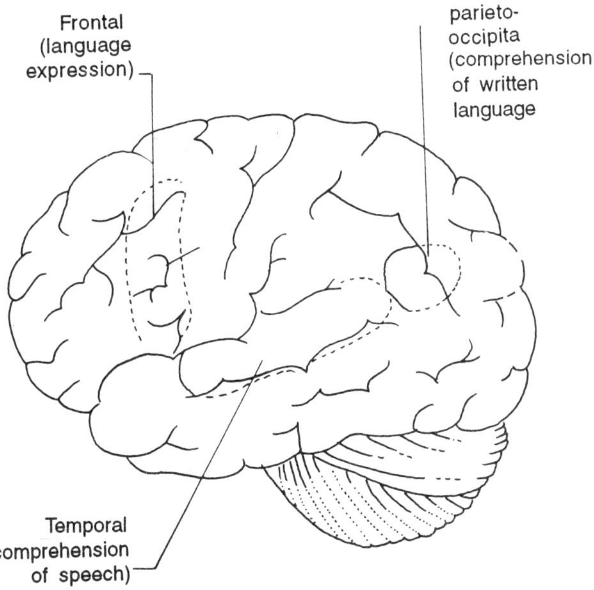

Fig. 4.12. Cortical areas concerned with language. One area in the frontal lobe is responsible for the motor aspects of language production: a second area in the temporal lobe is responsible for the comprehension of spoken language; while a third area on the boundary between the parietal and occipital lobes is responsible for comprehension of written language. Damage to any one of these areas produces characteristic language deficits.

written and spoken language. Motor aphasias, like sensory aphasias, can involve a deficit either in written or in spoken language; a patient with a motor aphasia can comprehend both spoken and written language but has difficulty expressing language. The areas responsible for the motor aspects of language are located in the frontal lobes just anterior to the motor areas.

Although, in a child, both cerebral hemispheres have an equal potential to develop language, language functions in most adults are largely limited to the left hemisphere. For this reason the left hemisphere has been termed the 'dominant hemisphere'. It has become clear, however, that although the right hemisphere has only limited language capability it has other capabilities absent in the left hemisphere; thus, it seems that the cerebral hemispheres are specialised in such a way that the left hemisphere takes over most of the language functions, while the right hemisphere predominates in functions such as the analysis of spatial relationships in the external environment and of musical forms. In normal individuals information can be exchanged between the two hemispheres via the corpus callosum, a large tract of nerve fibers joining the two cerebral hemispheres. This allows the two hemispheres with complementary specialisations to cooperate with each other.

It is hard to define precisely the role of the anterior pole of the frontal lobes. Damage to these lobes has little effect on intelligence, although it can cause some change in character and impair memory. One of the most striking effects of damage to this area is loss of anxiety which would appear in normal individuals under certain conditions. For this reason, operations have been performed in which connections are severe between the anterior pole of the frontal lobes and the remainder of the brain (prefrontal leucotomy) of patients suffering from acute states anxiety.

5

Cranial Nerves

Cranial nerves are those arising from brain. There are ten pairs of cranial nerves in lower vertibrates (Aminiotes) and twelve pairs in higher vertibrates (Amniotes). Those nerves are given below:

1. Terminal Nerve (0)

The terminal nerve arises from the cerebral hemispheres in the region of the medial olfactory tract and extends to the snout region in close association with, but independent of, the olfactory nerves.

It possesses one or more ganglia and is of doubtful function, being described as sensory by some investigators, as part of the autonomic system by others.

2. Olfactory Nerve (I)

The olfactory nerve is peculiar in that its fibers arise from cells of the olfactory epithelium. The dendrites of these cells have thickened endings which are exposed on the surface of the epithelium. The unmyelinated neurites making up the nerve have only a short distance to run to reach the olfactory bulb of the brain. In cyclostomes, which have only a single nasal sac, the olfactory nerves are paired as usual, indicating that the single organ represents a fusion of what was formerly two sacs.

In the skull of most vertebrates the olfactory nerve passes through a single foramen on either side to reach the brain, but in many of the higher animals it consists of a brushlike bundle of non-medullated fibers, *fila olfactoria*, that penetrate the skull separately through the pepperbox-like pores of the cribriform plate of the ethmoid bone. Thus, in man, instead of a single pair of olfactory nerves, it would not be entirely incorrect to say that there are at least twenty pairs.

3. Optic Nerve (II)

The optic nerve is not a true nerve but rather a *tract* of the brain both in development and structure. In development an evagination from the diencephalon forms the retinal layer of the eyeball. Then some of the retinal cells send their neurites back to the brain as the optic nerve, which therefore connects two parts derived from the embryonic central nervous system, the retina and the diencephalon. The fibers which make up this nerve, like most fibers in nerve tracts, are myelinated but without any neurolemma.

Upon reaching the ventral side of the diencephalon the fibers decussate, in the optic chiasma, before passing into the brain. The crossing of the fibers is complete except in the higher mammals in which the fibers from the nasal half of the eyeball cross while those from the temporal half do not. In man, therefore, the fibers from the left halves of the two eyes go to the left side of the brain, those from the right halves to the right side of the brain. This arrangement develops in association with improvement in binocular vision. After passing through the chiasma region, the fibers continue as the *optic tracts* each of which, after running over the outer surface of a cerebral peduncle, sends fibers into three parts of the brain, the *lateral geniculate body*, the *anterior colliculus*, and the region just anterior to the latter.

In these three pairs of regions the fibers of the optic tract synapse with neutons which relay the impulses to several different parts of the brain. From the lateral geniculate bodies the relaying fibers run chiefly to areas of visual sensation in the occipital cerebral cortex. The anterior coliculi, which receive fibers from the occipital cortex as well as the

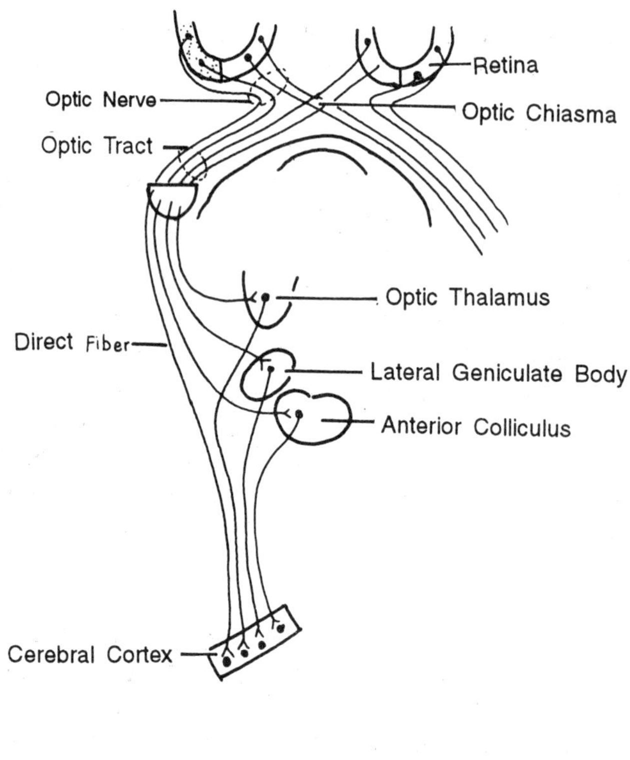

Fig. 5.1. Optic chiasma and tracts of man.

optic tracts, relay messages to the nuclei of the several cranial nerves which control the movements of the eyeballs and also of the head. Fibers from the area just in front of each anterior colliculus carry impulses which eventually reach the intrinsic muscles of the eyeball.

The intricate optic pathways of mammals have evolved from a relatively simple plan in lower vertebrates. In fishes most of the optic-tract fibers run into the optic lobes. In reptiles optic lobes continue to be highly important relaying centers in the optic pathways, but some optic fibers terminate in the diencephalon where they synapse with

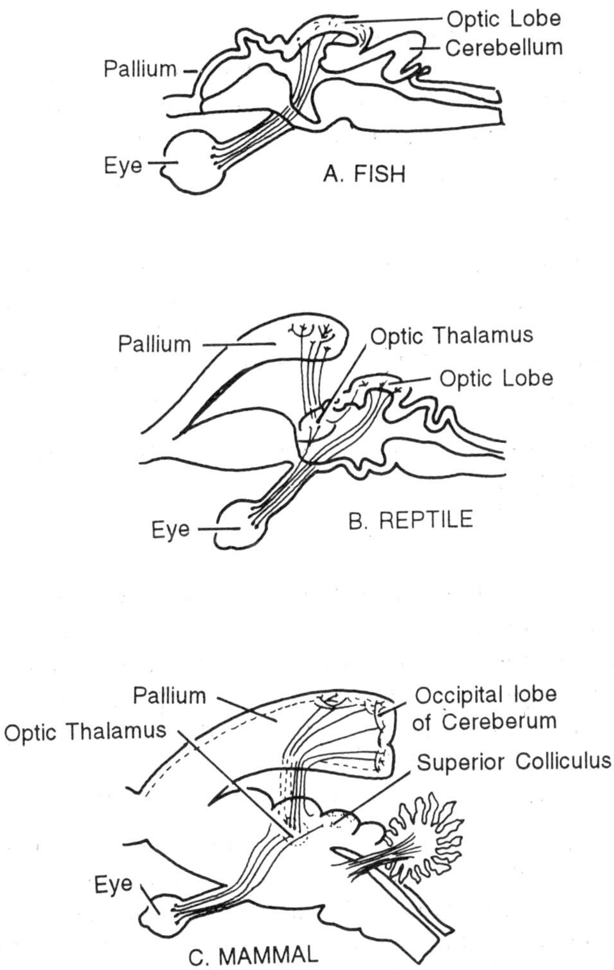

Fig. 5.2. Evolution of the optic tracts. A, fish; B, reptile; C, mammal. The dorsal part of the mesencephalon, which is the primitive visual center, becomes a relay center in mammals. In the latter group the definitive visual centers are in the occipital lobes of the cerebrum.

neurons leading to the cerebral cortex, which is definitely present in these animals. In mammals relatively few primary optic fibers go to the metencephalon, most of them terminating in the lateral geniculate bodies of the diencephalon.

4. Eye-Muscle Nerves (III, IV, VI)

The nerves of the eyeball muscles have much in common, being efferent somatic nerves associated with the three pairs of myotomes that remain in the head region. The oculomotor (III) and the trochlear (IV) arise from the mesencephalon, while the abducens (VI) comes from the myelencephalon. No cranial nerves take their origin from the metencephalon.

The most important nerve of the eye muscles is the *oculomotor*, which supplies not only the *inferior oblique* and three of the *rectus* muscles, namely, *superior, inferior*, and *internal*, but also the *levator palpebrae* that lifts the upper eyelid, as well as the intrinsic *iris* and *ciliary* muscles of accommodation within the eyeball itself.

The *trochlear* supplies the *superior oblique* muscle. The two trochlears decussate in the anterior medullary velum.

The *abducens actuates* the *lateral*, or *external rectus* muscle. It also sends a branch to the *retractor bulbi*, a muscle derived from the external rectus, which pulls back the eyeball as the name implies. This muscle is present in all tetrapods except ophidians and primates. The *nictitating membrane*, or third eyelid of reptiles, birds, and some mammals, is also supplied by the abducens nerve.

All three of these nerves are now believed to include proprioceptive sensory fibers from the structures which they supply.

5. Trigeminal Nerve (V)

The *trigeminal nerve* comes off dorso-laterally from the anterior region of the medulla is close association with the VIIth and the VIIIth cranial nerves, constituting together a most important group for the supply of the head. It has a strong dorsal root and a lesser ventral root and is one of the largest of the cranial nerves. It is the great sensory nerve of the head carrying nearly all of the general somatic sensory fibers from the surface of the head to the brain. The cell bodies of these fibers are located in the *Gasserian ganglion* of the dorsal root, one of the largest of all the ganglia associated with cranial nerves.

The trigeminal nerve is so called because of its three component branches, the *ophthalmic, maxillary*, and *mandibular*. It was probably formed by the joining of two original dorsal root nerves, the ophthalmic being the remains of one, and the maxillary and mandibular of the other. According to this interpretation the corresponding ventral root nerves are the oculomotor and the trochlear.

In fishes the ophthalmic, which is sensory in all animals, supplies the skin of the snout and dorsal part of the head. In mammals it is distributed to the nose, orbit, forehead, and top of the head. The maxillary, which is also sensory, goes to the teeth of the upper jaw, the upper lips, and the cheeks. The *mandibular* is mixed, being composed of: (1) sensory fibers from the teeth and skin of the lower jaw and also the skin of the side of the head; and (2) motor fibers which innervate the mandibular group of branchiomeric muscles.

The mandibular branch also includes proprioceptive sensory fibers coming from the muscles of mastication which it supplies. These proprioceptive neurons have their cell bodies in the mesencephalic nucleus of this nerve. In this respect they are unique, for the sensory neurons of all other vertebrate nerves have their cell bodies in ganglia, outside of the central nervous system. It will be recalled, however, that amphioxus has no ganglia, all of the cell bodies being within the central nervous system.

The maxillary branch may be regarded as the *pretrematic* nerve anterior to the mouth, and the mandibular branch, the corresponding *posttrematic* nerve posterior to the mouth. This pre- and posttrematic arrangement on either side of a pharyngeal opening, like mouth, spiracle, or gill slit, is repeated in other cranial nerves.

6. Facial Nerve (VII)

The VIIth nerve, or *facialis*, undergoes much modification as the result of evolutionary emergence from water to land life, owing to the loss of the lateral-life organs and, in higher mammals, to the development of the mimetic musculature of the face. The cell bodies of its sensory fibers are in the *geniculate ganglion* which in the lower vertebrates in often fused with the Gasserian ganglion of the Vth nerve.

In fishes and urodeles several dorsal branches of this nerve serve chiefly as sensory pathways from the lateral-line organs. These branches are lacking in anurans and higher vertebrates.

The ventral branch of the VIIth nerve forks into two trunks in fishes, the *palatine* and *hyomandibular*, which are respectively the pretrematic and posttrematic nerves of the spiracular opening.

In mammals the pretrematic branch is probably represented by the *chorda tympani*, a small nerve which runs through the middle-ear cavity. It will be recalled that this cavity corresponds to part of the spiracular passageway of fishes. The chorda carries fibers from the taste-buds on the anterior two-thirds of the tongue. It has also been joined by autonomic fibers associated with the sublingual and submaxillary glands. The post-trematic portion becomes the group of nerves which supply the hyoid-arch group of branchiomeric muscles, including the extensive muscles of facial expression in man.

7. Acoustic Nerve (VIII)

The *acoustic*, or *auditory, nerve* is a very short sensory nerve which does not emerge from the skull .It divides into two branches, the vestibular and cochlear, that go respectively to the semicircular canals and to the auditory mechanism (cochlea) of the internal ear. Each branch has a *ganglion* of similar name. As the semicircular canals aid in maintaining equilibrium, some of the fibers of the vestibular nerve run directly to the cerebellum, the main equilibrium center of the brain. Impulses from the cochlea, like those from the eye, are distributed through various parts of the brain. After being carried to the restiform body they are relayed to: (1) the auditory center in the cortex of the temporal lobe of the cerebrum; (2) the posterior colliculus, a center for reflexes initiated by sound; (3) other centers in the brain including those of the several motor nerves.

8. Glossopharyngeal Nerve (IX)

The *glossopharyngeal nerve,* primarily associated with the third splanchnocranial arch, forks around the first functional gill slits of fishes and sends a branch into the pharynx. Frequently it also has a small branch associated with the lateral-line system. Its sensory fibers have their cell-bodies located in the *petrosal ganglion.*

In mammals the sensory components are connected with the taste buds of the posterior third of the tongue, and general sense organs of this region and the neighboring portions of the pharynx. Most of its efferent fibers supply pharyngeal muscles derived from the group originally associated with the third visceral arch; a few synapse with autonomic fibers running to the parotid gland.

9. Vagus Nerve (X)

The *vagus nerve,* as the name implies, "wanders" to many parts of the body. It is apparently a composite of several segmental nerves. In fishes it splits into two main trunks, *lateral* and *visceral.* The lateral trunk, which is sensory, supplies some of the lateral-line organs of the head and extends along the side of the body as the nerve of the lateral-line canal. The visceral trunk, after giving off mixed *branchial* nerves to the remaining gill arches, continues posteriorly carrying visceral afferent and efferent fibers to the heart, the blood vessels, and the digestive tract and its derivatives as far as the posterior end of the small intenstine. The cell-bodies of the visceral afferent fibers are in the *nodosal ganglion.*

In strictly land vertebrates, with the loss of the lateral line system and the gills, most of the nerves connected with these structures disappear. Motor fibers of the branchial nerves persist, however, to innervate striated muscles of the pharynx and larynx. The main visceral trunk, which runs to the internal organs, retains its importance, carrying both sensory fibers and efferent fibers which connect with the autonomic nervous system.

In cyclostomes the vagus includes many somatic sensory fibers from the skin of the posterior part of the head. In fishes and amphibians these outaneous fibers are limited to the dorsal portion of this region, while in higher forms they are associated with the skin of the external ear.

10. Spinal Accessory Nerve (XI)

The spinal accessory nerve, found only in amniotes, is composed entirely of visceral efferent fibers. Part of these fibers, arising from the posterior portion of the medulla and running to join the vagus, are probably represented in lower vertebrates by posterior rootlets of the vagus. The others, arising by a series of rootlets from the anterior cervical region of the spinal cord, are thought to correspond to spino-occipital nerves of lower

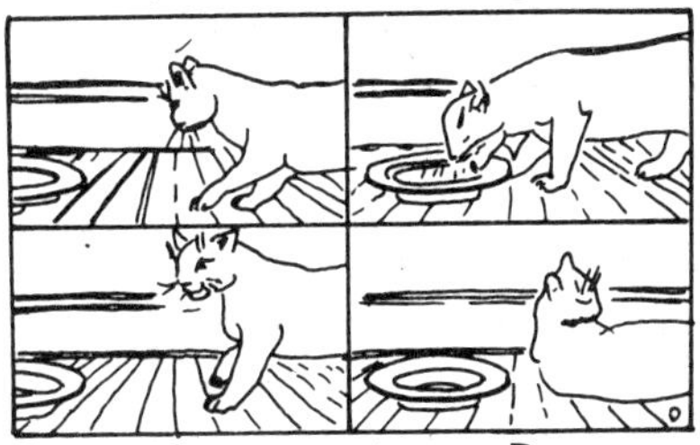

Fig. 5.3. The function of the cranial nerves. A, smelling and seeing (I, II); convergence and accommodation (III); depression of eyeballs (III, IV); mastication (V); salivation and tasting (VII, IX); swallowing (X, XII); tongue movements (VII). c, a moment of vigilance, with outward rolling of the eye (VI); facial and ear movements (VII); listening (VIII). D, digesting (X). The only omission is the spinal accessory (XI), supplying certain neck muscles which may have been used various times in this sequence.

forms. These fibers of spinal origin innervate the trapezius and sternocleidomastoid muscles. The fibers which join with the vagus are distributed with it to the striated muscles of the pharynx and larynx and to the autonomic nervous system.

11. Hypoglossal Nerve (XII)

The *hypoglossal nerve* is made up of somatic motor fibers which innervate the muscles of the tongue. Although it is found only in amniotes, it probably corresponds to some of the spino-occipital nerves of fishes.

The Autonomic Nervous System

Much of the routine work of the body, particularly of the circulatory and respiratory apparatus, of the viscera, and of the smooth muscles, is regulated by the general visceral efferent component of the nervous system, called by Langley the *autonomic nervous system.*

The autonomic portion of the peripheral nervous system is closely related anatomically to the spinal nerves and certain cranial nerves. Furthermore, nerve centers controlling the activity of autonomic neurons are located in the central nervous system. Consequently, all parts of the nervous system are so intimately bound together both structurally and functionally that none of its major constituents can be considered independently of the others.

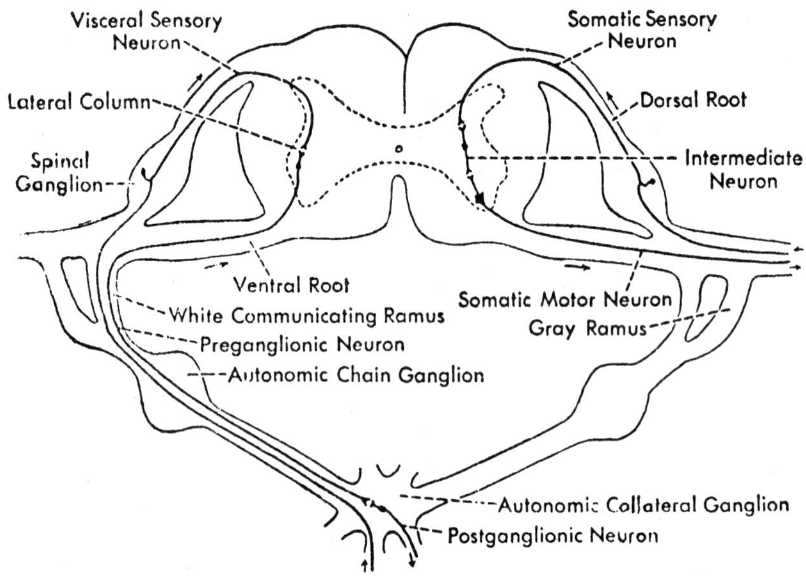

Fig. 5.4. Reflex pathways in the peripheral nervous system. Somatic reflex are on the right; an autonomic reflex are on the left. Arrows indicate courses of nerve impulses.

The autonomic portion of the peripheral nervous system is composed of efferent neurons which send impulses to smooth muscles and glands in all parts of the body. It regulates the function of structures which are under involuntary control. The muscle of the heart, although striated, is not subject to voluntary control, and it, too, is innervated by autonomic fibers. The proper function of this part of the nervous system is necessary for regulating such activities as rate of heart-beat, respiratory movements composition of body fluids, constancy of temperature, secretion of various glands, peristalsis, and other vital processes.

The complex connections of the autonomic neurons add to the difficulties embodied in an understanding of its structure most investigations have been carried out in mammals, and in man in particular. It will best serve our purpose first to discuss the autonomic system in man and then to make comparisons with other vertebrates.

It will be recalled that the cell bodies of the somatic motor neurons of cranial and spinal nerves are located in the ventral somatic motor column of gray matter of brain or spinal cord. Their medullated axons continue without interruption to the effector organ. A different pattern obtains in the autonomic system, in which efferent impulses must travel through two neurons, *preganglionic* and *postganglionic*, before they can bring about an effect.

The system is composed of these two types of neurons and a number of ganglia which serve as relay centers. The cell bodies of the preganglionic neurons are located in the visceral motor column of gray matter in the central nervous system. Their medullated fibers pass to outlying ganglia. These fibers make up the visceral motor components of certain cranial nerves and of spinal nerves. In the latter they are constituents of the white visceral rami. Postganglionic neurons have gray, sparsely medullated, or nonmedullated axons. The cell bodies of these neurons which are derived from neural-crest cells, lie in outlying ganglia which are often located at some distance from the central nervous system. It is here that the preganglionic fibers form synapses with the dendrites of postganglionic neurons. The axons of the postganglionic neurons are the ones which are distributed to smooth muscles, cardiac muscle, and glands in various parts of the body.

Although the peripheral autonomic system is essentially an efferent system, some authorities claim that certain visceral afferent fibers should be included. Such fibers pass from visceral organs up the dorsal roots of the spinal nerves to connect with the central nervous system.

Three large masses of nervous tissue, called ganglionated plexuses, are located near the vertebral column in the thoracic, abdominal, and pelvic regions. They are known as the *cardiac, coeliac,* or *solar,* and *hypogastric plexuses.* Each is composed of an intricate meshwork of nerves and ganglia containing visceral afferent fibers and visceral efferent fibers of the autonomic system. The cardiac plexus is situated near the base of the heart. The large coeliac, or solar, plexus is located at the upper level of the lumbar region and surrounds the roots of the coeliac, superior mesenteric, and inferior mensenteric arteries. A heavy blow stimulating the solar plexus affects almost all parts of the body. The hypogastric plexus, in the region where the sacrum joins the last lumbar vertebra, is composed of fibers distributed to the pelvic viscera.

The autonomic portion of the peripheral nervous system is divided into two main parts, the sympathetic and parasympathetic systems. The postganglionic fibers of both are, in most cases, distributed to all the involuntary structures of the body. The two systems, in general, work antagonistically. Whereas the one system (sympathetic) functions in such a manner as to strengthen an animal's defenses against adverse conditions by an expenditure of energy, the other (parasympathetic) is concerned with processes which tend to conserve and restore energy. Moreover, the manners in which these two systems bring about their effects differ for the most part. In both cases the postganglionic fibers give off chemical substances which, in the last analysis, bring about the effects. Post-ganglionic sympathetic fibers (except those going to the sweat glands and uterus, which cause vasodilatation) produce a hormone, formerly called *sympathin,* now known to be a catecholamine named *norepinephrine.* The same amine, in different concentration, along with epinephrine, is produced by the medulla of the adrenal gland. For this reason, postganglionic sympathetic fibers of this kind are usually spoken of as *adrenergic fibers.* Postganglionic parasympathetic fibers, and those postganglionic sympathetic fibers supplying the sweat glands and uterus, liberate a chemical called acetylcholine and are frequently referred to as *cholinergic fibers.* Preganglionic fibers of

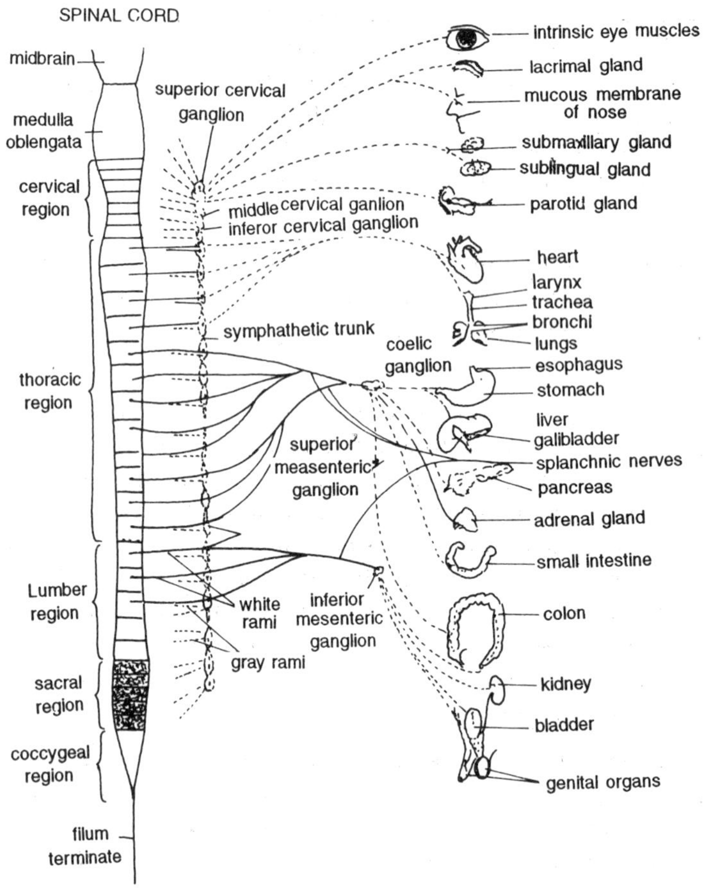

Fig. 5.5. Unilateral diagram of essential parts of sympathetic nervous system of man. Preganglionic fibers are shown in solid lines; postganglionic fibers in dotted lines.

both sympathetic and parasympathetic nerve are also considered to be cholinergic since they liberate acetylcholine at the synapse. Epinephrine. or norepinephrine and acetylcholine have opposite effects upon smooth muscles and glands. This further emphasizes the basic dual nature of the autonomic portion of the peripheral nervous system.

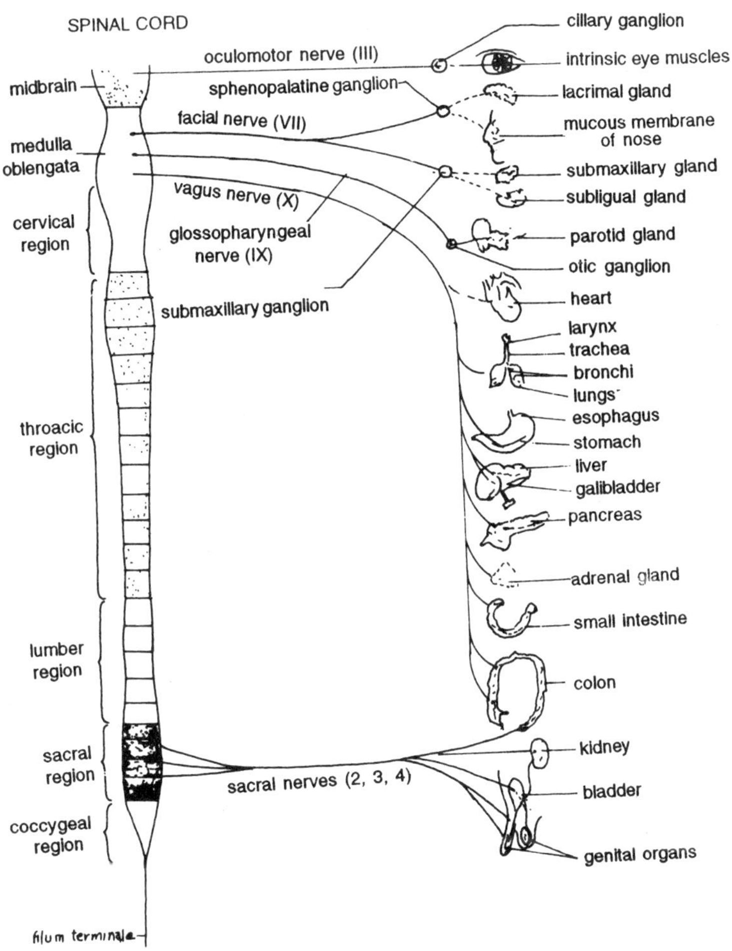

Fig. 5.6. Unilateral diagram of essential parts of parasympathetic nervous system of man. Preganglionic fibers are shown in solid lines; the very short post-ganglionic fibers in dotted lines.

Sympathetic Nervous System. Since the preganglionic fibers of the sympathetic nervous system connect to the spinal cord only in the thoracic and lumbar regions, the term *thoracolumbar outflow* is often applied to this portion of the autonomic system.

On either side of the ventral part of the vertebral column lies a *long sympathetic trunk,* extending from the foramen magnum to the coccyx. The trunk even enters the cranial cavity through the *carotid canal* in the temporal bone. At fairly regular intervals each sympathetic trunk bears enlargements known as the *chain ganglia*. Groups of these ganglia at the anterior end of the sympathetic trunk have fused, forming three large masses, the *superior, middle,* and *inferior cervical ganglia*. The latter is located near the point of junction of the last cervical and first thoracic vertebrae. The chain ganglia are numbered according to the vertebrae opposite which they lie, but fusions may occur obscure their segmental character. The inferior cervical ganglion on each side is frequently fused with the first thoracic ganglion, forming a *stellate ganglion*. In man there are cross communications between the number portions of the sympathetic trunks.

The white visceral rami of all the thoracle spinal nerves and the first, second, and third lumbar are partly composed of preganglonic fibers which connect with the corresponding chain ganglia. They may terminate in the ganglion at the point where they enter or may send fibers up or down the sympathetic trunk for some distance. Other preganglionic fibers pass without synapses through ganglia of the sympathetic trunk and form connections with one or more of three large, *prevertebral ganglia* of the coeliac plexus, located in the abdominal region in front of the lumbar vertebrae. A cording to definition, prevertebral ganglia are sympathetic ganglia of the thorax and abdomen other that those of the sympathetic trunk. The prevertebral ganglia of the coeliac plexus include the *coeliac, superior mesenteric,* and *inferior mesenteric ganglia*. The nerves leading to these ganglia from the sympathetic trunk are called the splanchnic nerves.

From the chain ganglia and prevertebral ganglia arise sparsely medullated, or non-medullated, postganglionic fibers which are distributed to the various structures in the body under involuntary control. A gray visceral ramus comes from each chain ganglion of the sympathetic trunk, whether or not a white visceral ramus is present. The postganglionic fibers of which the gray rami are composed are distributed via the dorsal and ventral rami of spinal nerves to the skin of the head, trunk, and limbs, where they supply smooth muscles in the walls of blood vessels. The arrector pili muscles, and skin glands. Other postganglionic fibers from the cervical ganglia at the anterior end of the sympathetic trunk pass to the intrinsic muscles of the eye, lacrimal glands, mucous membrane of the nose, palate, and mouth, and to the submaxillary, sublingual, and parotid salivary glands. From the inferior cervical ganglion and the first few chain ganglia in the thoracic region arise postganglionic fibers going to heart, larynx, trachea, bronchi, and lungs. The coeliac and superior mesenteric ganglia are the points of origin of postganglionic fibers which supply esophagus, stomach, small intestine, and the first part of the large intestine, as well as liver, pancreas, and blood vessels of the abdomen. The inferior mesenteric ganglion sends postganglionic fibers to the remainder of the large intestine and to the urogenital organs.

Preganglionic fibers pass directly to the medulla of the adrenal gland. This ectodermal, glandular structure, derived from neural-crest cells, is composed of specialized, or modified, sympathetic ganglionic cells which are homologous with postganglionic sympathetic neurons.

Function of the Sympathetic System. The action of the sympathetic neurons on the structures supplied by them has been the subject of many investigations. Among the reactions brought about by stimulation of the sympathetic systems are (1) constriction of cutaneous blood vessels, causing pallor; (2) contraction of arrector pili muscles, causing goosefiesh and making the hair stand erect; (3) secretion of sweat glands (cold sweat); (4) dilatation of the pupil permitting more light to enter the eyeball; (5) reduction in amount of saliva secreted so that but small quantities of a thick; mucinous secretions are given off; (6) acceleration of heartbeat; (7) dilatation of the bronchi; (8) relaxation, or inhibition, of the smooth muscles of the digestive tract, causing a temporary cessation of peristalsis; (9) relaxation of bladder musculature; (10) lengthening of the urethral musculature (11) increase in blood sugar; (12) rise in blood pressure; (13) increase in number of red corpuscles in the blood stream; and (14) decrease in clotting time of blood.

The above reactions, when considered together are those usually associated with pain, fear, and anger. They serve the body in a beneficial capacity in times of danger or when it is in an "aggressive" state. Many individuals, under conditions of extreme fear, may void urine involuntarily. This would seem to be paradoxical in light of the above. In such cases, however, certain reflexes, referred to as conditioned reflexes, usually established in early life, may bring about a reversal of reactions which normally occur in the aggressive state. Punishing or hurting a child in an effort to train it in toilet habits may be basically responsible for such poor conditioning.

Injection of epinephrine, a hormone of the medulla of the adrenal gland, causes effects which appear to be identical with those brought about by stimulation of the nerves of the sympathetic system. The hormone presumably acts upon the structures supplied by sympathetic nerve endings. Under normal circumstances the adrenal medulla secretes only insignificant amounts of epinephrine into the bloodstream. In times of stress, however, significant amounts may be liberated and the action of the hormone reinforces that of the sympathetic system so that maximal efficiency results. This action of epinephrine has been called the "emergency mechanism" of the body, for during times of stress the body is thus better adapted for self-preservation.

The adrenal medulla and its secretion are not essential to life. Sympathetic effects may be secured after removal of the adrenal medulla. It has already been indicated that stimulation of sympathetic postganglionic fibers (with the exception of those supplying the sweat glands and uterus, which are cholinergic) induces them to secrete norepinephrine. Epinephrine and norepinephrine are relatively stable compounds (catecholamines) which, circulating in the bloodstream, will simultaneously stimulate all structures (except sweat glands and uterus) supplied by the sympathetic system. Although these substances act rapidly, the effects lasts for only a short time.

Other tissues, known as *chromaffin tissues*, located in various parts of the body, also secrete norepinephrine. They like the adrenal medulla, are actually modifications of sympathetic ganglionic cells.

Parasympathetic Nervous System. The term *craniosacral outflow* is frequently used to designate the complex of preganglionic fibers of the parasympathetic nervous system. The term is appropriate, since only certain cranial and sacral spinal nerves are involved.

Four cranial nerves are composed, at least in part, of preganglionic parasympathetic fibers. They are oculomotor (III), facial (VII), glossopharyngeal (IX), and vagus (X) nerves. The ganglia in which they terminate are situated close to, or in, the organs supplied by this system. Hence the preganglionic fibers are rather long, and the postganglionic fibers are very short. The preganglionic parasympathetic components of the oculomotor nerve terminate in a *ciliary ganglion,* about the size of the head of a pin, situated in the back part of the orbit. Here they synapse with postganglionic fibers which pass to eyeball, supplying the sphincter muscle of the iris as well as the ciliary muscles.

The facial nerve contains preganglionic fibers which pass either to the *sphenopalatine* or to the *submaxillary ganglion* in the head region. In the sphenopalatine ganglion located close to the sphenopalatine foramen, certain fibers of the facial nerve synapse with postganglionic neurons, the fibers of which pass to the facrimal gland, mucous membrane of the nose, palate, and upper part of the pharynx. Certain fibers of the chorda tympani branch of the facial nerve are preganglionic fibers which pass to the small submaxillary ganglion situated just above the submaxillary salivary gland. Short postganglionic fibers arising in the submaxillary ganglion are distributed to the submaxillary and sublingual glands.

An *otic ganglion,* located close to the foramen ovale of the sphenoid bone, receives preganglionic fibers of the glossopharyngeal nerve. Postganglionic fibers pass to the parotid gland and mucous membrane of the mouth.

The preganglionic fibers of the vaguserve, like those of the other three cranial nerves forming part of the parasympathetic system, terminate in ganglia, but the ganglia are very small and are located in the walls of the structures which they supply. It is believed that those of the esselagus, stomach, small intestine, and upper part of the large intestine connect with the *plexuses* of *Auerbach* and *Meissner*. From these plexuses postganglionic fibers are distributed to the smooth muscles and glands of the alimentary tract. Other parasympathetic fibers of the vagus innervate the heart, larynx, trachea, bronchi, lungs, blood vessels of abdomen, liver, gallbladder, and pancreas.

The part of the parasympathetic system known as the *sacral outflow* is composed of efferent fibers which course through the white visceral rami of the second, third and fourth sacral nerves, which together form the *pelvic nerve*. These preganglionic fibers, like those of the vagus, pass directly to the structures which they supply, to terminate in ganglia in, or very near, the organs. The pelvic nerve suppliers, the lower part of the large intestine, kidneys bladder, and reproductive organs. Postganglionic fibers within these organs are relatively short.

Function of the Parasympathetic System. Stimulation of the various components of the parasympathetic system brings about effects which are, in general opposite to those secured by stimulating the sympathetic nerves supplying the same organs. Among these reactions are (1) dilation of blood vessels (except the coronary vessels of the heart); (2) constriction of the pupil; (3) increase in salivary and gastric secretion; (4) constriction of bronchi; (5) contraction of walls of the digestive tract, bringing about peristalsis and other types of the contractions; (6) contraction of bladder musculature; (7) shortening of the uren thral musculature; and (8) dilation of blood vessels of the external genital organs.

The above reactions, when considered as a group, are those associated with comfortable or pleasurable sensations in the body and those which conserve energy. They form the mechanism of normal functions when the body is in a "receptive" state.

It has already been mentioned that the parasympathetic system brings about its effects by the liberation of a chemical substance, acetylcholine, at the terminal nerve endings of the postganglionic fibers. Acetylcholine may also be produced in other parts of the body besides the parasympathetic nerve endings. It is an unstable chemical substance, quickly rendered inactive in the body by an enzyme, acetylcholinesterase, the action of which is measured in thousandths of a second. Hence its effect is limited to the immediate region in which it is produced. It cannot affect parts of the body at any distance from the point of secretion or liberation. For example, when a savory odor induces the parasympathetic system to bring about muscular contractions of the stomach, it does not at the same time cause a desire to void, nor does it cause the pupils to constrict. The changes in the body associated with sexual stimulation, such as erection and glandular secretion, are the result of stimuli affecting the parasympathetic fibers of the sacral outflow which are distributed to the genital organs.

Hypothalamus. It has been amply demonstrated that the hypothalamus is a region of great importance in connection with the proper functioning of the autonomic nervous system. It is here that the nerve centers controlling the sympathetic and parasympathetic systems are located. Neurosecretory cells supplying the posterior lobe of the pituitary are also connected with this portion of the diencephalon. It is in the hypothalamus that the autonomic system forms connections with all the other nervous tissues of the body and is thus influenced by every external and internal change. The possible role of the hypothalamus as an endocrine organ has already been mentioned.

The stable nature of the internal environment of the body, referred to as homenostasis is controlled by hypothalamic nuclei. Such phenomena as constancy in amount of blood sugar, the part played by the sweat glands in regulating body temperature, composition of body fluids, and rate of heartbeat under different conditions are regulated and integrated in the hypothalamus.

Lesions of the hypothalamus are believed to be associated with such abnormal conditions as *diabetes insipidus* and *adiposogenital dystrophy*.

Autonomic System of Lower Chordates. The general scheme of arrangement of the autonomic system in tetrapods is similar to that of man. The lower vertebrates show a progressive complexity of autonomic system as the evolutionary scale is ascended.

If a peripheral autonomic system is actually present in amphioxus, it is apparently represented by the parasympathetic system alone. It will be recalled that in amphioxus dorsal and ventral spinal nerve roots remain separate. Visceral motor neurons course through the segmentally arranged dorsal spinal nerves directly to the visceral organs, where they form synapses with cells making up a nervous plexus. No intervening ganglia or relay-type connections are discernible. In cyctostomes segmental sympathetic ganglia are present, but these are not connected, nor are sympathetic trunks to be found. In lampreys, as in amphioxus, the dorsal and ventral spinal nerves do not unite. Preganglionic sympathetic fibers emerge from the spinal cord through the dorsal spinal nerves. In the hagfishes, in which the roots do unite, these fibers apparently pass through the ventral roots. A parasympathetic system appears for the first time in lampreys since visceral motor branches of the vagus nerve (X) terminate in the walls of the heart and gut. The hagfish heart apparently lacks vagal innervation. The autonomic system is much better developed in elasmobranches. Sympathetic and parasympathetic components are clearly demarcated. The sympathetic elements are confined to the abdominal region, there being no cranial sympathetic nerve fibers. It seems that no sympathetic nerve fibers innervate the heart of fishes. Nevertheless, it has been shown that catecholamines cause an increase in the rate and force of the heartbeat in elasmobranchs and teleosts but not in the hagfish. It seems that regulation of the rate of heartbeat in fishes lacks the precision of that found in tetrapods. The consecutive sympathetic ganglia are sometimes joined by lateral connectives, but, in general the sympathetic strands dorsal to the body cavity have a rather diffuse arrangement. All sympathetic ganglia connect with spinal nerves by white visceral rami, and each ganglion is closely associated with a small mass of chromaffin tissue. Parasympathetic fibers of the vagus pass to esophagus and stomach but do not seem to go to the intestine or urogenital organs. Parasympathetic fibers are also present in the oculomotor (III), facial (VII), and glossopharyngeal (IX) nerves. In teleosts, the autonomic system shows a still greater advance and considerable similarity to that of tetrapods. The sympathetic ganglia on each side are connected by a longitudinal trunk, forming a chain. This extends from the first spinal nerve to the region of the first hemal arch. The two trunks come together and fuse into a single strand between the kidneyes, but diverge again posteriorly, becoming paired at the level of the first hemal arch. Parasympathetic components seem to be confined to the oculomotor and vagus nerves. The Dipnoi also have a pair of longitudinal sympathetic trunks, but segmental swellings, or ganglia, are inconspicuous or absent, although they are joined by metameric white visceral rami. The oculomotor and vagus nerves apparently contain parasympathetic fibers. In urodele amphibians the condition is similar to that of teleosts except that the sympathetic system is divided into cephalic, cervical, abdominal, and caudal regions. White visceral rami form connections in all but the cephalic region. Only cranial parasympathetic fibers are present, and these seem to be confined to the oculomotor and vagus nerves. In anurans, for the first time, a sacral outflow appears, in addition to the usual cranial parasympathetic fibers. The autonomic system in caecitians has not been extensively studied. A typical sympathetic system is present, but little is known about the parasympathetic system.

6

Physiology of Nervous System

Nerve Cells

Nerve cells or neurones are specialised for receiving and transmitting electrical signals, often working over long distances. Classically the neurone can be considered to consist of a receiving zone, a conducting zone and an output zone. The dendrites of neurones act as receiving zones and are contacted by other nerve cells at junctions known as synapses. Signals which are sufficiently strong to excite the neurone pass down the conducting portion of the cell, the axon, and finally reach the output zone of the cell, the nerve terminals, which make synaptic contact with other cells. Each neurone has an enlarged portion, the cell body, in which the nucleus is located. Figure 6.1 shows the structure of a spinal motor neurons. This type of neurone is directly responsible for the activation of muscles and so the synapses formed by motor neurone terminals are upon muscle fibers. Recently, however, the division of neurones into receiving, conducting and output zones has become blurred, since it has become apparent that the dendrites of a number of different types of neurone are capable not only of receiving signals from other neurones, but can also transmit signals themselves to other cells. Therefore, some dendrites can be involved with transmitting as well as receiving information.

The structure of different types of neurone can vary considerably, so that the size of the dendritic tree relative to the length of the axon and the number of terminals can be large or small. Depending upon the type of neurone, the axon can be a number of metres long or as short as a fraction of a millimetre. The position of the cell body of a neurone can also vary.

Satellite Cells

Although in the majority of descriptions of the nervous system most attention is paid to neurones, they are, in fact, outnumbered approximately 10:1 by satellite cells: these, although smaller than neurones occupy about half the volume of the central nervous system (CNS). Satellite cells within the CNS are termed neuroglia or simply glia and, like neurones, are embryologically derived from neural ectoderm. Glia can be classified into the following types: oligodendrocytes, astrocytes and ependyma. Oligodendrocytes and astrocytes are found both in the grey and white matter of the

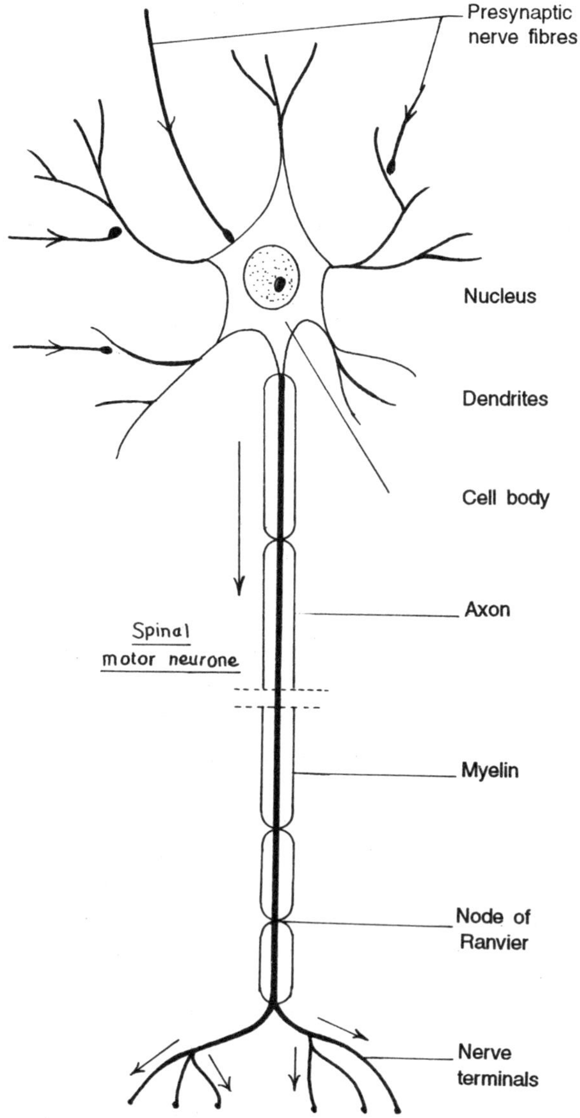

Fig. 6.1. Spinal motor neurone. The terminals of presynaptic neurones form synapses upon the cell body and dendrites of the motor neurone. Impulses are conducted along the axon, which is surrounded with myelin formed by Schwann cells. The motor neurone nerve terminals form synapses upon skeletal-muscle fibers.

CNS, although oligodendrocytes are found predominantly in the white matter. Ependyma are found on the inner surfaces of the CNS, lining the cerebral ventricles.

A major function of at least some oligodendrocytes is to form myelic around the larger nerve fibers of the CNS. This role is similar to that of Schwann cells in the peripheral nervous system, although the embryological origins of Schwann cells and

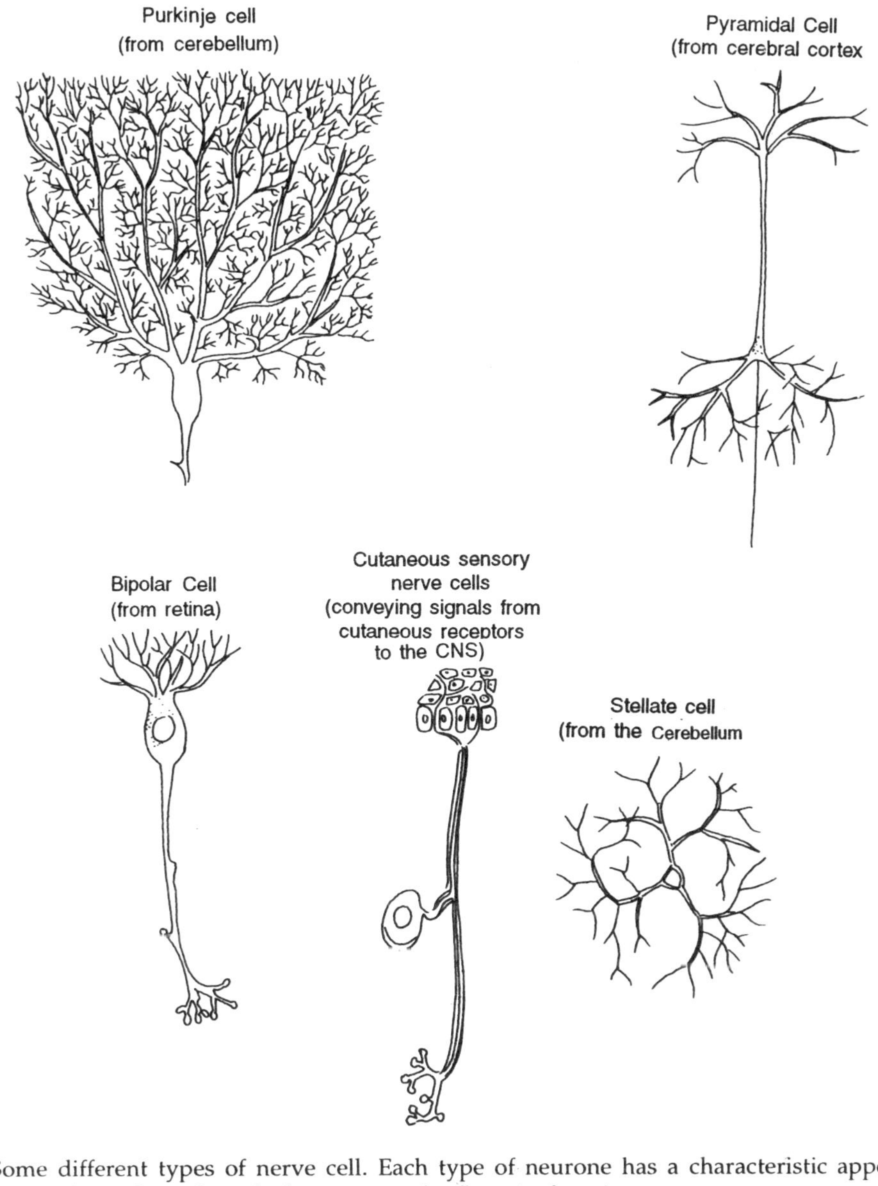

Fig. 6.2. Some different types of nerve cell. Each type of neurone has a characteristic appearance which distinguishes it from that of other types and reflects its function.

glia are different. Other functions of glia are not so clearly defined; it has been suggested that they may supply nutrients to neurones, provide them with mechanical support, and may also be involved in the control of the fluid-bathing neurones. In addition to true glia the CNS contains 'microglia'. These are not true glia since they invade the CNS during foetal life and are of mesodermal origin. These cells may be important following damage to the CNS, since they become phagocytic and may remove tissue debris.

Synapses

Synapses, the junctions between neurones, can be divided into two basic types, electrical and chemical, depending upon whether the effects of activity in one neurone (the presynaptic neurone) are passed on to the postsynaptic neurone directly by the flow of current or indirectly by the release from the presynaptic neurone of a chemical known as a transmitter substance which effects the activity of the postsynaptic neurone.

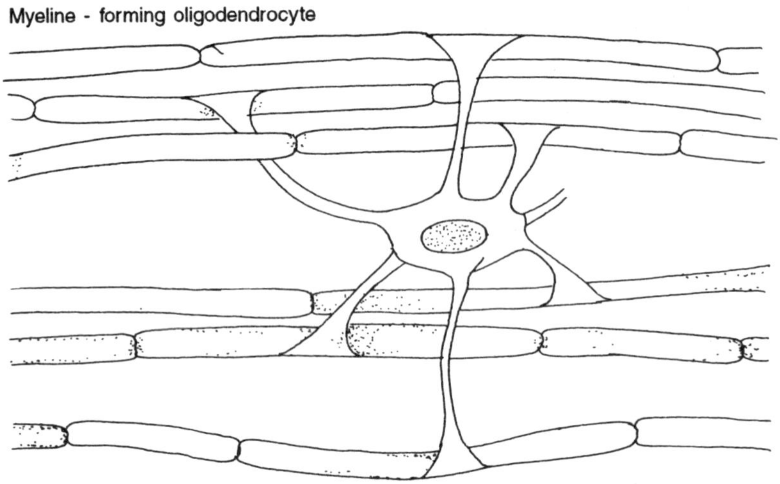

(a)

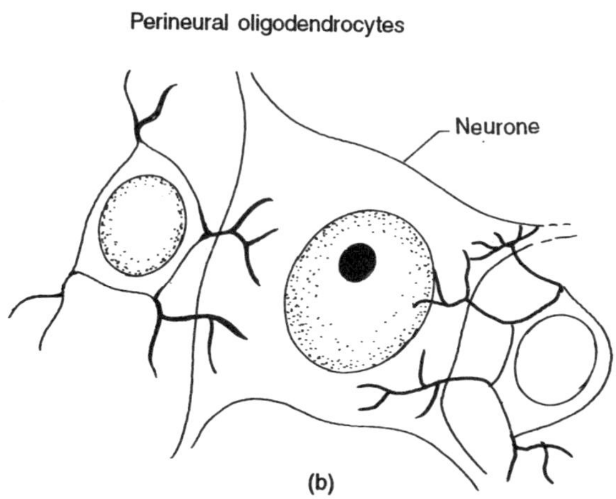

(b)

Fig. 6.3. Satellite cells. (a) Myelin-forming oligodendrocytes are found mainly in white matter of the CNS where they wrap around and ensheath axons; (b) perineuronal oligodendrocytes are closely associated with the cell bodies of neurones; (c) astocytes have many branches, some of which may terminate on neurone cell bodies and others which may contact blood capillaries; (d) ependyma line the ventricular system of the brain; (e) microglia appears to act a scavengers, especially after damage to the CNS.

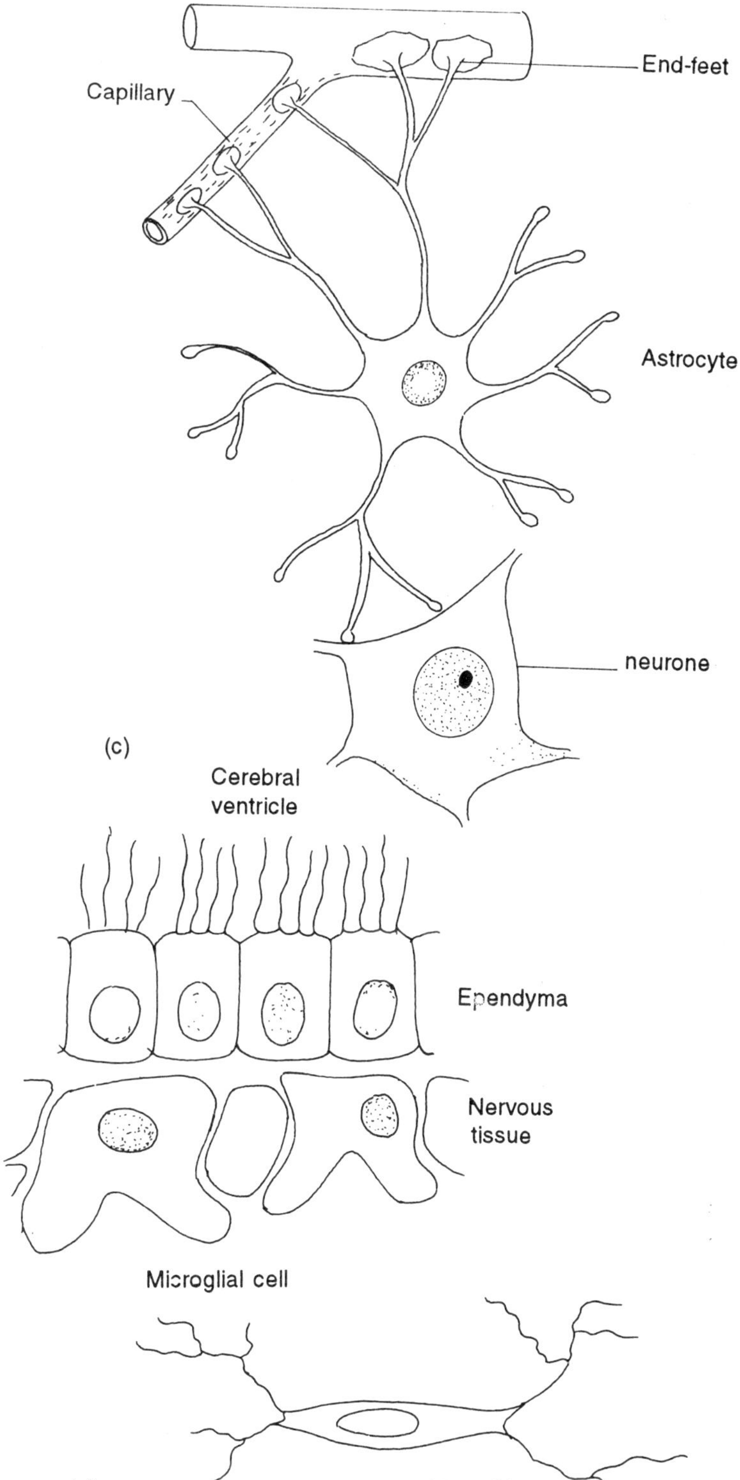
End-feet
Capillary
Astrocyte
neurone
(c)
Cerebral
ventricle
Ependyma
Nervous
tissue
(b)
Microglial cell
(e)

Fig. 6.3. (Contd.)

Electrical Synaptic Transmission

The nerve impulse travels along an axon by means of local current which depolarise the region of the axon in front of the impulse. At the terminals of such an axon, the local currents may flows and depolarise the postsynaptic neurone if two conditions are met. For there must be a low resistance to current flow between the prepostsynaptic neurones. Second, there must be only a relatively small of current through the external solution in the gap between the pre- and postsynaptic membranes. If these conditions are met transmission may be electrical, if not, potential changes in the presynaptic neurone can only be passed on to the postsynaptic cell indirectly through the action of a synaptic transmitter substance.

It is now known that transmission across a number of synapses is mediated electrically. Electrical transmission is correlated with the presence of gap junctions between neurones. At these junctions, the membranes of the electrically coupled cells come very close together and are separated by a gap of only 2 nm (instead of the 20-nm gap seen at chemically mediated synapses).

Until recently electrical transmission was considered relatively rare and unimportant in the vertebrate CNS. However, careful observation has led to an increase in the number of electrical synapses which have been demonstrated in vertebrates. Such transmission has been neglected largely because the existence of a synapse in a given CNS pathway has often been detected either by observing a delay in conduction (transmission across chemical synapses is associated with a delay of about 0.5 msec) or by modifying synaptic transmission with drugs. Electrical synapses have no synaptic delay and are resistant to most drugs and therefore can easily escape detection.

Physiology of Nerve

The nerves which we dissect and study are bundles of processes from nerve-cells. Each cell gives off a long process or axis-cylinder which is the essential conducting medium, but some nerves, the medullated nerves, have a surrounding myelin sheath which stains with osmic acid, and outside this another thinner sheath, the neurolemma. Non-medullated nerves have no medullary sheath. On section a nerve is somewhat reminiscent of a compound electric cable, the fibers of which are insulated from each other and which are bound together into bundles.

Nerve-fibers vary very much in size, a fact which is related to their function, as the larger fibers of the order of 15-19 μ, which are found in the spinal nerves supplying the voluntary muscles, conduct impulses most rapidly. Smaller fibers, which may be I.8 μ to 3.6 μ, exist in the autonomic part of the nervous system. They carry messages to the viscera or internal organs and for the most part are of the non-medullated variety.

Investigation of the Functions of a Nerve

There are two main methods by which the functions of a nerve may be ascertained: (1) section, and (2) stimulation.

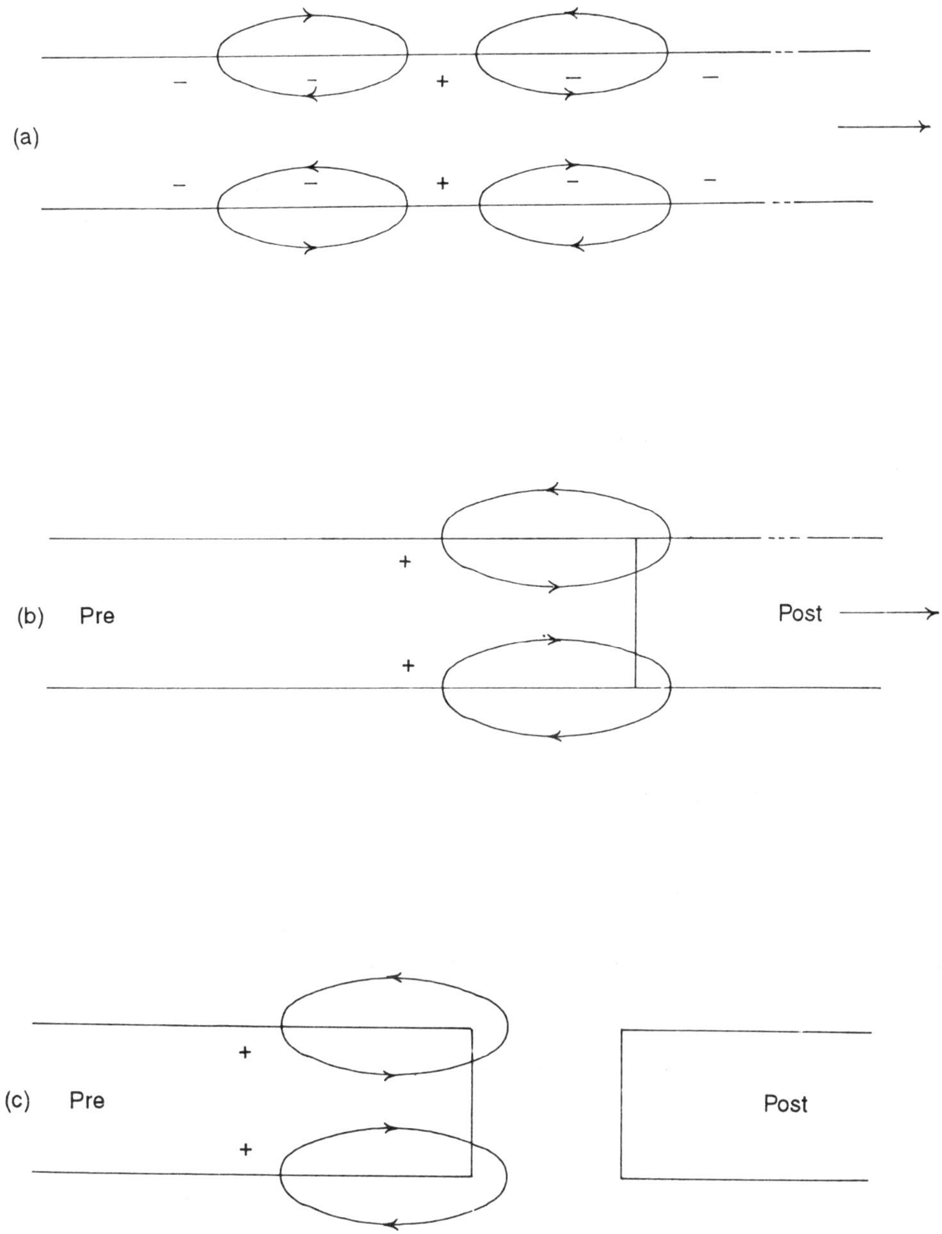

Fig. 6.4. Flow of electrical signals in nervous tissue. (a) The nerve impulse is transmitted along an axon by flow of current away from the act vezone; this depolarises and excites the adjacent regions of the axon. (b) If the electrical resistance between two cells is low and their membranes are close together, current can flow from one cell to another and produce excitation. (c) If the gap between two cells is large, current will flow into the intercellular space and there can be little or no direct flow of current from the presynaptic to the postsynaptic cell; under these circumstances excitation must be mediated through a chemical transmitter substance.

Section.— If a nerve is cut the loss of function that ensues may be observed. Thus, if a motor nerve is cut, motion of the muscles it supplies can no longer be produced by activity of the nerve-centre; the muscle is paralysed. If a sensory nerve is cut, the result is loss of sensation in the part from which it comes.

Stimulation.— In a cut motor nerve, stimulation of the central end (i.e., the end still connected with the central nervous system) produces no result; stimulation of the peripheral end produces a nervous impulse which excites the muscles to contract. In a cut sensory nerve, stimulation of the peripheral end has no result, but stimulation of the central end causes a sensation usually a painful one, and also reflex actions.

Degeneration of Nerve

When a nerve is cut, there are other results than the loss of function just mentioned; for, even though the nerve is still left within the body with a normal supply of blood, it becomes less and less irritable, till at last it ceases altogether to respond to stimuli.

The part left connected to the parent cell, usually in the central nervous system, remains almost normal; but the peripheral end undergoes what is called, after the discoverer of the process, *Wallerian degeneration*. In the medullated fibers the axis-cylinders fragment and the medullary sheaths break up into droplets of myelin. These changes appear between the first and third days after the section D, the small fibers in general showing the earliest changes; they may readily be detected by staining the myelin droplets black with osmium tetroxide (Fig. 6.6). Initially the changes occur autolytically, but later the droplets are digested and further broken up by the Schwann cells and, in the larger nerves, by invading macrophages. Most of the debris is removed within a month. At the same time, particularly between the fifth and ninth days of degeneration, there is a multiplication of Schwann cell nuclei. In the non-medullated fibers the fragmented axons are digested by the Schwann cells alone. The endoneurial tubes, which in the normal nerve surround each fiber, remain patent during degeneration, though they shrink in diameter. There is a steady increase in the amount of endoneurial collagen from about the beginning of the second week of degeneration onwards. Except for precocity in the immediate neighbourhood of the wound, the degeneration occurs simultaneously throughout the whole extent of the peripheral stump of the nerve.

Forty-eight hours after section, cholinergic nerves cease to be able to synthesise acetylcholine but they can still conduct.

Reaction of Degeneration.— When the nerve to a muscle becomes injured or impaired the excitability of the muscle is for a short period increased but later a reduced excitability occurs. This is because nerve has a much shorter chronaxie than muscle and can therefore be excited by currents of shorter duration and less strength. Normally, when a muscle is stimulated it is really being stimulated partly by its nerves, but when these degenerate through being separated from their parent cells by injury or disease, a much stronger or prolonged stimulus is needed to excite the muscle itself which has a much longer chronaxie.

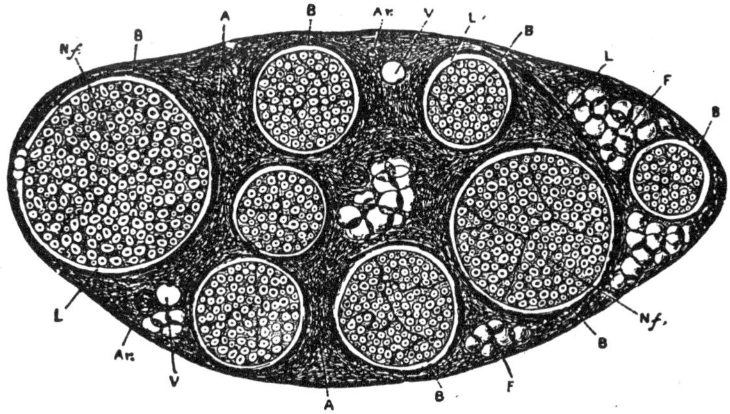

Fig. 6.5. Transverse section of the sciatic nerve of a cat, about X 100. It consists of bundles (funiculi) of nerve-fibers ensheathed in a fibrous sheath, epineurium, A; each bundle has a special sheath (not sufficiently marked out from the *epineurium* in the figure) or *perineurium* B; the nerve-fibers Nf are separated from one another by endoneurium; L, lymph spaces; Ar, artery; V, vein; F, fat. Somewhat diagrammatic.

When therefore the motor nerve is degenerated, the muscle also loses all its power of response to currents of very short duration such as those produced by an induction coil. As the nerve is in the actual process of degenerating, however, and for reasons not completely understood, the muscle is in a state of "irritable weakness," in which a weaker constant current stimulates the muscle more than in the normal state, but the contraction is propagated more slowly than when the nerve-fibers are intact. There is also a qualitative as well as quantitative change. In health the first contraction to occur on gradually increasing the strength of the current is at the negative pole, when the circuit is closed (Pflüger's law), and a stronger current is required before closure-contraction occurs at the positive pole. But in the morbid state we are discussing, closure-contraction may occur at the positive pole more readily than at the negative pole, i.e. A.C.C. is greater than K.C.C.

The reaction of degeneration is of considerable importance in medical and surgical diagnosis as it is a convenient objective method of demonstrating whether or not the nerve supply to a muscle is intact. The sluggish reaction to a constant current is specially characteristic of degeneration which does not appear for some time after voluntary movement is lost. These changes are developed after a week or ten days, but after a longer period of months the muscles lose their power of contracting altogether. Gradually the disused muscles themselves degenerate and waste away.

After nerve degeneration, muscles become abnormally sensitive to acetylcholine and to the depressant effect of potassium. These may be the results of permeability.

Regeneration of Nerve-Fibers

The histological appearance of a degenerated nerve indicates that there is a breakdown not only in an anatomical sense but in a chemical sense also. As degeneration proceeds, frozen sections made after formal fixation gradually lose the birefringence which is characteristic of normal myelin. The first changes can be detected six to twelve hours after the nerve has been cut, and provide a very delicate test of early degeneration. Staining reactions also change, though these are not consistently visible until at least two days after the nerve has been cut. The reactions most commonly employed are those originating from the technique of Marchi. Intact medullar sheaths blacken in osmium tetroxide (in virtue of the contained phosphatides) but not if the nerve is treated with an oxidising agent (potassium bichromate in Marchi's method), which is usually mixed with the osmium tetroxide. Degenerated medullary sheaths on the contrary blacken even in the presence of an oxidising agent. In the later stages of degeneration the Marchi reaction is not obtained, because the broken-down globules have by that time been absorbed.

After a nerve has been divided, function may be restored by axis-cylinders sprouting from the central stump of the cut nerve, entering and growing down the degenerate peripheral stump, and re-establishing connection with the receptors and effectors. There was formerly much controversy about the origin of the new axis-cylinders, many workers holding that they were formed *in situ* in the peripheral portion. Modern silver methods of staining the young axis-cylinders, however, show clearly that they come from the central stump, and this is supported by observation on living material, which is possible in tadpoles (Williams, Speidel).

All recent work has indeed confirmed the older work in this respect, notably that of Halliburton, who showed that the regeneration of nerve could be prevented by putting a gutta-percha cap on the central stump. He and Mott also showed that if after regeneration the nerve be cut again more peripherally degeneration occurs only on the peripheral side of the second cut.

The work especially of J.Z. Young and of Abercrombie indicates that the following changes occur.

The outgrowth from the central stump, which occurs mainly from the beginning of the second week after the lesion onwards, takes place by an outflow of the material of the axis-cylinders, so that the latter shrink in diameter (Gutmann and Sanders). Each axis-cylinder as it flows out splits up into a large number (up to 50) of fine fibrils. Meantime the neurolemma cells of the peripheral end have been very active.

Ramifying chains of Schwann cells grow out from the cut surface of the peripheral stump, and are responsible for bridging most of the gap between the two stumps; but they can only reach the sprouting axis-cylinder fibrils and Schwann cells of the central stump (which by themselves do not grow far) if the gap is not too large. Once the regenerating axis-cylinder fibrils meet these chains of Schwann cells they grow rapidly and with little deviation along their surfaces, and are hence directed into the peripheral stump. In the peripheral stump the regenerating fibrils extend rapidly (the fastest at the

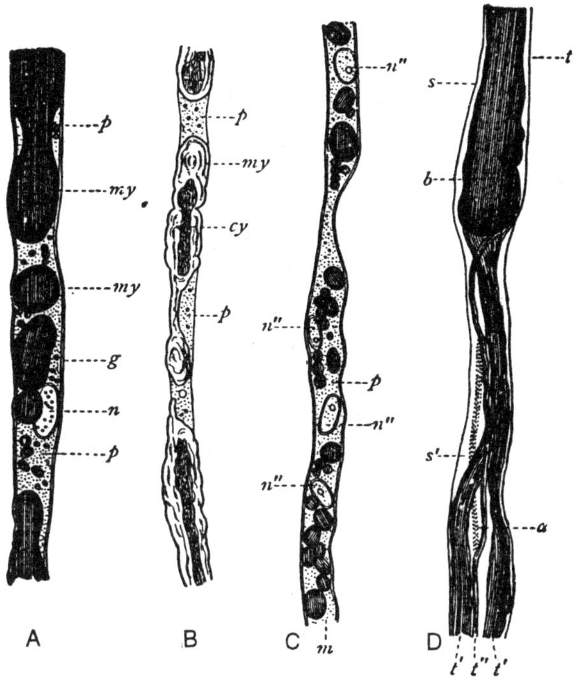

Fig. 6.6. Degeneration and regeneration of nerve-fibers. A, nerve-fiber, fifty hours after operation; *my*, medullary sheath breaking up into myelin drops; *p*, granular protoplasm; *n*, nucleus; *g*, primitive sheath or neurolemma. *B*, nerve-fiber after four days; *cy*, axis cylinder partly broken up and enclosed in portions of myelin. C, a more advanced stage in which the medullary sheath has almost disappeared; numerous nuclei, *n''*, are seen. D, commencing regeneration; several fibers (*t'*, *t''*) have sprouted from the somewhat bulbous cut end (*b*) of the nerve-fiber; a, an axis cylinder which has not yet acquired its medullary sheath; *s*, *s'*, primitive sheath of the original fiber.

rate of about 3½ mm. a day) down the persistent neurolemma tubes, which are more or less filled with proliferated Schwann cells. The regenerating fibrils are thus led to the places previously innervated by the nerve. Each neurolemma tube receives several of the regenerating fibrils; there may be 25 in the larger tubes.

Functional recovery depends on the re-establishment of correct peripheral connections for an adequate number of fibrils. The fibers must further return to approximately their correct diameters, on which depend their conduction velocities. In crossing the gap between central and peripheral stumps the regenerating fibrils inevitably become muddled up, and whether they both find tubes which permit them to expand to their right diameter and reach appropriate end-organs depends apparently on chance. The large number of fibrils into which an original axis-cylinder splits as it regenerates greatly increases the probability that each axis-cylinder will eventually establish at least one connection with an appropriate end-organ *via* an appropriate tube. The large number of new fibrils in each tube are later gradually reduced to few or one. Those which fail to make any peripheral connection apparently disappear; and some of those which make inappropriate connections may also be eliminated. But many inappropriate connections, as well as multiple connections of a single axis-cylinder (resulting from the branching during regeneration) persist. And since in these circumstances relearning seems to be impossible, perfect functional recovery after a nerve has been completely divided probably never occurs. If a nerve has only been crushed, in such a way that the neurolemma tubes remain intact, muddling of the axis-cylinders cannot occur in the injured region, and recovery of function may be complete.

The intrinsic fibers of the central nervous system which have no neurolemma seem to have only a small capacity for sprouting after injury; in the adult brain perhaps none at all. Further, the absence of Schwann cells and of neurolemma tubes means that even should sprouting occur (as for instance in the regeneration of a dorsal root) there are not pathways to encourage and direct the growing axis-cylinders.

Regeneration leads to a complete recovery of function on the average in from three to twelve months, depending on the length of the nerve and provided the muscles have been prevented from degenerating by electrical stimulation and massage. It grows at about the rate of 1 mm. per day. Sensation returns by stages, crude sensation returning earlier than finer detailed sensation, but the exact cause of this is still under discussion. Reviews on the subject have been made.

Nerve Crossing

It has been found possible to attach the centre end of one nerve to the peripheral end of another and to secure complete regeneration of the peripheral end and its function. This was well shown by the experiments of Kennedy and of Langley. The former cut in a dog's thigh the nerves supplying the flexor and the extensor muscles, and sutured them together crosswise. Regeneration of structure and restoration of function occurred as quickly as when the central ends were united to the peripheral ends of their own proper nerves. On examining the cortex of the brain in those animals in which nerve-crossing had been accomplished, it was found that stimulation of the region which in a normal animal gave flexion now gave extension of the limb, and vice versa.

A series of equally important experiments was carried out by Langley, in which he showed that the nerves that supply involuntary muscle behave in the same way. These nerve-fibers will, under certain experimental conditions, terminate by arborising round other nerve-cells than those with which they normally form connections (synapses). It will be sufficient to give one typical experiment. If the vagus nerve is cut across in the neck, its peripheral end degenerates downwards; if the cervical sympathetic is cut across

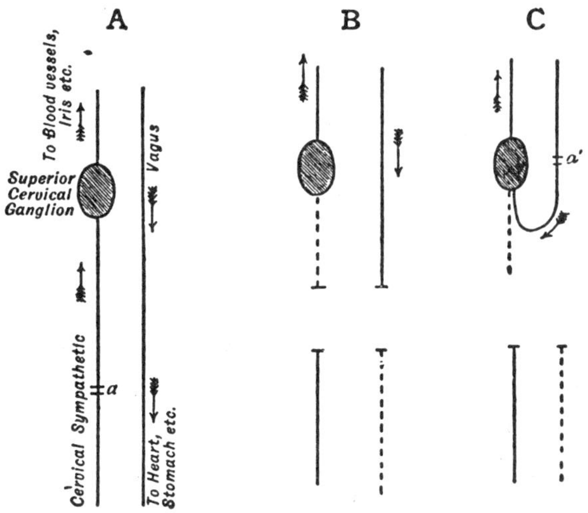

Fig. 6.7. Diagram to illustrate Langley's experiment on vagus and cervical sympathetic nerves. In A, the two nerves are shown intact; the direction of the impulses they normally carry is shown by arrows, and the names of some of the parts they supply are mentioned. In B, both nerves are cut through. The degenerated portions are represented by discontinuous lines. In C, the union described in the text has been accomplished, and stimulation at the point *a'* now produces the same results as were in the intact nerves (A) produced by stimulation at *a*.

below the superior cervical ganglion, its peripheral end degenerates upwards, as far as the ganglion. If subsequently the central end of the cut vagus is united to the peripheral end of the cut sympathetic, in the course of some weeks the vagus fibers grow into the sympathetic and form synapses round the cells of the superior cervical ganglion, and stimulation of the united nerve now produces such effects as are usually obtained when the cervical sympathetic is irritated; for instance, dilatation of the pupil, raising of the upper eyelid, and constriction of blood-vessels of the head and neck.

Such experiments as these are important because they show that though the function of various nerves may be so different (some being motor, some inhibitory, some secretory, some sensory, etc.) what occurs in the nerve trunk itself is always the same; the variation of action is due to difference either in the origin or distribution of the nerve-fibers. The familiar illustration in which nerve trunks are compared to telegraph wires is a helpful one. The destination of a certain group of telegraph wires may be altered, and the alteration may produce different consequences at various places; the electric change in the wires would, however, be the same throughout. So the nerve impulse is always the same sort of molecular disturbance; if it is made, as in the experiment just described, to go by a wrong channel, it produces just the same results as though the impulse had reached its destination by the usual channel.

Refractory Period of Nerve

Until 0.015 of a second after stimulation the excitability of the nerve is decreased; indeed, for 0.003 second it will not respond at all (absolute refractory period). The excitability returns to normal or slightly above, but later there is a period of subnormal responsitivity corresponding to the period of positive after-potential. This period is held by Gasser to explain the phenomenon of inhibition and to be fundamental to the normal activity of the nervous system.

These facts in relation to excitability tell us that only about 2000 impulses can pass along a large mammalian nerve per second and then only for a short time.

The Nature of the Nerve Impulse

Nerve like muscle, exhibits resting (injury) and action potentials. The former is most easily demonstrated in the giant nerves of the squid.

The action potential is propagated at the same rate as the impulse, it is present in every nerve that conducts and is depressed by all agents which depress conduction. Its size may be taken to represent strictly the size of the impulse; indeed, so closely related is the change of potential to the impulse that many believe it to be the nerve impulse itself, and certainly all recent evidence supports this view.

The action potential may be shown if one electrode is placed on the nerve and the other earthed and the nerve stimulated by applying to it a hot wire to avoid electrical complication. An initial abrupt and large negative wave, which may be as much as from 25 to 50 millivolts, is recorded. This is known as the spike. It not only falls off rapidly but is followed by waves of negative and positive after-potential. Its general form is not unlike that already figured for the action potential of muscle, but the spike is sharper and larger.

The electrical changes are now thought to be dependent on a sudden movement of ions, for if the nerve is placed in a solution deficient in sodium, the action potential disappears, while it is increased if the outside sodium is increased. In the active nerve potassium in similar circumstances moves outwards more slowly.

It seems probable that a difference between the concentration of ions, especially those of sodium and potassium, on each side of the surface membranes is maintained by an expenditure of energy, for the potential disappears if the nerve is deprived of oxygen. The process is indeed reminiscent of the back E.M.F. which is produced by the accumulation of ions of the electrodes when a current is passed through salt solution. The action potential is of very special importance.

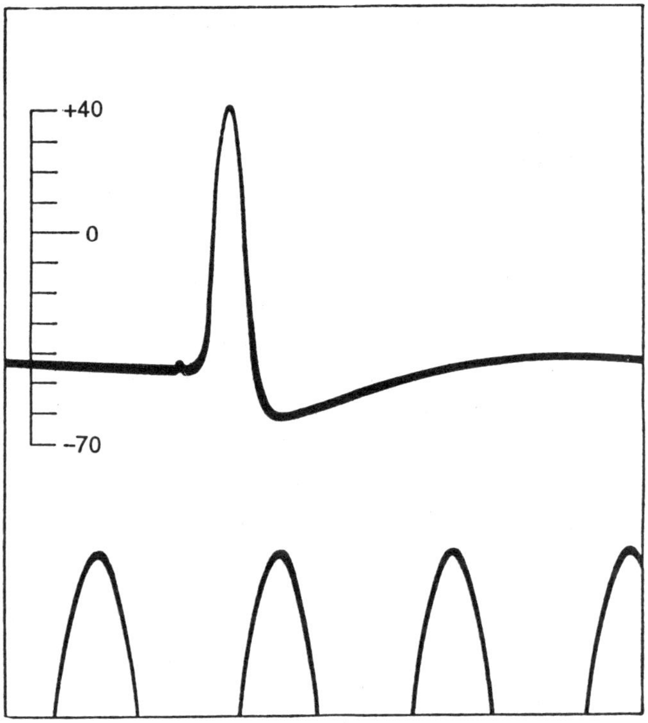

Fig. 6.8. Action potential recorded between inside and outside of axon. The marker below 500 cyc./sec. The vertical scale indicates the potential of the internal electrode in millivolts, the sea water outside being taken as at zero potential.

Lillie has made an interesting model which in many ways imitates the conduction of a nerve impulse. If a piece of iron wire is placed in a solution of nitric acid with a specific gravity over 1.2, a thin film of oxide is formed on its surface which protects it. If now the wire is "stimulated" at one end by the usual means, it becomes black at that place and effervesces for a short period. The activation propagates itself to the other end at about the same rate as a nerve impulse and the wire cannot be activated again for a given space of time, i.e., it has a refractory period and gives all the phenomena which are found in nerve, except of course its vital reaction, e.g., to drugs. The wire exhibits the all-or-none law, has a strength-duration curve, and is blocked by a constant current like a nerve.

Lillie's experiment goes far to support the view that the nerve-impulse is a changed of potential due to depolarisation which passes down the surface of the axis-cylinder and which gives rise to the spike just described. We can also imagine how it is produced. If, for example, the surface of the nerve-fiber at rest consisted of a monomolecular film of fatty acid and was positively charged while its interior was maintained negative by the oxidation processes going on—a state commonly found in living things—it would be conceivable that any physical disturbance of the surface, such as that brought about by stimulation, would bring about a depolarisation or equalisation of potential between the surface and the interior which would spread to the adjacent polarised region. An alternative view is that the action potential, once set up, acts as a stimulus to adjacent parts after the manner of a train of gunpowder or a chain of condensers. There is indeed no end to the ingenious ideas of this kind which have been put forward by the electrically minded.

It is important to emphasise that whatever the nature of the nerve impulse, the impulse is self-propagating, somewhat like the combustion in a train of gunpowder when ignited, although admittedly this convenient analogy is a very crude and erroneous one. Adrian has shown that if the conductivity of a nerve be locally damped down by placing a segment in a chamber of alcohol vapour, the impulse, as soon as it reaches an undamped region, flares up to its original strength as judged by its effect on the attached muscle or the extent of the electrical change set up.

At the same time it must be understood that a nerve is not merely a conductor of impulses as a wire is of an electric current. A nerve impulsse travels relatively slowly and it depends on the vital activity of the nerve, for it is abolished by cold, by CO_2, and by anesthetics. It may also be blocked by pressure and by the passage of a constant current which presumably acts by setting up a movement of ions. How all these facts are related to each other is not yet known, but it can be imagined that many procedures

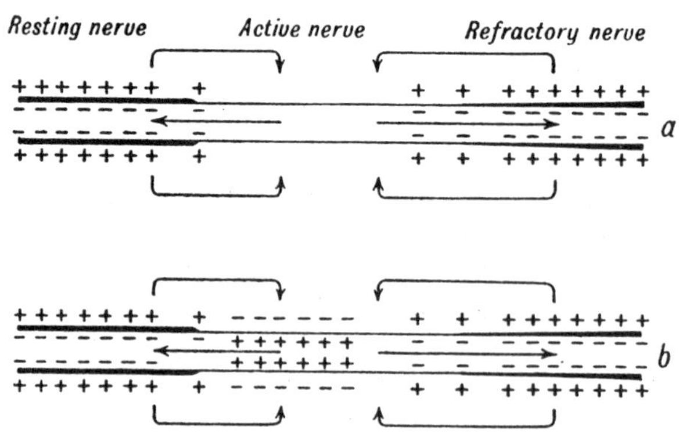

Fig. 6.9. Diagram illustrating (a) classical and (b) revised concepts of nervous activity.

interfere with the recovery of the resting potential, a process involving the expenditure of energy.

Chemical Changes.— It can be shown that nerve requires oxygen and emits minute quantities of carbon dioxide and ammonia; indeed, its requirements are almost identical with those of muscle. It uses glucose and its metabolism is doubled by activity. Its need for glucose is closely related to its need for potassium.

Thermal Changes.— By placing bundles of nerves on a thermopile it has been found that heat is produced when a nerve conducts and during recovery (A.V. Hill).

Chemistry of Nervous Tissues

Nervous tissues contain 65 per cent. to 85 per cent. of water. The first careful study of this subject we owe to Halliburton, who showed that grey matter contained a smaller proportion of solid (I6.5 per cent.) than white matter (30 per cent.). He showed that in the cerebral grey matter the percentage of protein in the solids was highest (51 per cent.) and consisted mainly of nucleo-protein.

Fat-like substances are also more abundant in non-medullated nerve than in medullated. In the former, as percentages of total solids, there occur cholesterol 47 per cent., lecithin 9.8 per cent., kephalin 23.7 per cent., and galactosides 6 per cent. Various salts and extractives are also present.

When a nerve degenerates the solids become less, in particular the phosphorus content decreases greatly in three weeks.

At the moment the chemistry of nerve tissue is a very academic subject, but there is no doubt of its great practical importance because we know that various parts of the nervous system respond very differently to drugs, a fact which must depend on chemical differences which are as yet unknown.

Direction and Velocity of the Nerve Impulse

Nerve impulse are normally conducted in only one direction: in efferent nerves from, in afferent nerves to, the nerve-centres, but if the nerve is stimulated in the middle instead of at one end, the electrical change (the evidence of an impulse) is found to be conducted towards both ends of the nerve.

A nerve impulse can, however, only pass in one direction across a synapse, that is only from axon to dendron or cell body. This is discussed later in relation to the structure and function of the synapse. It will also pass from one fiber to another if the latter is made abnormally excitable by reducing its calcium (Arvanitaki), but this does not normally occur in an intact nerve except after the nerve has undergone its final division (Kuhne).

In the frog, for instance, at ordinary room-temperature the velocity in motor nerves averages 27 metres per second. In warm-blooded animals it is 90-120 metres per second.

By taking a long piece of nerve, it is found that the impulses set up arrive at a given point at different times, and by studying fibers in detail it has been shown that large fibers conduct more rapidly than small. Three groups have been differentiated.

Group A fibers have velocities of 30-90 metres per second. They carry impulses to and from the muscles, impulses from the skin, sensations of touch and temperature, and impulsess of the para-sympathetic.

Group B have slower rates, 10-20 metres per second. They are sympathetic and convey impulses to the blood-vessels and glands.

Group C have still slower rates, 0.3-1.6 metres per second. These are concerned probably with crude sensations. Pain impulses are apparently carried by all fibers.

Some idea of the sensations which are carried by the different fibers is given by a study of the effects of pressure and cocaine. Cocaine blocks the smallest fibers first, and with this anesthetic sensations in man disappear in the order, cold, warmth, pain, pressure, while with pressure, due to a sphygmomanometer cuff, the order is pressure and cold, then warmth and pain. This may then be compared with the effects of these procedures on various nerves of anesthetised animals.

Afferent impulses, as measured by Gasser, travel at about a third of the rate of efferent impulses in the same reflex are.

Effects of Electric Currents on Excitability and Conductivity

If a constant current at about 2 volts is passed through a nerve and the excitability of the nerve tested by placing a pair of stimulating electrodes close to the positive (the anode) and to the negative (the kathode) wires, it is found that in the region of the anode the nerve is unexcitable, while in that of the kathode it is hyperexcitable. These conditions are known as *anelectrotonus* and *katelectrotonus* respectively. If then a constant current is passed through a nerve the nerve ceases to conduct (Bernstein) because of the area of anelectrotonus at the anode. Use is commonly made of this fact in physiological experiments as such a nerve-block is equivalent to nerve section with the advantage that it is only temporary.

This effect on a nerve must not be confused with the momentary stimulation of a nerve which may occur the moment the circuit is made or broken. At the make the stimulating electrode is the kathode, but at the break the stimulating electrode is the anode, facts of some importance in relation to reaction of degeneration in which the excitability is altered.

The Neuromuscular Junction and End-Plate Potential

It has now become apparent that the region of the neuromuscular junction is of great importance not only in relation to muscle but because many of its activities are very similar to those at the synapses between different nerve neurones.

A nerve fiber ends by losing its myelin sheath and breaking up into a number of branches in a spray-like manner in grooves on the surface of the muscle fibers which may be 50-100 in number. Details differ much in various animals. According to Couteaux, the fibers do not lose their neurolemmal sheath, as was thought. In the fiber immediately below the grooves is an area free from stripes which contains many nuclei and which is stainable with Janus green. In this area also he describes pallisades. The whole is the

End-Plate seen in ordinary sections. It does not wholly degenerate when the nerve is cut, and when the nerve is stimulated there is set up in it a negative end-plate potential which only differs from the action potential in being strictly localised to the end-plate region and non-conducted. In some muscles the nerve-endings occupy a very limited region. E.P.P. has probably the same fundamental basis as A.P., for one merges into the other; indeed, E.P.P. only becomes apparent when A.P. is abolished by small doses of potassium and by amounts of curare which abolish muscle contraction. Larger doses of curare and potassium abolish both. The end-plate acts as a detonator and is the starting-point of A.P. in the fiber and bears a striking resemblance to the auricular ventricular node of the heart.

Humoral Transmission

Evidence is now very complete that nerves do not act on tissues directly but through the agency of a chemical mediator, acetylcholine.

The first suggestion of the occurrence of such humoral transmission came from Loewi, who found that, when the frog heart is slowed by stimulation of the vagus nerve, a chemical substance is produced which will slow another heart perfused at pH 6.5. This is found to be due to the liberation of acetylcholine, a substance long known to slow the heart and to dilate blood-vessels. The action of the acetylcholine is prevented by the drug atropine, but it can be shown that it is still produced, for if the atropine is painted on the first heart only the second heart still slows when the nerve to the first is stimulated although the first does not. The drug eserine (physostigmine), on the other hand, prevents the destruction of the acetylcholine and prolongs its action.

Subsequently it was shown, especially by Dale and his co-workers Brown and Feldberg, that acetylcholine was released by the parasympathetic nerves is other parts of the body, and eventually Dale, Feldberg, and Vogt found that it was liberated by the stimulation of nerves in skeletal muscle.

Dale with his colleagues also showed that the injection of acetylcholine into the blood-vessel supplying a muscle causes it to twitch (actually a brief asynchronous tetanus) just like the stimulation of its nerves. In order to produce this result, however, the circulation must be arrested temporarily and the injection made at close range into the artery supplying it.

The treatment of the disease myasthenia gravis with eserine and prostigmine soon followed. Patients suffering from this fatal disease may be too weak to feed themselves, but the injection of prostigmine renders them almost normal for a few hours. Prostigmine and eserine also greatly potentiate the contractions produced by nerve stimulation of isolated muscles.

All these results appear to indicate that the acetylcholine is the essential transmitter, but if this is so it must be very rapidly destroyed after the contraction, indeed, within the refractory period of the muscle. An enzyme capable of carrying out such destruction has been discovered by Stedman and Stedman, and it can be shown to be inactivated by eserine and prostigmine.

It would seem that the acetylcholine does not act directly on the muscle-fiber but on its end-plate. This view is based largely on the fact that acetylcholine depolarises and thereby causes an electrical discharge of 40-80 volts from the electric organs of the fish torpedo, which are enlarged end-plates originally derived from muscle but lacking the contractile element. The surfaces of the interface between a saline solution and a lipoid layer which gives a positive electromotive force may similarly be depolarised when very small amounts of acetylcholine are added to the saline solution.

According to present views, then, there is first an all-or-none process in nerve, followed by two variable processes, the liberation of acetylcholine and the production of end-plate potential which if large enough sets up a propagated action potential which determines the actual fibers excited. Finally there is an all-or-none contraction of the muscle-fiber.

There is, however, much debate regarding the exact role of the acetylcholine, it may be that it facilitates the electrical change or that the amount at the end-plate determines the actual fiber excited. Thus individual fibers may be rested if activity of the unit is continued.

It now seems likely that many of the phenomena which we have noted in relation to muscle are explicable as due to the accumulation of acetylcholine at the nerve-endings, especially the effects of summation, the genesis of tetanus and, as we shall see, neuromuscular fatigue.

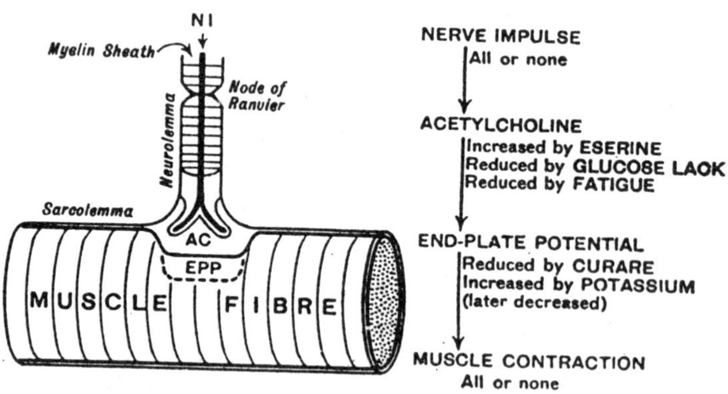

Fig. 6.10. Diagram illustrating the chief features of humoral transmission. According to some histologists, the axis cylinder retains its sheath to its termination.

The *cholinergic nerves*, which liberate acetylcholine and possess cholinesterase which destroys it rapidly, have the power also of synthesising acetylcholine along the whole course of their fibers, but conduction of the impulse does not depend on this, for it still occurs forty-eight hours after the nerve is cut and the synthesis has ceased.

Some sympathetic nerves have also been shown to liberate a chemical substance *sympathin*, which has an action almost identical with that of nor-adrenaline and the opposite action to acetylcholine.

Finkleman demonstrated that when a piece intestine contracting rhythmically in a trickle of oxygenated saline is inhibited by stimulating its attached splanchnic nerve, there passes into the saline a chemical substance like adrenaline, which inhibits the movements of another piece of intestine. Later, Cannon brought forward evidence to show that, when blood-vessels are caused to constrict by nerves, a similar substance is produced which acts like adrenaline on the heart. Such nerves have therefore been called *adrenergic*.

Chemical Synaptic Transmission. In this type of transmission between nerve cells a substance, termed a chemical transmitter substance, is released by a nerve impulse from the terminals of a presynaptic neurone. The transmitter substance diffuse across the synaptic gap and, by interacting with specific molecules (receptors) in the postsynaptic membrane, brings about a change in its permeability to certain ions. Depending upon the ions whose permeability is increased, the postsynaptic membrane potential can be either depolarised (made less negative) or hyperpolarised (made more negative). The direction of the shift in membrane potential will determine whether the synapse has an excitatory or inhibitory action on the excitability of the postsynaptic neurone. So far, because of technical difficulties, only a few transmitter substances have been identified with certainty. These include acetylcholine (ACh), adrenaline (epinephrine), noradrenaline (norepinephrine) and gamma aminobutyric acid (GABA), although there are other likely candidates, such as dopamine, 5-hydroxytryptamine (5-HT, serotonin) and glutamic acid.

Figure shows the structure of the chemical synapse as it appears under the electron microscope. The features of different chemical synapses are relatively constant. The presynaptic terminals contain mitochondria, microfilaments, smooth endoplasmic reticulum and aggregates of vesicles close to the synaptic cleft. The vesicles vary between about 50 and 500 nm diameter at different junctions and may have dense cores. (Dense cored vesicles are found in terminals known to release catecholamines such as noradrenaline). the pre- and postsynaptic cells are separated by a gap or synaptic cleft of approximately 20 nm.

The transmitter substance is stored in the presynaptic terminal within the synaptic vesicles. When a nerve impulse arrives at the presynaptic terminal it causes an influx of calcium ions, which triggers the release of transmitter substance into the synaptic cleft. For this to occur some of the vesicles in the terminal fuse with the surface membrane of the terminal and release their contents, the vesicles are then thought to be pinched off from the surface membrane for refilling with transmitter substance in a recycling process.

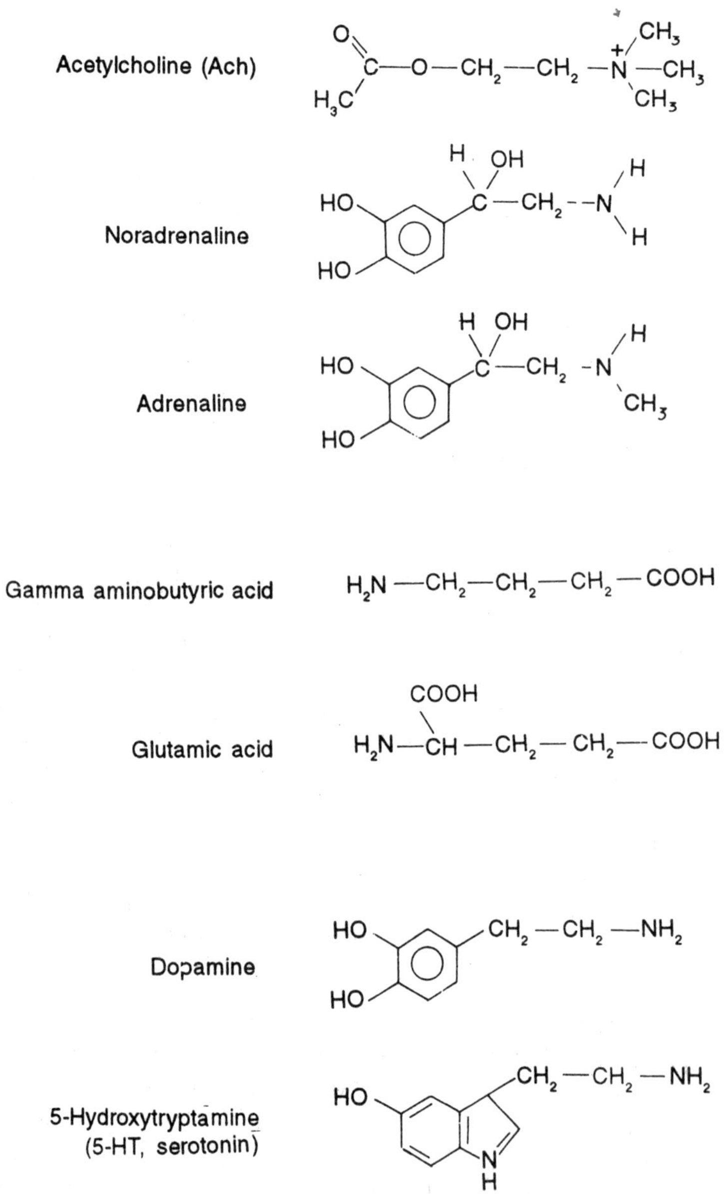

Fig. 6.11. Chemical transmitter substances. Acetylcholine, adrenaline, noradrenaline and gamma aminobutyric acid are known to be transmitter substances; glutamic acid, dopamine and 5-hydroxytryptamine are likely candidates.

Although nerve terminals are capable of synthesising some materials, such as the transmitter substance ACh, they are ultimately dependent on the transport of materials, such as enzymes from the cell body of the neurone, since nerve terminals themselves contain no ribosomes and so are incapable of protein synthesis.

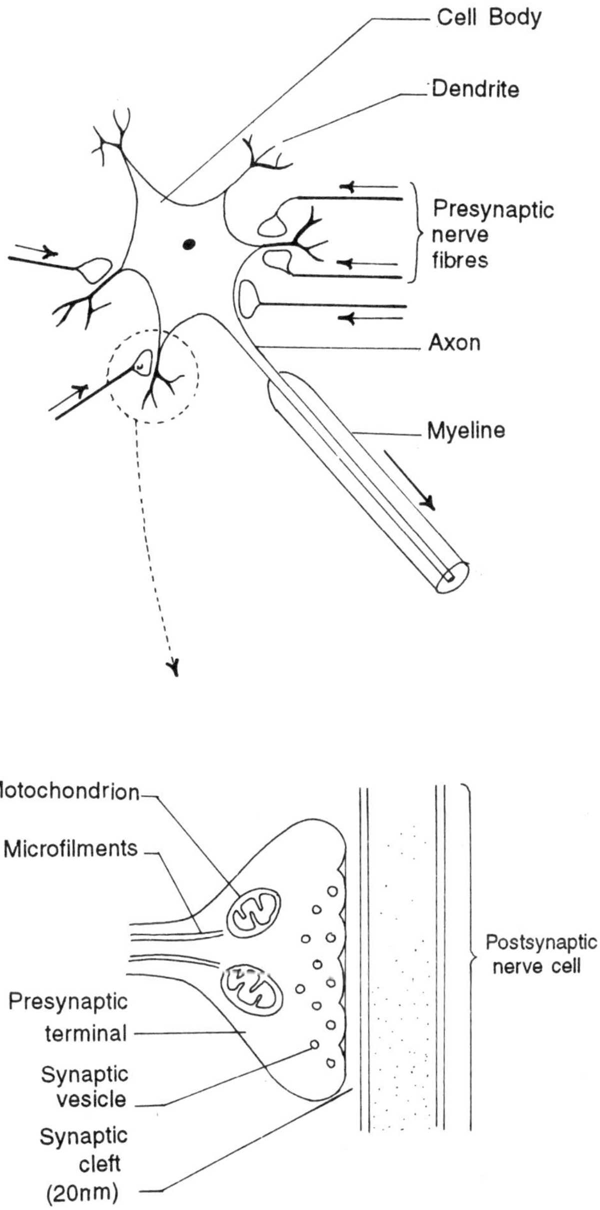

Fig. 6.12. Chemical synapse. (a) Presynaptic nerve fibers form terminal buttons on the cell body and dendrites of a neurone. (b) The presynaptic and postsynaptic membranes are separated by a 20-nm gap. Terminal buttons normally contain mitochondria, microfilaments and synaptic vesicles. The synaptic membranes are frequently thickened and modified.

On the outer surface of the postsynaptic membrane are situated receptor molecules, which can interact specifically with a given transmitter substance. This interaction in turn triggers specific changes in the permeability of the postsynaptic membrane. At

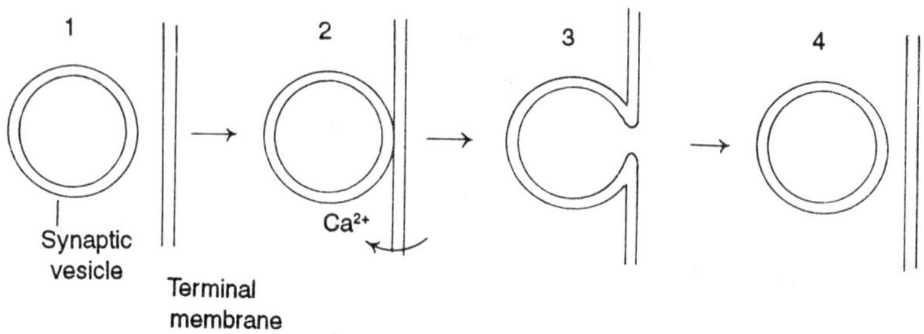

Fig. 6.13. Release of chemical transmitter substance. (1) Some synaptic vesicles come to lie close to the synaptic membrane. (2) Some calcium ions enter the presynaptic nerve terminal during an impulse; this triggers fusion of vesicles with the synaptic membrane. (3) The vesicle opens to the exterior and releases transmitter substance into synpatic cleft. (4) The vesicle then separates from the synaptic membrane and is ready to be refilled with transmitter substance.

excitatory synapses this consists of a simultaneous increase in permeability of the postsynaptic membrane to sodium and potassium. The equilibrium potential for sodium is about + 50 mV, while that for potassium it is about — 100 mV; the increase in the permeability of the membrane to sodium and potassium induced by the transmitter substance drives the membrane potential towards a level intermediate between the equilibrium potentials for each ion (approximately — 10 mV). The neuronal membrane has, however, a relatively high resting potassium permeability which partially 'short-circuits' the effects of the transmitter substance. This tends to 'clamp' the membrane potential and to limit the amplitude of the response to only a few millivolts depolarisation. This depolarising response to an excitatory transmitter substance is known as an excitatory post-synaptic potential (e.p.s.p). The amplitude of e.p.s.p.s. produced by successive presynaptic action potentials may fluctuate. Such amplitude variations are not continuously graded, but vary in steps. For this reason the amplitude of e.p.s.p.s. is said to alter in a 'quantal' fashion. This occurs because the transmitter substance is released in 'packets' rather than as individual molecules. Each 'packet' of transmitter substance is thought to correspond to the release of the contents of a single synaptic vesicle. The number of vesicles released by each presynaptic impulse fluctuates and gives rise to the quantal jumps in the amplitude of e.p.s.p.s. At synapses in the mammalians CNS there is an interval of about 0.5 msec between the arrival of the impulse at the presynaptic terminal and the onset of the postsynaptic response. This is known as the synaptic delay and results mainly from the time taken for the presynaptic impulse to trigger release of the transmitter substance.

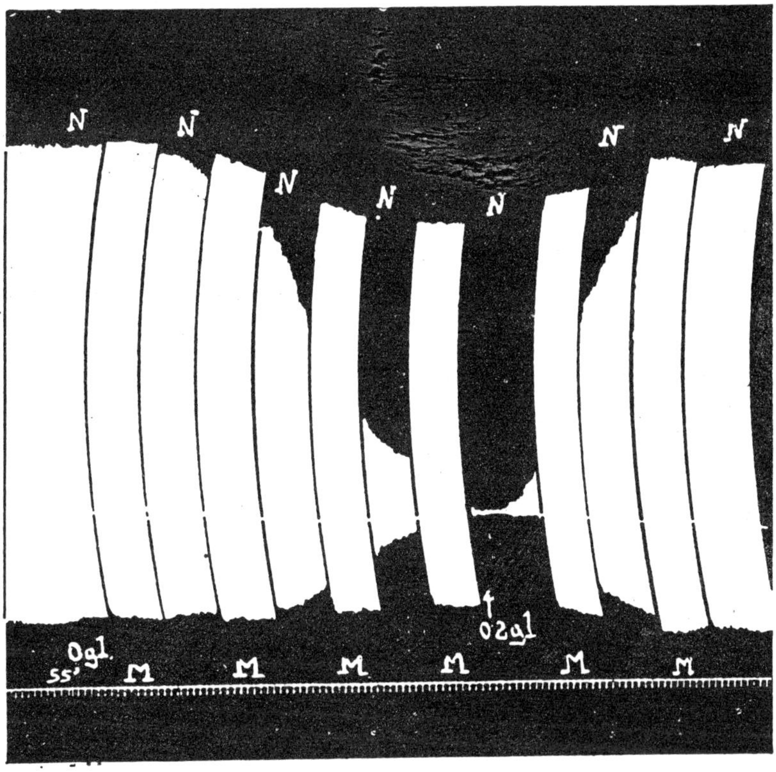

Fig. 6.14. Neuromuscular block in phrenic diaphragm preparation such as produced by lack of glucose which prevents acetylcholine synthesis or by the addition of curare. Muscle (M) and nerve (N) were stimulated in groups alternately, the muscle with a long-duration stimulus (2000 microseconds) and the nerve with a short 200 microseconds duration stimulus. Lack of calcium produces a similar block.

From the above description, it may be seen that the e.p.s.p. differs from the nerve impulse first in that the increase in membrane permeability to sodium and potassium is simultaneous and not sequential. In addition, the e.p.s.p. is local and not regenerative and is not followed by a refractory period. Thus, postsynaptic potentials themselves are not propagated along the axon of a neurone. Normally a single e.p.s.p. produces insufficient depolarisation to exceed the threshold for action potential generation. For this reason it is necessary for several e.p.s.p.s. to add together (summate) in order to evoke an action potential. If the e.p.s.p. showed a refractory period summation of successive e.p.s.p.s. would be impaired.

The Phrenic Diaphragm Preparation, etc.

This preparation has assumed a unique importance in the study of neuromuscular transmission. The rat, kitten, mouse, or guinea-pig is killed and the front of the thorax skinned. A piece of costal margin is cut away and with it a piece of diaphragm with its phrenic nerve attached. The rib margin is tied to a suitable fixture of perspex or glass in which electrodes are attached so that the muscle can be stimulated through its nerve or directly. The preparation must be kept at about 37°C. in nutrient solution such as that of Tyrode, and aerated with 95 per cent oxygen and 5 per cent CO_2. The apparatus used for intestine may be adapted. The preparation is of special value because it is so thin and therefore can be adequately oxygenated and acted upon rapidly by a wide variety of substances.

Such a preparation if stimulated rhythmically at about 6 per minute shows the action of eserine and adrenaline in enhancing the response to nerve stimulation, and of curare preventing neuromuscular transmission. It can also be shown that neuromuscular transmission depends on an adequate supply of glucose and of calcium.

The Action of Curare, the South American arrow poison, was until recently a physiological curiosity, but now the substance has been used to facilitate muscular relaxation during anesthesia. It prevents the action of acetylcholine and reduces end-plate potential so that after its use it is impossible to cause contraction of affected muscles by stimulation of their nerves, although they will contract if stimulated directly. In large doses it causes death by paralysing the respiratory nerves, but its action is rapidly antagonised by eserine. A number of other drugs have a curare-like action, notably choline and large doses of acetylcholine.

It has now been found possible to utilise a large number of muscles without dissecting out the nerve, and taking advantage of the fact that if the muscle is stimulated by currents of short duration, e.g., 200 micro-seconds, the stimulation is really through the nerve elements and its effects are abolished by curare. Stimulation of muscle may then be effected by using currents of 2000 microseconds.

Fatigue

We are all familiar with the fact that when a muscle is used too much it becomes fatigued and we cease to be able to make it contract any longer. This problem is of such obvious importance that it has been made the subject of much study and it has become apparent that the fatigue may be localised in several regions according to the tissue we study. It may be in the central nervous system, at the nerve-endings, or in the muscle itself, and experiments indicate that nature has provided several mechanisms by which the muscle is protected against exhaustion.

If a nerve-muscle preparation be stimulated frequently through its nerve, at first the contractions improve, each being a little higher than the preceding; this is due to the *beneficial effect of contraction*. Then the contractions get less and less. But what is most noticeable is that the curves are much more prolonged: the latent period is longer, the period of contraction longer, and the period of relaxation very much longer. This condition is known as *contracture*, and the original base-line may not be reached by the time the next stimulus arrives. In the last stages of fatigue, contracture passes off. Contracture is often absent in fatigue of mammalian muscle.

When a nerve-muscle preparation has been fatigued by stimulation through the nerve, it is found that the muscle will still contract if stimulated directly, and this raises the question whether the nerve or the nerve-ending is the seat of the fatigue. That the nerve is not fatigued may be shown by the following experiment. A temporary block is applied to the nerve between the point of stimulation and the muscle. For blocking, a piece of ice or a galvanic current may be used. The nerve is not stimulated for a period much longer than that which would be necessary to cause fatigue if contraction were occurring. During such a period the nerve, if fatigable, must have become fatigued, but it is found that immediately the block is removed the nerve conducts quite normally.

From the above experiments it has been concluded that, since neither the nerve nor the muscle have been fatigued, the seat of this fatigue must be in the region of the nerve-endings.

The evidence is now very complete that this fatigue is in fact due to an exhaustion of the humoral transmitter or its precursor, but depressor substances such as choline and potassium may also be liberated. By studying the end-plate potential when the nerve is stimulated by two successive stimuli, it has been found that in fatigue this potential at first becomes increased for a fraction of a second and later there is a depression lasting several seconds. The facilitation would account for the initial increase which precedes fatigue. It appears to occur at the nerve terminals themselves since it can be shown to occur during the action of curare, but the depression is apparently due to lack of stimulation of the end-plate by acetylcholine.

From these results it becomes obvious why curarised muscle, or one deprived of glucose to reduce acetylcholine synthesis, is more easily fatigued than a normal muscle. Normally, however, acetylcholine is liberated greatly in excess of that necessary for the stimulation of the end-plate.

It must be understood that there is also a purely muscle fatigue which can be produced in a curarised or denervated muscle, but this is very exhausting and is normally prevented by the block at the neuromuscular junction.

The *relative absence of fatigue* in a nerve, as in the heart, is probably due to the fact that it is not acting continuously but intermittently, and during the resting period, although this is extremely short, it is able to recover. It is interesting to note that, as would be expected from the large heat production, crab nerve is fatigued comparatively quickly (Hill).

This is not to say that other nerves are absolutely unfatigable. After prolonged stimulation a diminished irritability, reduced current of action, and increased refractory phase is obtainable, but in spite of these changes a nerve will still continue to conduct. It is as if there was some form of adaptation to fatigue. Oxygen-want may make a nerve capable of carrying only occasional impulses.

Fatigue of Voluntary Movement

The foregoing suggests that local poisoning is responsible for fatigue, and in support of this, Mosso showed that the blood of a fatigued animal caused fatigue if injected into the blood of another.

It has, however, been shown that if the circulation to a part is cut off the liability to fatigue is not so great as would be expected (Reid). Other factors must be considered.

By the use of the ergograph (Mosso, Waller), it has been shown that the state of the brain and central nervous system generally is an important factor in fatigue.

One of the most striking of Mosso's experiments illustrates in a very forcible manner the fact that the central nervous system is more easily fatigued than muscle. A person goes on lifting a weight until, under the influence of the will, he is unable to raise it any more. If then, without waiting for fatigue to pass off, the nerves going to the finger muscles are stimulated artificially by induction shocks, the muscles once more enter into vigorous contraction.

It may be that the "fatigue" which occurs in central synapses is a result of the formation of fatigue products locally or the exhaustion of central cells. This has been supported by the finding that in fatigue the Nissl granules of the nerve-cells, which usually stain well with methylene blue, are absent or are represented by a diffuse blue haze (chromatolysis). It has, however, been suggested that something of the nature of a central inhibition results from impulses which pass up from the active muscles themselves. It appears that normally we are capable of using only a certain proportion of the muscle-fibers at one time, because inhibitory impulses are set up by the pressure on the sensory nerve-endings, the spindles of the muscles, and pass into the central nervous system. The excessive strength which can be exercised by a madman or individual under severe stress may in part be due to his bringing into use more fibers that can be used normally. This lengthening reflex which presumably prevents muscles from being torn from the bones can be demonstrated in a cat whose cerebrum has been removed.

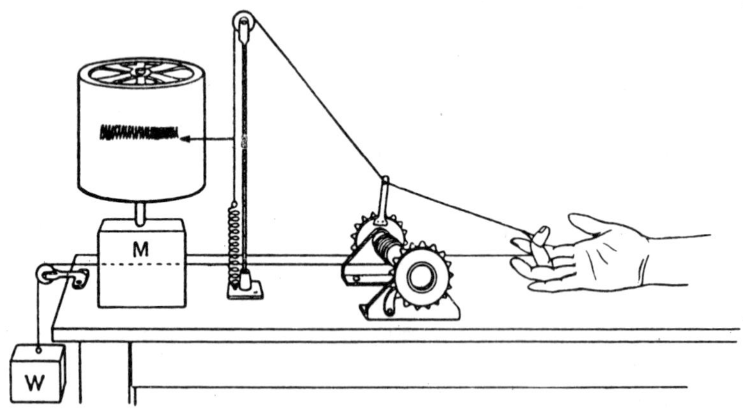

Fig. 6.15. A simple ergograph. The subject pulls with his finger at a rate set by a metronome. The work done may be calculated from the record on the drum or by the height to which the weight (W) is raised. Two bicycle free-wheel mechanisms make robust ratchets.

The Sensation of Pain in Muscle. The pain which results when a muscle is exercised, especially if its blood supply is defective, has been specially studied by Lewis because it throws light on the very intense pain which occurs when the arteries to the heart are occluded. This pain is one of the most severe known to man. It has been found that the intensity and duration of pain, when produced in the arm of man, are increased if the blood supply is occluded by a sphygmomanometer cuff. It is therefore suggested that a chemical substance is produced which stimulates the sensory nerve-endings. It may be lactic acid which, as we have seen, is at least partly responsible for local fatigue. The subject is discussed later in regard to that of Sensation.

Rest Pauses. It may be shown on an isolated muscle of by means of the ergograph that is not economical to fatigue a muscle to its limit and that to get the maximum work out of it in a given time there should be rest pauses. The pauses should, as far as possible, be evenly distributed.

A good example was given by Myers. If in an ergograph experiment the finger makes 30 contraction in 60 seconds with a certain load, two hours' rest is necessary for complete recovery. If, on the other hand, the finger makes 15 contractions in 30 seconds with same load a rest of only half an hour is necessary. Hence in a two-hour period of work the second arrangement would give double the output of work.

These facts, which were extensively studied in munition works especially by Vernon from 1914 to 1918, have a wide application to work generally, as they not only give more leisure to the worker but increase the quantity and quality of the work done. Experiments on the learning of poetry by students, and on rats learning to get out of a maze, suggest that it is probable that the necessity for rest pauses applies to mental work also.

General Fatigue

In addition to the fatigue described above there is a fatigue which depends on more general states such as the total amount of energy in the body. It is possible, too, that fatigue products may circulate in the blood, for we have seen that local fatigue is the result in part of the accumulation of such products which are normally washed away in the blood-stream. We know, too, that in exercise lactic acid passes into the blood-stream and is excreted in the urine as lactate. Workers on the subject of industrial fatigue have shown that a great deal can be done to eliminate this by the avoidance of all unnecessary movements, by reducing the total amount of muscle used, e.g., by not using the large muscles of the trunk and legs and by making continued smooth movements instead of a series of new movements which waste energy in overcoming inertia and viscosity.

Many mental factors also tend to affect fatigue, notably incentive, boredom, and general conditions of work, especially the temperature and humidity of the air. Most are familiar with the bracing effects of dry, cool air and the enervating action of a hot, moist atmosphere.

The factor which is really important is the cooling power of the air which is determined by the kata-thermometer introduced by Leonard Hill. This is essential an alcohol thermometer. It is heated to 100^0 F. and the observer takes the time for it to fall to

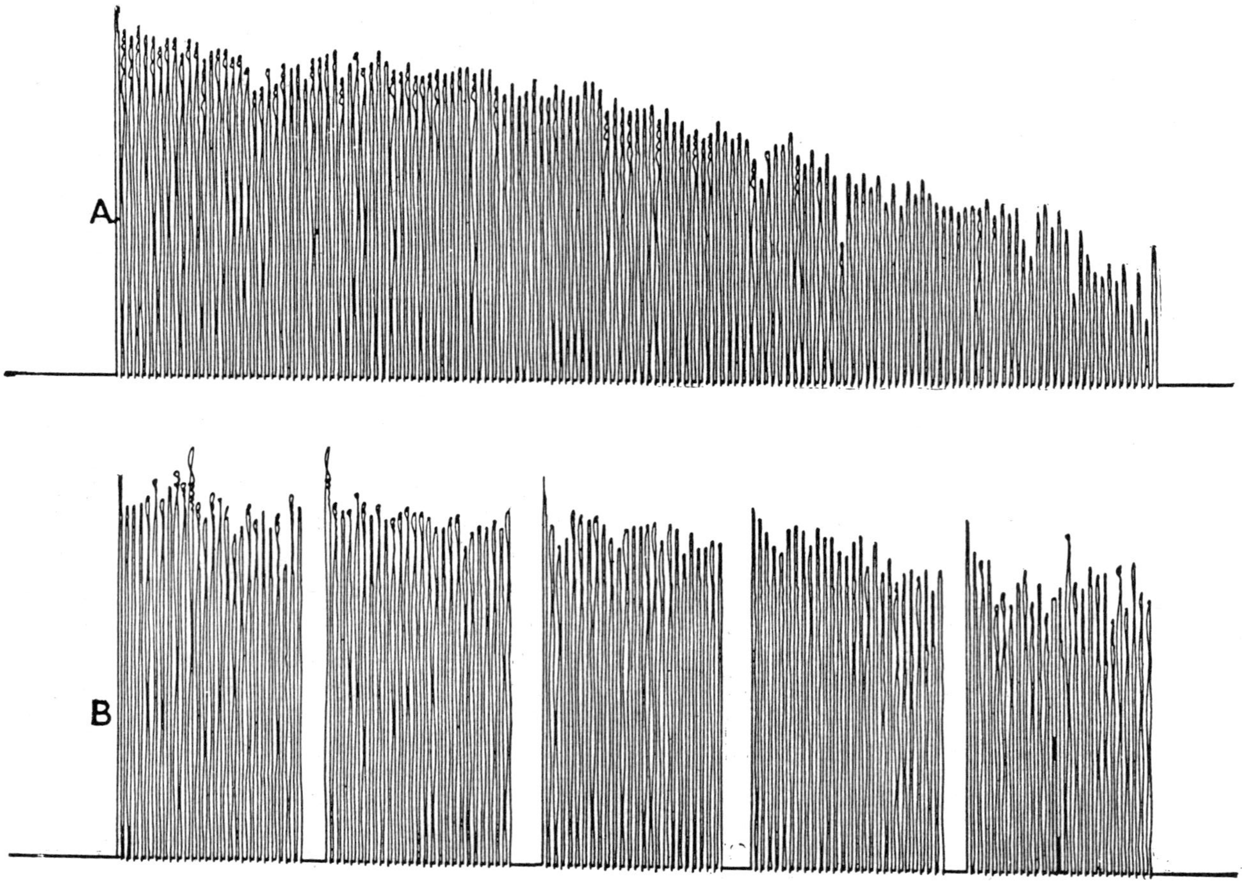

Fig. 6.16. A shows fatigue of an ordinary voluntary muscle of a finger, doing work on an ergograph at the rate of 48 contractions per minute. In B the subject worked for the same length of time—three minutes—but took four rest periods of five seconds each. In A the amount of work done was I.80 kilogram-metres. In B the amount of work done was 2.23 kilogram-metres.

95°. It may be used like a wet-bulb thermometer by covering it with a wet cloth. The cooling power of the air depends on its temperature, humidity, and movement. A gentle breeze of 100 feet per minute with a temperature of 72° F. will cool as much as a temperature of 60° will if there is no air movement. Hence the power of draughts in producing chilling of the body and the benefit of fans. The optimum working temperature, as judged by the accident incidence in factories, appears to be from 60° to 65° F.

Physiological Organisation of Spinal Motoneurones. Spinal motor neurones are arranged in such a way that their position in ventral horn of the spinal cord is related to the muscles they innervate. Thus motor neurones that supply the muscles of the arms (these neurones are located in the cervical segments of the spinal cord) are organised so that motor neurones supplying the upper arm are near the midline, while those supplying the arm extremities are located at the lateral edge of the ventral horn. In addition, motor neurones are segregated so that flexors lie dorsal to extensors. This type of organisation in which there is a spatial separation of cells supplying different parts of the body is quite common throughout the CNS. (cf. Somatic sensory and motor areas of the cerebral cortex.)

Concepts of the physiological organisation of motor-neurone pools have changed in recent years. It is well known that the force of contraction is a given muscle can be graded both by increasing the impulse frequency in individual motor neurones and by recruiting successively more motor neurones with increasing demand. At one time it was thought that the order of recruitment of motor neurones supplying a given muscle was dependent upon the source of the stimulus. It has become apparent, however, that, with increasing demand the order in which motor neurones to a given muscle are

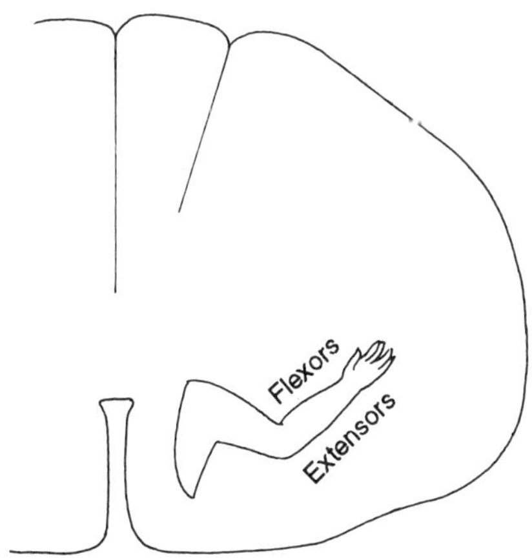

Fig. 6.17. Cross-section of a cervical segment of the spinal cord showing functional arrangement of spinal motor neurones. (The arms are innervated by motor neurones located in the cervical segments of the spinal cord.) Motor neurones supplying the arm extremities are located at the lateral margin of the ventral horn: motor neurones innervating the upper arm are at the medial margin of the ventral horn. Extensor motor neurones are found ventral to flexor motor neurones (after Netter).

recruited is always the same no matter what the driving stimulus. The smallest motor neurones to the muscle are always activated by the weakest stimuli. With increase in stimulus strength motor neurones of progressively increasing size become active. This system is efficient, since the smallest motor neurones and the muscle fibers they innervate are well adapted to sustained activity. Small motor neurones also innervate fewer muscle fibers than do large motor neurones. Thus, when only a low level of force output is required from the muscle small motor neurones are first brought into play. These activate only a relatively small number of muscle fibers and so generate relatively low muscle forces, making it possible to perform delicate manipulations. Because motor neurones are organised in this way a number of older concepts (such as occlusion, fractionation and subliminal fringes) can no longer be applied to groups of motor neurones supplying particular muscles.

Reflex Activity of the Spinal Cord. Responses to many stimuli can be made without the need for conscious control of movement. Thus, if one's hand touches a hot object the hand is removed before we have had time to appraise the situation; only after the hand has been removed do the conscious actions take place. The initial response is quite similar from one individual to another, while the responses which follow may vary a

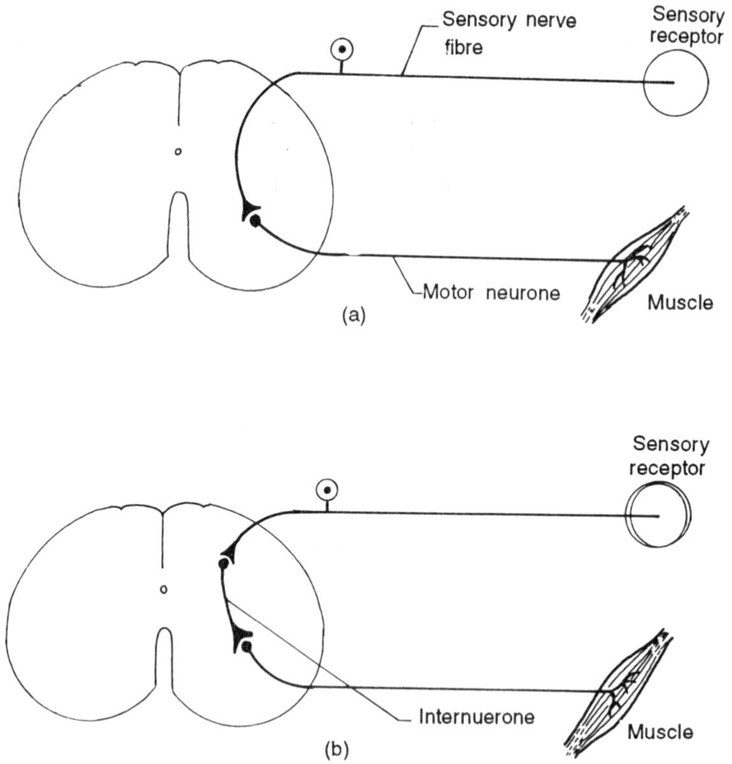

Fig. 6.18. Spinal reflexes. (a) Monosynaptic reflex. Sensory nerve fibers make direct connections with spinal motor neurones. (b) Polysynaptic reflex. At least one interneurone is interposed between the sensory nerve terminals and the motor neurones.

great deal! The initial, stereotyped response is an example of a reflex action. There is a wide range of reflexes of varying complexity. The simplest is the monosynaptic reflex. In this type of reflex stimulation of a sensory receptor produces a burst of impulses in a sensory nerve which synapses directly upon and activates motor neurones in the spinal cord. The motor neurones, in turn, cause muscular contraction and movement. This type of reflex is termed monosynaptic since it involves only one synapse within the CNS. In actual fact two synapses are involved, as motor neurones activate muscle fibers via nerve-muscle synapses. Reflexes involving more than one central synapse are termed polysynaptic reflex. Other more complex reflexes may involve more than one spinal segment and are known as intersegmental reflexes.

In any reflex there is a delay (the reaction time) between the stimulus and the muscular response. Contribution to this delay is the time taken for conduction along nerve fibers to and from the CNS transmission across the central and nerve-muscle synapses and activation of the contractile apparatus of the muscle fibers. This delay is approximately 20-24 milliseconds for the monosynaptic knee-jerk reflex.

Muscle Spindles. If a normally innervated muscle is stretched it generates tension to resist the applied movement; this is known as stretch reflex and is monosynaptic. The sensory receptor responsible for this reflex is the muscle spindle. This consists of several muscle spindle are different from 'normal' muscle fibers, being thinner and having many nuclei aggregated about half way along their length. These specialised muscle fibers of the spindle are termed intrafusal muscle fibers, while 'normal' muscle fibers which are responsible for developing the force of a muscle are known as extrafusal muscle fibers. Unlike extrafusal muscle fibers the muscle fibers of the spindle have a sensory innervation. Some terminals of the sensory nerve fibers coil around the nucleated portion of the muscle fibers and are known as primary or annulospiral endings. This type of sensory ending gives rise to large Group IA afferent nerve fibers. A second type of sensory ending, the secondary of flower-spray ending, gives rise to smaller Group II afferent nerve fibers; in the following description these will be ignored and the role of the annulospiral endings only discussed. In addition to these sensory endings the spindle muscle fibers, like the extrafusal muscle fibers, have a motor innervation. The motor innervation of intrafusal fibers is by small neurones—the motor neurones—whereas that of the extrafusal fibers is by large neurones—the α-motor neurones.

Muscle spindles lie within the body of muscles, among and parallel to extrafusal muscle fibers. If the whole muscle is stretched the fibers within the muscle spindle are stretched; this excites the sensory nerve terminals and produces a burst of impulses in the sensory-nerve fibers. If, on the other hand, the extrafusal muscle fibers contract and cause shortening of the whole muscle, the spindle is no longer stretched and the frequency of impulses in the sensory-nerve fibers falls. The sensory-nerve fibers from the spindle may produce impulses while the muscle is at its resting length. Therefore, the impulse frequency in the sensory nerves from muscle spindles may be increased by stretching or decreased by shortening the muscle.

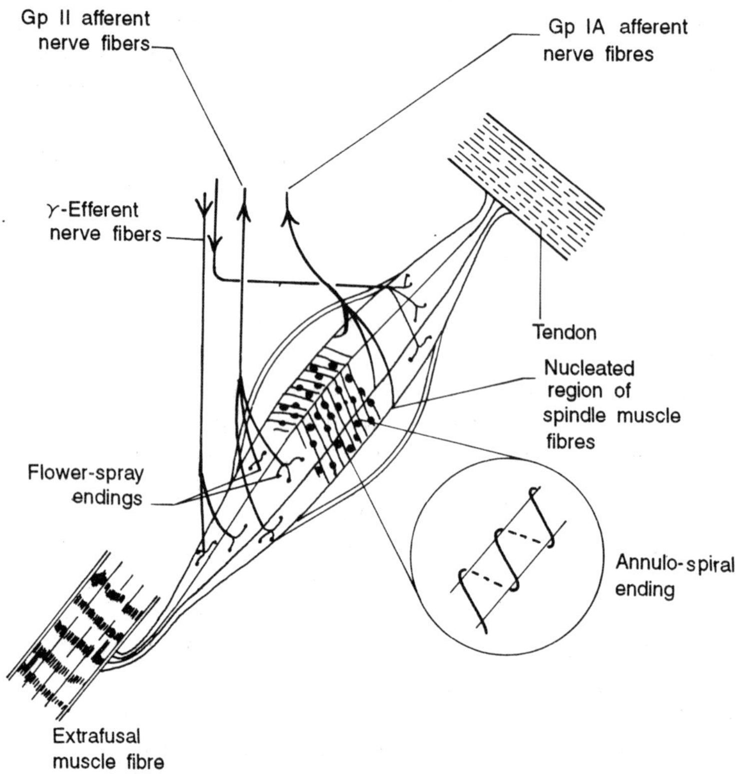

Fig. 6.19. Muscle spindle.

The sensory nerves from a muscle spindle enter the spinal cord to form excitatory synapses on α-motor neurones of the same segment; these motor neurones in turn innervate extrafusal muscle fibers near to the original muscle spindle. This circuit, consisting of muscle spindle and adjacent muscle fibers together with their connecting nerves, is the basis of the monosynaptic stretch reflex. When a muscle is stretched the impulse frequency in sensory-nerve fibers from its muscle spindles increases. This leads to excitation of α-motor neurones supplying the muscle which has been stretched. This muscle then contracts, relieves the tension on the spindle muscle fibers and allows the impulse frequency in the muscle-spindle sensory nerves to fall back to a lower level. The α-motor neurones are now no longer excited and contraction stops.

Muscle spindles not only produce monosynaptic excitation of α-motor neurones to their own muscle, but simultaneously cause reflex inhibition of α-motor neurones to antagonist muscles. This is produced by the activation of interneurones which inhibit the antagonist motor neurones. This inhibition of antagonist motor neurones facilitates

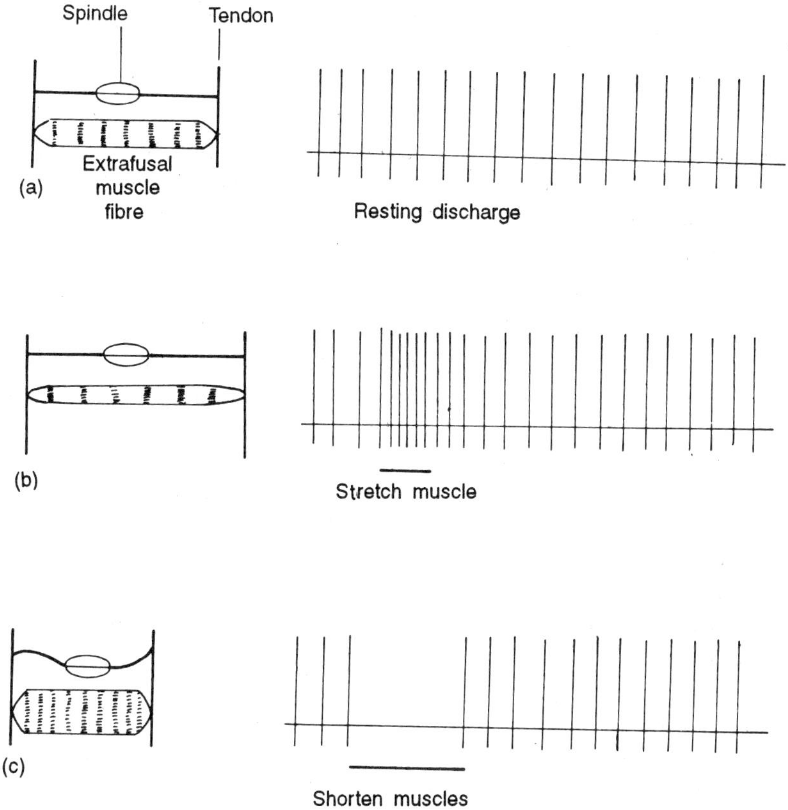

Fig. 6.20. Activation of muscle spindles. (a) When the muscle is relaxed, the sensory-nerve fibers of the muscle spindle produce a resting discharge of impulses. (b) If the muscle spindle is stretched, the central portions of the spindle muscle fibers are put under tension and their sensory-nerve terminals stimulated. (c) If the muscle contracts (and shortens), the tension of the central regions of the spindle muscle fibers is reduced and the impulse frequency in their sensory-nerve fibers falls.

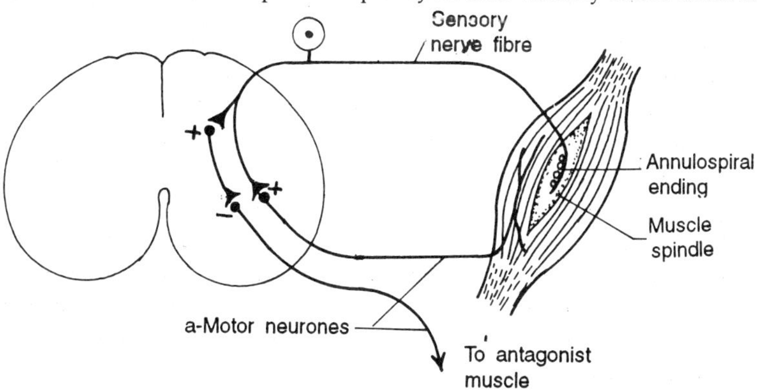

Fig. 6.21. Muscle spindle reflexes. When the annulospiral endings of a muscle spindle are stimulated a burst of nerve impulses travels to the spinal cord; the sensory-nerve fibers form excitatory synapses upon motor neurones supplying the muscle containing the activated spindle. Thus, impulses in the sensory-nerve fibers of a muscle spindle produce muscular contraction via a monosynaptic reflex-the stretch reflex. In addition to monosynaptic activation of motor neurones to their own muscle, the spindle sensory-nerve fibers also produce inhibition of motor neurones to antagonist muscles.

shortening of synergistic* muscles during the stretch reflex. The arrangement whereby opposing effects are produced in neurones with antagonistic functions is known as reciprocal innervation and is found commonly in reflex and other actions of the CNS.

An example of the stretch reflex is the knee-jerk reflex, in which the patellar tendon is tapped with a hammer. This rapidly stretches the thigh muscle (and the spindles within it) and produces a knee-jerk by stimulating contraction of the thigh muscles via their motor neurones.

Role of γ-motor Neurones. The muscle spindle is extremely sensitive to length changes of its muscle; if it merely responded passively to muscle stretch, however, it would only be capable of working effectively over a narrow range of muscle lengths. γ-Motor neurones innervating the spindle muscle fibers allow the muscle spindle to work over a wide range of muscle lengths without loss in sensitivity. Activation of γ-motor neurones causes contraction of each end of the intrafusal muscle fibers. The middle, nucleated portion of the fibers (on which the annulospiral endings are located) is not contractile. Therefore, contraction of each end of the spindle muscle fibers stretches the central portion of these fibers and excites the sensory-nerve endings. This causes shortening of the muscle by reflex stimulation of α-motor neurones: this is, turn, relieves the tension on the sensory endings of the spindle. If the level of activity in the γ-motor neurones becomes still higher, the ends of the spindle muscle fibers contract further and the sensory endings of the muscle spindle produce even stronger reflex muscular contraction. Thus, the range of muscle length over which a muscle spindle is responsive can be adjusted by altering the level of activity in γ-motor neurones. In this way the spindle is enabled to be highly sensitive to changes in muscle length by altering the range over which it works. This is in fact, just one example of the way in which the CNS can send impulses to a peripheral sense organ and thus modify its sensitivity to sensory stimuli.

Commands from the brain usually produce simultaneous activation of α- and γ-motor neurones. If only α-motor neurones were activated by such commands, shortening of the muscle would take the load off the spindles and make them insensitive to length change. Instead the fibers of the spindle shorten along with the extrafusal muscle fibers and so keep the spindle in their range of maximum sensitivity. This simultaneous activation of α- and γ-motor neurones also means that compensations can be rapidly made to adjust for different loads on the muscle. For example, if a heavy weight is to be lifted activation of the a-motor neurones may be insufficiently strong to life the weight; therefore, the muscle does not shorten. The spindle muscle fibers, however, have been simultaneously activated by the γ-motor neurones; because the muscle is too heavily weighted to shorten this produces a burst of impulses in the sensory-nerve fibers from the spindle. This in turn, increases the excitatory drive upon the α-motor neurones supplying the muscle (via the monosynaptic stretch reflex) and leads to an increase in the force generated by the muscle.

Information about muscle length provided by muscle spindles does not reach the level of consciousness. We have other types of sensory receptor which allow us to be aware of the position of different parts of the body relative to each other.

---

* *Synergistic muscles (or motor neurones) work together to produce a movement around a particular joint; antagonistic muscles (or motor neurones) have opposing actions.*

Golgi Tendon Organs. We have seen that muscle spindles provide the CNS with information about muscle length. Information about muscle tension is provided by another type of sensory receptor, the Golgi tendon organ. The Golgi tendon organ consists of branched nerve endings embedded in the tendon of a muscle. Golgi tendon organs are supplied with Group IB sensory nerve fibers. When the muscle tendon is put under strain the nerve endings of its Golgi tendon organs are stimulated. In this way, the CNS receives information about the force generated in a given muscle. If this force becomes so great that it may cause tissue damage, the Golgi tendon organs can mediate a protective reflex which inhibits the activity of motor neurones to the muscle with which they are in series; this results in a sudden loss of muscular tension. Thus, if an excessively heavy weight is applied to a muscle, the stretch reflex mediated by muscle spindles is overridden; the muscle no longer opposes extension and damage is prevented. Sensory-nerve fibers

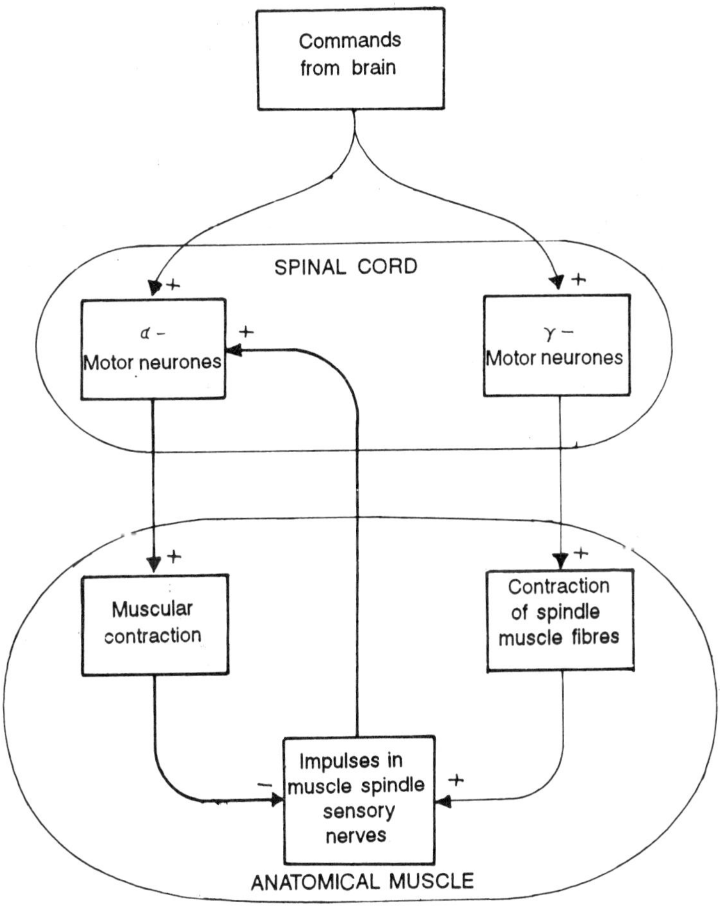

Fig. 6.22. Effect of the motor supply to muscle spindles. When stimulated by signals form the brain γ-motor neurones cause shortening of spindle muscle fibers; this causes excitation of their sensory nerve terminals. In this way modification in the level of activity in γ-motor neurones allows muscle spindles to work over different ranges of muscle length by altering the length of thier muscle fibers.

from Golgi tendon organs, on entering the spinal cord, form synaptic connections with interneurones which inhibit motor neurones supplying their muscle (Fig. 6.24).

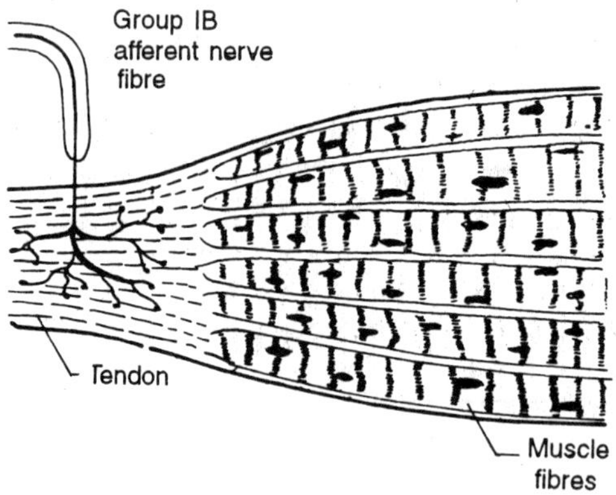

Fig. 6.23. Golgi tendon organ. Golgi tendon organs are located within the tendons of muscles and consist of many-branched nerve terminals; they respond to tension in the muscle. Different Golgi tendon organs have different thresholds and so work over different ranges of muscle tension.

The Golgi tendon organ, like the muscle spindle, does not provide us with conscious awareness about the state of out muscles, but instead function at the subconscious level.

Other Reflexes. In the above descriptions we have seen that reflexes can mediate rapid responses which would be delayed if it was necessary to consciously decide what

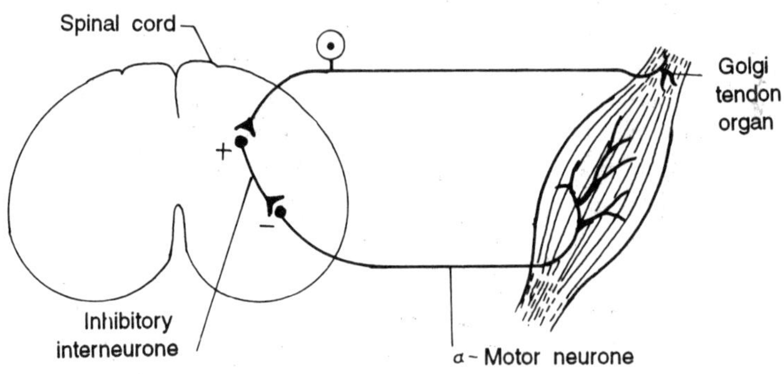

Fig. 6.24. Golgi tendon organ reflexes. Sensory-nerve fibers from Golgi tendon organs form synaptic contacts with interneurones in the spinal cord. These interneurones inhibit motor neurones supplying the muscle to which that Golgi tendon organ is attached.

action to take. This allows us to devote our conscious thoughts to fewer matters while routine movements are delegated to automatic mechanisms.

The reflexes mediated by muscle spindles and Golgi tendon organs serve to illustrate some of the basic features of reflexes; however, there is a wide variety of reflexes of greatly varying complexity. Thus, if we move our bodies we have to make a large number of postural adjustment in order to maintain balance; these adjustments are largely produced by coordinated reflexes mediated by different types of receptor including the eyes and the vestibular apparatus of the inner ear as well as by muscle spindles and Golgi tendon organs.

7

Reflexes

It has already been stated that the reflex may be considered the physiological unit of the nervous system. It has been usual to classify reflexes anatomically according to the amounts of the nervous system which they involve, but it is really best, however, to classify them physiologically, which is also their order to phylogenetic appearance.

1. *Protective Reflexes.*— These are seen in all animals and protect the animal from injury by withdrawing the stimulated part. Most involve the spinal cord but some the brain stem. They are brought into operation by harmful stimuli.

2. *Antigravity Reflexes* maintain the rigidity of the limbs against the force of gravity. They involve the spinal cord and the medulla.

3. *Righting Reflexes* adjust first the position of the head to the earth's surface, then the position of the trunk to the head, and the position of the limbs to the body. These reflexes involve the spinal cord, medulla, and mid-brain. Like the antigravity reflexes they are brought about by proprioceptive stimulation from the body itself, especially from the muscles and tendons.

4. *Conditioned Reflexes* result from experience. The significance of the sensory stimulus depends on the circumstances in which the stimulus was previously experienced. Here the cerebrum, as well as the lower parts of the nervous system, are concerned.

The discovery of reflex action was made by Marshall Hall (1833), a physician in London, who during his lifetime never received adequate recognition of his work. The antigravity reflexes were first described by Sherrington, in 1898. He was originally a bacteriologist, but subsequently became Professor of Physiology at Liverpool and later at Oxford. He and his pupils made a study of spinal reflexes generally. The righting reflexes were elucidated chiefly by Magnus, Professor of Pharmacology in Utrecht, while the importance of the conditioned reflexes was first appreciated by Pavlov in Moscow.

Protective Reflexes

The simplest form of reflex activity known is the axon reflex, which does not involve the central nervous system and is concerned with the protection of the skin. If an irritant, e.g., a mustard plaster or croton oil, is applied to the skin, a reddening due to dilatation of blood-vessels is produced. If the nerve-supply is cut, as is sometimes done by surgeons to relieve pain, e.g., in neuralgia of the 5th nerve, the reddening on application of the irritant can be obtained for a few days but is no longer possible after the peripheral fibers have degenerated. This demonstrates the dependence of the action on a local nervous mechanism, apparently in the peripheral part of the axon: the axon appears to divide, giving a branch to the skin and another to the wall of a blood-vessel. It may be, however, that the sensory impulse somehow passes to vasodilator fibers which we know are distributed from the sensory posterior nerve-roots.

The *Spinal Protective* reflex is the simplest form of reflex involving the central nervous system. It depends on the co-operation of a receptor organ, an afferent sensory nerve, a chain of nerve-cells in the spinal cord, an efferent motor nerve, and an effector organ, the whole constituting the reflex arc.

Although a spinal reflex is usually described, it must be understood that reflexes of this type are obtained from cranial nerves—notably the corneal reflex by which the eye is protected.

The reflex activities of the spinal cord may be studied in a *spinal animal*, i.e., an animal in which the brain has been destroyed or the spinal cord cut across in the cervical region. In the case of a mammal, artificial respiration is necessary since the respiratory centre is cut off, unless the section is made below the origin of the phrenic nerves.

The simplest way to produce a typical spinal mammal is to clamp the vertebral and the carotid arteries and allow time for the anesthesia to pass off.

A cat so operated upon, after a short period of shock has passed off, assumes a characteristic position of flexion; it curls up. If a limb is pinched or pricked it is at once withdrawn (flexion withdrawal reflex). This is obviously a defence reflex to remove the limb from the injuring force or noxious stimulus. Sometimes the stimulus throws the whole animal into extreme flexion (mass reflex).

After a period of absence of reflexes following operation a spinal animal may show extensor reflexes also.

After destruction of the brain of a frog the shock of the operation renders the animal for a variable time motionless and irresponsive to stimuli, but later on it gradually assumes a position which differs but little from that of a conscious animal. If thrown into water it will swim; if placed on a slanting board it will crawl up; if stroked on the flanks it will croak; if it is laid on its back, and a small piece of blotting-paper moistened with acid is placed on the skin, it will generally succeed in kicking it off; if a foot is pinched it will draw the foot away; if left perfectly quiet it remains motionless.

The occurrence of many protective reflexes in man similar to those in animals are facts of everyday experience. The flexion withdrawal reflex may be elicited during ordinary sleep or light anesthesia. It is also obtained in individuals suffering from paralysis due to injury to the pyramidal tracts and who may be unable to move the part voluntarily.

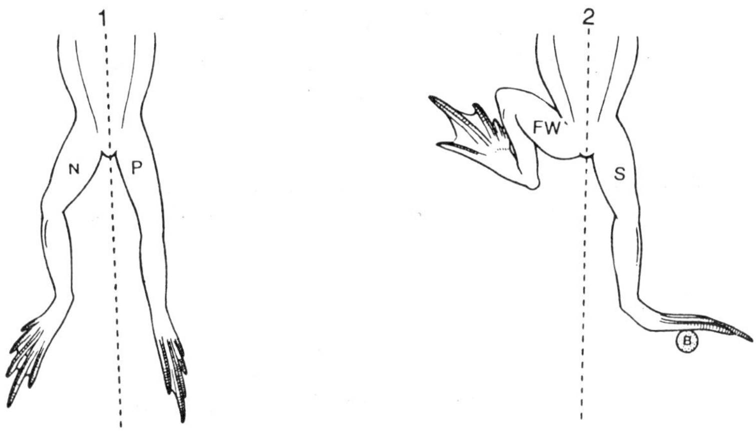

Fig. 7.1. Reflexes in the frog (diagrammatic). In I the normal reflex tone N of the legs as indicated by the partial flexion at the knee is seen. This is absent if the spinal cord is destroyed, P. In 2 is seen the flexion withdrawal reflex. FW is the response to a harmful stimulus and the thrust reflex S to a blunt object, B.

Extensor Antigravity Reflexes

These reflexes are most conveniently seen in an animal whose brain stem has been cut across just above the pons (see Decerebrate Animal), but they are also obtained from a chronic spinal animal, that is, an animal whose spinal cord has been cut across some time previously and in which the shock of the section has passed off. Normally the activity of the reflexes is reduced by the activity of the cerebrum, hence the necessity for its removal.

The pathways on which they depend are similar to that of the simple spinal arc, but in addition there are pathways to (spino-vestibular) and from (vestibulo-spinal) Deiters's nucleus, i.e., the lateral vestibular nucleus in the upper part of the medulla.

The reflexes which keep the legs of the animal straight in standing are normally found, as would be expected, in the extensor muscles, and are stretch reflexes. They may be demonstrated by stretching a muscle, as by sudden bending of the leg, or by tapping a tendon. As these facts suggest, they are set up by impulses from the muscles themselves, and this is proved by the fact that they are abolished by section of the posterior roots through which the impulses from the muscles pass. Moreover, if a muscle is denervated and attached to a lever by which its tension may be measured, it is found that when

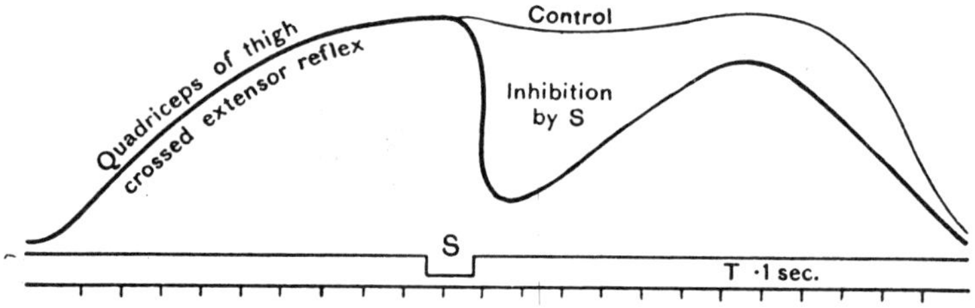

Fig. 7.2. Records showing inhibition of the crossed extensor reflex in the cat.

stretched it develops much less tension (not more than 20 per cent., due to its elasticity) than when its nerves are intact. The reflex is not abolished by local anesthesia of the tendon. Many reflexes of this type occur, but the thrust reflex and crossed extensor reflex may be taken as examples. They are also the bases of the postural reflexes which are discussed in a later section.

The thrust reflex is seen if a sudden force is applied to the foot so as to bend the leg. This causes the quadriceps extensor in the front of the thigh to contact and the limb to straighten. The importance of this reflex in propelling the body forward in walking is obvious.

The crossed extensor reflex is seen in the quadriceps extensor of the thigh when the corresponding nerve of the opposite side is stimulated. It, too, is part of the walking mechanism since the lifting of one leg requires increased contraction of the muscles of the other to maintain the weight of the body. The crossed extensor reflex is dramatically inhibited by stimulation of a sensory nerve of the same side.

Difference between the Flexor and Extensor Reflexes.— Flexor reflexes, being protective, are more immediate and rise to a maximum more rapidly than extensor reflexes which rise slowly. In so doing they are said to demonstrate recruitment as they apparently bring into action more neurones and muscle fibers as the stimulus is kept up. This is possibly an adaptation to the load to be borne and appears to be a "self-braking" action is such reflexes, for if the afferents of the executant muscles are cut the contraction is speeded up. Extensor reflexes show a long after-discharge, presumably because of their reaching their maximum slowly.

In the extensor reflexes the slow-acting red muscles play a predominant part, but white fibers may also be used. It is this use of the red muscles which makes the extensor reflexes less liable to fatigue; indeed, a single unit may go on discharging at a slow rate, 5-8 per second indefinitely.

The Sensory Nerve-endings in Muscle

From what has been said of the extensor reflexes it is evident that there are important sensory nerve-endings in muscle and allied tissues. These were found histologically by Ruffini (1898) and by Golgi. They are studied in relation to Sensation in general later.

The Properties and Characteristics of Reflex Arcs

Reflex arcs have certain characteristics which may be seen in the study of the spinal reflex. These are of importance, as there is reason to believe that similar characteristics are exemplified in higher arcs also. Most of these characteristics, it will be seen really depend on the properties of the region of the synapse; indeed, much of our knowledge of this region has been obtained from the study of reflexes. The synapse is discussed in a separate section.

Resistance.— If the time which a reflex ought to take be calculated from our knowledge of the rate of the nerve impulse as conducted by nerve-fibers, it is found that the actual time taken is appreciably longer. This extra time or central *reflex time* has presumably been spent in traversing the central nervous system and especially in passing across the synapses or junctions between one neurone and another. It has been calculated that the time lost at a synapse is 0.002 sec. The more synapses the more the time lost.

Effect of Repetition of Stimulus.— Once a reflex has been evoked it is found that it becomes, up to a point, increasingly easy to elicit it, and the reduced reflex time becomes lessened. This is known as facilitation. This fact is of obvious importance in relation to increase of skill in various manual occupations. Beyond this point, however, fatigue may readily set in. This must occur on the central part of the arc, at the synapse, since nerve is not fatigable in the ordinary sense; it is found that when fatigue is present and a reflex can no longer be elicited, the muscle concerned can still be made to contract through its nerve or through another afferent nerve. Fatigue of a spinal reflex appears to be recovered from with remarkable speed, provided the blood circulation is good.

Summation.— Although a stimulus may be insufficiently strong to elicit a response, the repetition of the stimulus may be effective. The fact suggests that there is an accumulation of excitatory states centrally or peripherally at the point of stimulation. Thus it may be possible to bring about a response with two separate subliminal stimuli, each of which is insufficient; or, if each is sufficient, the total effect will be greater than with each independently.

Summation of Chemical Stimuli is well illustrated by Turck's method. If a number of beakers of water are prepared, acidulated with 1, 2, 4, etc., parts of sulphuric acid per 1000, and the tips of a spinal frog's toes are immersed in the weakest, the frog does not at first respond, but in time the cumulation or summation of the sensory impulses causes the animal to withdraw its feet. If this is repeated with stronger liquids in succession, the time that intervenes before the muscles respond becomes less and less.

This method also serves to test reflex irritability when the frog is under the influence of various drugs.

Dependence on Oxygen.— We have noted that fatigue may set in if a stimulus is too often repeated. If, however, the oxygen supply is deficient, it sets in more readily. Synapses are apparently particularly sensitive to the effects of oxygen-want. A fall of blood-pressure markedly depresses the reflexes, which disappear in man when the mean arterial pressure drops below 50 mm. Hg. It is possible that the height of the blood-pressure is of considerable importance in relation to nervous activity, but it is extremely difficult to obtain data on this point.

Dependence on Carbon Dioxide.— Some reflexes arcs, e.g., those concerned with posture, require carbon dioxide as is shown by the fact that if the carbon dioxide is washed out by over-ventilation the reflexes disappear. It is probable that in part at least this apparent dependence on carbon dioxide is really that this gas facilitates, as we have seen, the unloading of oxygen from the blood.

Spread.— The effect of a given stimulus which is capable of evoking a reflex depends very largely on its strength. A relatively weak stimulus may cause a simple response confined to one limb, but a stronger stimulus may spread not only to the opposite side by also to the adjacent segments of the cord, bringing about a generalised movement. It appears likely that in the first instance the afferent impulses take the easiest path, which suggests that the resistance of the synapses in the various paths may vary appreciably. It is considered that such a grading of synapses may play an important part in the general activity of the nervous system.

Local Sign.— If a portion of the body be stimulated, e.g., the flank pinched, it is observed that the reflex is definitely purposeful and the movement is directed towards the removal of the stimulation. Thus a piece of blotting-paper soaked in dilute sulphuric acid and placed on the flank of a decapitated frog is removed by the reflex activity of its hind foot.

Unidirectional Conduction.— We have noted that a nerve impulse may be carried in both directions along a nerve. In a reflex arc the impulse can go in one direction only.

Inhibition.— One reflex can inhibit another, the reflex more important for the welfare of the animal predominating. This we have already seen in relation to the crossed extension reflex. It is also evident in regard to the scratch reflex in which one protective reflex predominates over another. The inhibition of a sneeze by firm pressure on the upper lip is a similar phenomenon.

The Nature of the Reflex Response.— If a motor nerve is stimulated by a single shock the resulting response is a muscular twitch. If a tetanising current of short duration is applied to a motor nerve all the muscle-fibers supplied contract at once and the tension rises and falls abruptly. If, however, the same stimulus is used to actuate it reflexly the rise and fall of tension are more gradual as more nerve and muscle units come into action and are released. This is specially well seen in the antigravity reflexes and is very characteristic of reflex action. It should perhaps be added that in order to demonstrate

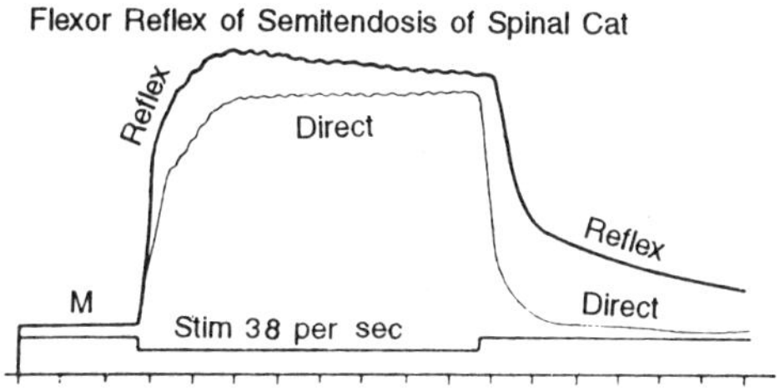

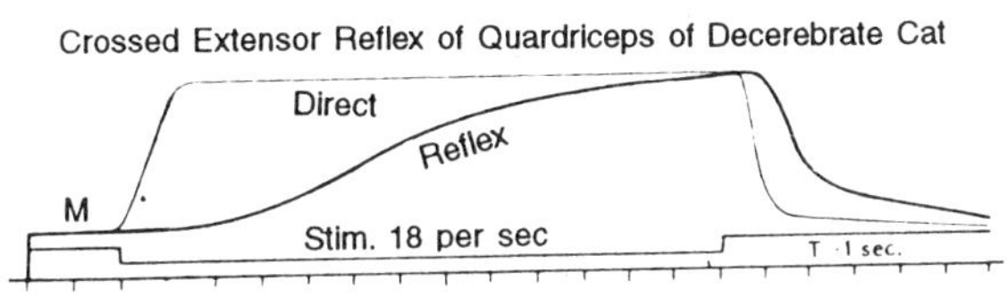

Fig. 7.3. Upper—a typical flexor response. Lower—a typical extensor response.

such rapid changes it is necessary to use a photographic recording system as the inertia of an ordinary lever system is too great. The movement or other activity produced reflexly does not cease directly the stimulus is removed, but continues for a time after cessation of stimulation. This phenomenon is called after-discharge, and is one of the most striking features of reflex action.

If during tonic contraction an inhibitory afferent nerve is stimulated, the contraction at once becomes less, but the muscle again contracts the moment the inhibitory stimulus is removed, often to a larger extent than before. This is known as rebound, but is a very variable phenomenon.

There is considerable overlapping reflexes.

It will be realised that many of the characteristics of reflexes depend on the synapses concerned.

Action of Drugs on Reflexes

Reflexes are enhanced by strychnine and diminished by bromide, which apparently acts on the resistance of the synapse. It is of interest that these drugs are used commonly in medicine, strychnine to enhance and bromide to depress the activity of the nervous system. Nicotine first stimulates cells of the autonomic system and then paralyses the transmission of impulses at the synapses in autonomic ganglia, but does not affect spinal reflexes.

The Tendon Reflexes in Man

The tendon reflexes of man are of special interest and importance because of the easy method by which they can be studied and because their absence or exaggeration is often an indication of the presence of injury or disease of the spinal cord. In this connection it is the purely spinal component of the reflexes which is of most importance, although as we have seen in relation to the extensor reflexes generally, they are really but part of a more elaborate antigravity mechanism with pathways to and from Deiters's nucleus in the medulla. Thus the reflex, although described as a spinal reflex, is really a fractionated antigravity reflex. In each case it is brought about by stimulating the nerve-endings in the tendon mechanically. It will be realised that physiologically this is a very abnormal stimulus.

The knee-jerk.— The quadriceps muscle is slightly stretched by putting one knee over the other; a slight blow on the ligamentum patellae causes a movement of the foot forwards. The reflex is present in health.

The ankle-jerk is one of importance, for in such diseases as locomotor ataxia (tabes), in which the tendon reflexes are lost, it usually disappears before the knee-jerk. It is best elicited if the patient kneels with one knee upon a cushioned chair, whilst standing on the other leg by the side of the chair. The calf muscles of the kneeling leg are thus slightly stretched by the weight of the foot, and a sharp tap upon the tendo Achillis elicits the jerk.

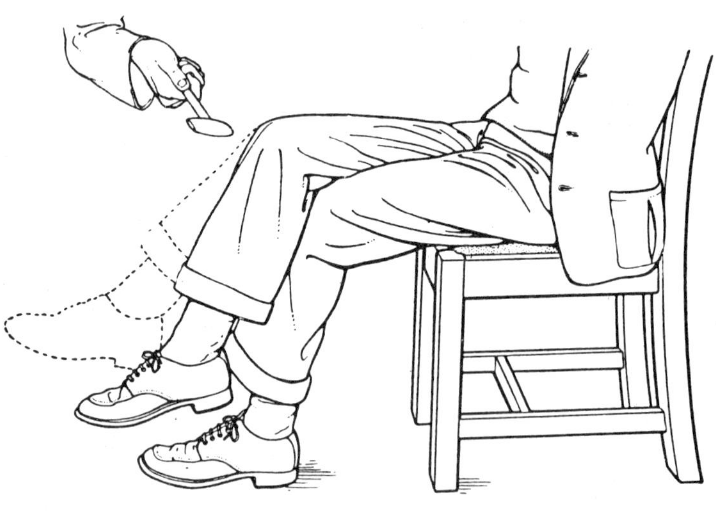

Fig. 7.4. The taking of the knee-jerk.

Jerks of the biceps, triceps, and supinator of the upper limb may also be elicited in a similar way, but they are not normally so active. The jaw-jerk, which causes the open lower jaw to close sharply when its point is tapped, is only present when the path to the motor nucleus of the 5th nerve is involved.

Ankle-clonus.— This is elicited as depicted in the next figure: the hand is pressed against the sole of the foot, the calf muscles are thus put on the stretch and they contract, and if the pressure is kept up a quick succession or clonic series of contractions is obtained. This is not readily obtained in health.

The exact course of the reflex are concerned in the knee-jerk has been worked out by Sherrington in the monkey. The nerve-fibers are mainly those which pass (1) to and from the extensors by the anterior femoral nerve, and (2) to and from the hamstrings by the sciatic nerve. The fibers which supply the extensor arise from the spinal nerve-roots which in man correspond to the 3rd and 4th lumbar; the hamstring supply is from the 5th lumbar and 1st and 2nd sacral roots.

Lombard's experiments upon the knee-jerk indicate that it is sometimes more readily obtained even in the same person than at other times. It varies with changes in mental activity, and during sleep may be entirely absent. It is increased and diminished by whatever increases or diminishes the relative state of irritability of the nervous system as a whole.

Closely related to this is the phenomenon known as *reinforcement of the knee-jerk,* which was first described by Jendrassik in 1883, and has since been studied by numerous observes. The extent of the jerk may be increased if at the time the patellar tendon is struck a strong voluntary contraction, such as clenching the fists or the jaw, is made by the individual. In many normal persons the knee-jerk is difficult to elicit, but it must never be regarded as absent until reinforcement has been tried. After the reinforcing action has occurred it is followed by an interval in which the knee-jerk is lessened (inhibition or negative reinforcement).

Absence of Reflexes.— The tendon reflexes must obviously disappear if any part of the arc on which they depend is destroyed. Disease or injury of the afferent nerve, efferent nerve, or spinal grey matter abolishes them. Thus they cannot be obtained in locomotor ataxy (damage to the posterior nerve-roots), or in infantile paralysis, also known as anterior poliomyelitis (damage to the anterior horns of grey matter). This absence of the reflexes is therefore an important diagnostic sign of disease of the spinal cord or of the nerve-roots. Especially is this so if the tendon reflexes which are usually elicited are affected, but the superficial reflexes are more variable and may be unobtainable even in the absence of nervous disease.

Alteration of the Character of the Reflex.— This is well seen in the case of the knee-jerk. In lesions of the pyramidal tracts as in the decerebrate animal the knee-jerk is too well sustained, but on the other hand in cerebellar disease the leg falls quite limply. The normal is midway between the two. These facts indicate that the knee-jerk is intimately related to higher mechanisms. It is indeed a fractionated stretch reflex or part of the more complicated reflex by which we stand.

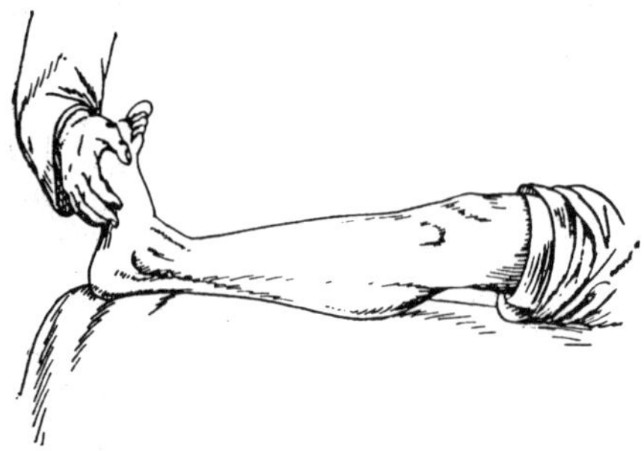

Fig. 7.5. Ankle-clonus.

The Influences of the Higher Centres on Lower Reflex Arcs.— If in the frog experiments, the cerebrum only is destroyed and the optic lobes left intact, the reflex reactions are found to be appreciably slower, thus showing the inhibitory effect of the remaining parts of the brain.

In man, this influence is of considerable clinical importance in the diagnosis of nervous disease, in which an exaggeration of the reflexes may, in certain circumstances, be considered to indicate that the higher centres have been cut off, e.g., by damage to the motor tracts. The state thus produced is that of the chronic spinal animal in which the shock of the operation has passed off. Research suggests that the exaggeration is essentially the result of the cutting off of the impulses which pass down the rubrospinal tracts, but as these tracts lie in close association with the pyramidal tracts in the cord, conditions which affect one tract commonly affect the other. The reflex may be exaggerated in any condition which increases the irritability of the nervous system.

The effect of reinforcement referred to above is a closely allied phenomenon, but a generally accepted explanation has not yet been found. On the other hand, we are familiar with the fact that reflexes may be largely inhibited by volition, e.g., sneezing. Cranmer, when burnt at the stake, held his hand in the fire till it was consumed.

The Plantar Reflex.— We have seen in the frog experiment described above that two reflexes may be produced by stimulation of the foot. Two similar reflexes are seen in man: the *withdrawal reflex*, involving fanning of the toes and dorsiflexion of the great toe (extensor plantar response); and the *thrust reflex*, involving flexion of the toes (flexor plantar response). Normally they are elicited by two distinct varieties of stimulation, but, as a result of walking, the protective withdrawal reflex is in partial abeyance and a *gentle* scratch of the sole of the foot with the finger-nail causes flexion of the toes. In disease of the pyramidal tracts, however, or in very deep sleep, whether normal or produced by a narcotic, when local protection is more essential, the withdrawal reflex is more prominent and such stimulation causes extension of the toes, especially the great toe. This is an important diagnostic sign of interference with the pyramidal tract

(Babinski's sign); or in some persons it may be the result of fatigue of the higher centres. American workers have put forward evidence that the fanning component is the result of interference with the extra-pyramidal system from the red nucleus.

The Superficial Reflexes

These reflexes are probably protective in nature. They are obtained by a gentle stimulation, such as a touch on the skin; the muscles beneath are usually affected, but muscles at a distance may be affected also; for example:

(*a*) *Gluteal reflex:* a contraction in the gluteus when the skin over it is stimulated.

(*b*) *Cremasteric reflex:* a retraction of the testicle when the skin on the inner side of the thigh is stimulated.

(*c*) *Abdominal reflex:* a contraction of the muscles of the abdominal well when the skin over the side of the abdomen is stroked; the upper part of this reflex is a very definite contraction at the epigastrium, and has been termed the epigastric *reflex*.

(*d*) A series of similar reflex actions may be obtained in the muscles of the back, the highest being in the muscles of the scapula.

These reflexes commonly disappear if the pyramidal tracts are destroyed, but they are so variable normally that little is known regarding the exact pathways on which they depend. In animals some of them appear to play a part in the driving off of flies.

The Visceral Reflexes

The Spinal grey matter contains centres which regulate the operation of many involuntary muscles. Some of these centres are:

The *cilio-spinal* centre which controls the dilation of the pupil; it is situated in the lower cervical region, reaching as far down as the origin of the first to the third thoracic nerves.

Subsidiary vasomotor centres. The principal vasomotor centre is situated in the bulb, and subsidiary centres are scattered through the spinal grey matter.

Centres probably exist for all the muscular viscera, but particular study has been directed to those in the pelvis, and centres for *micturition, defaecation*, erection, and *parturition* are contained in the lumbo-sacral region of the cord. If the spinal cord is cut through above the situation of the centres, the result is, in general terms, that any influence of the higher (voluntary) centres over these actions is no longer possible. The actions in question are then simply reflex ones occurring after a period of shock unconsciously at certain intervals, and set in movement by the peripheral stimulus (distension of bladder, or rectum etc.).

Muscle Tone and the Postural Reflexes

In our consideration of the tendon reflexes we saw that certain reflexes occur when tendons are stretched by tapping or otherwise. These reflexes are, however, really part of a most elaborate mechanism by which the body maintains its posture an co-ordinates its muscular activities. The so-called "stretch reflex" is therefore of fundamental importance in the maintenance of posture.

Normally the muscles of the body, even when apparently at rest, are not fully relaxed, but are constantly maintained in a state of partial contraction. This state we know as *tonus*.

This may readily be seen in a decerebrate frog, which, if held up by the head, is seen to maintain its legs in a slightly flexed position. If, however, the anterior or posterior lumbar roots are cut, or the spinal cord in the lumbar region destroyed, the legs hang flaccid. It is evident from such experiments that the muscular tone which was present was dependent not only on impulses which pass out from the cord, but also on those which pass in by the posterior roots. Similarly, in man, if any condition is present which interferes with the spinal arc, either on the afferent or the efferent side, there is unusual flaccidity. On the other hand, if the pyramidal tracts are destroyed by disease there is found in association with the increased reflexes a marked rigidity of the lower limbs due

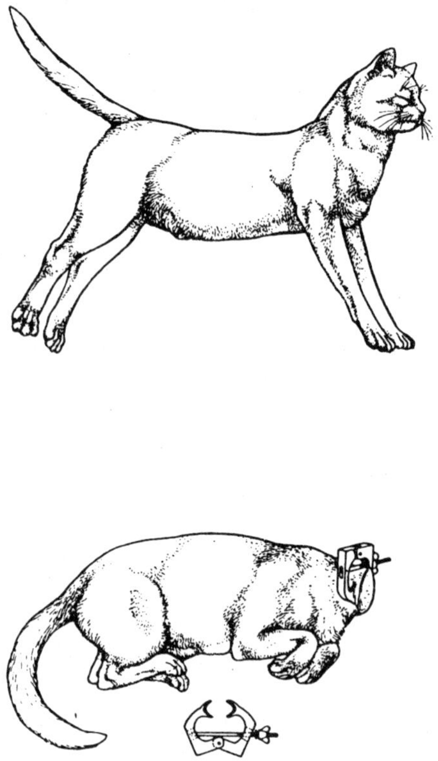

Fig. 7.6. The upper drawing shows the posture of a mid-brain animal in decerebrate rigidity. The lower shows the posture of a spinal cat, with head removed. A clamp (McDowall) is applied to the vertebral arteries, the carotid arteries being occluded. Artificial respiration is needed.

to increased tone of the extensors. Generally we may say that loss of reflexes is associated with loss of tone and increase of reflexes with increase of tone.

We may arrive at some, as yet incomplete, explanation of these facts if we study the phenomenon of muscle tone in animals.

The Spinal Animal has already been studied. It has been seen that it is possessed of flexor tone and it shows an exaggeration of the protective flexor reflexes, and may, after a period of absence, also show tendon reflexes.

The Mid-Brain Animal.— If, however, the section is made through the mid-brain, through or just below the red nucleus, quite the opposite state of affairs is produced, namely, that first described by Sherrington as decerebrate rigidity, which is a state in which there is gross exaggeration of the antigravity reflexes. The condition has been much studied because of the light it throws on the mechanism of posture generally and on states of rigidity which occur in disease in man.

The Nature of the Rigidity.— Fundamentally the rigidity is due to a sustained exaggeration of the antigravity extensor reflexes already described and the result of stimuli which originate in the stretched tendons and muscles, which normally extend the limb. In this condition the limbs are fully extended and are rigid as the result of increased tone in the muscles of the back and neck, in the quadriceps, the extensor of the knee, and in the gastrocnemius at the back of the leg. There is produced, in other words, a condition of reflex standing, since all the antigravity muscles are contracted and the preparation can therefore maintain its own weight of placed on its feet, but cannot right its position if pushed over. The reflex paths concerned in the phenomenon may be investigated by studying the condition of the tone present in the quadriceps extensor of the knee. It is found that the maintenance of the tone depends on both the anterior and posterior roots (lumbar 5 and 6 in the case of the quadriceps in the cat), indicating that tonus is dependent on afferent impulses arising in the muscle itself. These impulses may be shown to depend on the slight stretch imposed on the muscle by its bony attachments from the tendency for the legs to bend, since, if the tendon is severed, the tonus and the impulses which are found by the electrical method to pass up its nerve at the rate of 15 per second at once disappear. Nor is the cerebellum concerned, for it can be removed without affecting the rigidity. That the skin is not involved is seen by the fact that decerebrate rigidity is fully present in a skinned limb. Impulses from the labyrinth are concerned in the neck and fore-limb rigidity.

The Central Mechanism Involved.— It is seen, however, that the central nervous system, as high as the pons, is concerned in the reaction, since destruction of Deiters's nucleus or section of the antero-lateral tract removes the rigidity. Thus we may conclude that this condition of decerebrate rigidity depends on a reflex arc, of which the afferent side is the afferent nerves from the muscles, the posterior roots, and the antero lateral tract, while the efferent side is the vestibulo-spinal tract from Deiters's nucleus (Bazett) is the upper medulla and lower pons, the anterior roots and the motor nerves to the muscles.

Normally it would seem that decerebrate rigidity is essentially a release phenomenon; that is, the reflex arc upon which it depends is released by the section from the influence of the higher centres. The higher centres concerned are the red nucleus and probably the cerebrum, for it has been found that careful destruction of the red nucleus only (Ranson) or section of the rubro-spinal tracts does not cause rigidity unless the pyramidal tracts are also cut, while stimulation of the latter causes the rigidity to disappear. Animals in which the cortex has been removed tend, too, to have some extensor rigidity, although the distribution of tone is fairly normal (Bard). It would seem then that impulses which travel down by the rubro-spinal and the pyramidal tracts compete with those from the vestibulo-spinal tracts for effects on the anterior horn cells of the spinal cord.

In man, states similar to decerebrate rigidity are met with in tumours involving the mid-brain and pyramidal tracts, but the legs, for various reasons, are more affected than the arms, which, indeed, may be flexed. In meningitis a condition almost identical with decerebrate rigidity may sometimes be seen; in this, retraction of the head is a marked feature.

In the cat it is easy to demonstrate the conversion of a decerebrate animal into a spinal animal by clamping the vertebral and carotid arteries. This procedure destroys Deiters's nucleus which, however, recovers again if the carotid is released. It is thus possible to reflex and extend the legs by clamping and releasing the carotid artery. Experimentally, decerebrate rigidity is absent if carbon dioxide is washed out by over-ventilation.

The Characteristics of the Rigid Muscles.— The contraction is a sustained contraction especially of the red fibers in muscle. It must then he looked upon as a form of tetanus which results from slow periodic discharges of certain motor-cells acting cyclically. It must be understood that the amount of muscular tension thus kept up is only a fraction of the maximum which can be produced by the same muscles, and the amount of oxygen required is only 25 per cent. above that required at rest. The liability to fatigue is, therefore, very little indeed; the rigidity can be kept up for many days. The reflexes are very resistant to inhibition and their rate of electrical discharge is very slow—5 to 8 per second. The posturing limb shows the phenomenon of plasticity, which tends to keep the limb in whatever position it is placed.

The degree of tone in posturing muscles is related to the body as a whole.

Reflex walking may be seen if a roller platform is moved along the feet of a suspended decerebrate animal; if the movement is rapid the carcase gallops, if slow it walks. (Graham Brown).

An interesting phenomenon of posturing muscle is the *lengthening reaction*. If the muscle is severely stretched it is felt to give way owing to a sudden disappearance of the tone as a result of inhibitory impulses which pass up from the muscle spindles. This reaction, together with fractionation, is important in preventing the tearing of muscles. It seems likely that the excessive strength of lunatics and of athletes trained for specialised events is somehow due to reduced lengthening reaction.

The Thalamic Animal.— If a section is made above the red nucleus, the postural reactions and balance of the animal are complete. For convenience the thalamus also is left intact in order that the animal shall be able to regulate its own body temperature. The animal possesses *righting reflexes*, that is, is capable of righting itself from any position in which it may be placed, although of course by the removal of the cerebrum it is deprived of all volition and is a mere automation. It can also walk about, but it does so stiffly because of the presence of the slight exaggeration of tone in the extensor muscles,

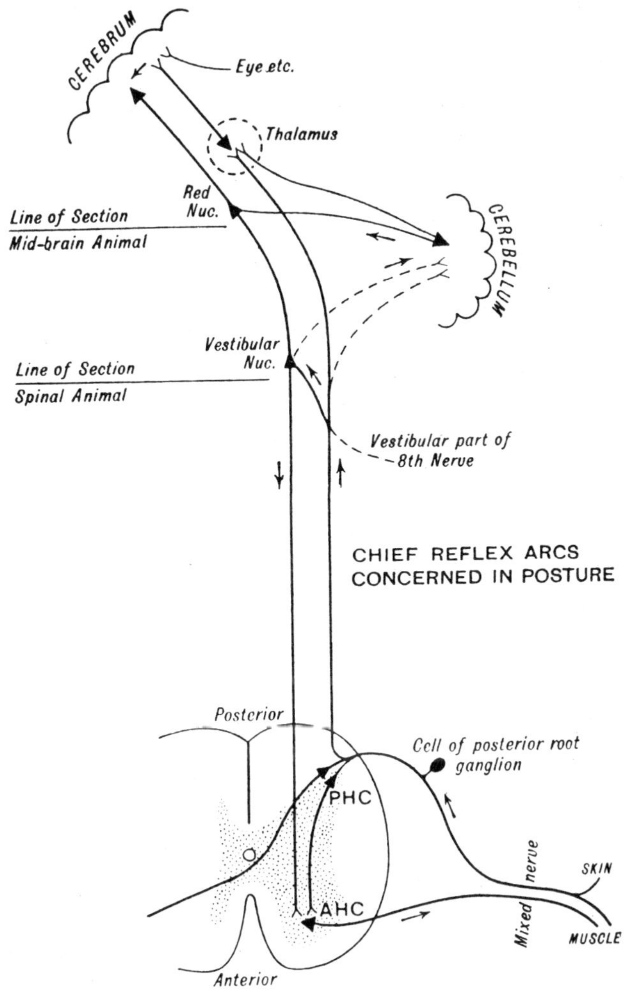

Fig. 7.7. The lower part of the figure shows a simple spinal reflex arc and the reflex pathways of the spinal animal. The upper part shows the arc responsible for decerebrate rigidity and the sources of the impulses from the red nucleus and the cerebrum which inhibit it. For convenience the vestibulo-spinal and pyramidal tracts are shown as fusing; also only one neurone is showing joining PHC and AHC. For simplicity also the sensory fiere entering the cord is shown dividing. The three branches are derived from three separate cells in the posterior root ganglion. Probably there is a chain of internuncial neurones with lateral connections at this point.

due to some release of the antigravity reflexes. If the animal is suspended there is an extensor rigidity not depending on stretch reflexes (Bard and Rioch).

Experiments on the decerebrate and thalamic animal, which we owe largely to the schools of Magnus in Utrecht and of Sherrington in Oxford, show that certain parts of the body bear a definite relation to each other in the maintenance of posture, and that when one part of the body is moved, a reflex alteration in tone changes the position of other parts of the body. Thus, if the neck is flexed, the fore-legs bend and the hind-legs extend, while the opposite occurs if the head is extended (i.e., a tonic work reflex occurs). Such movements, it is realised, take place together normally in the life of the animal when it is eating or looking up. Also if one leg is bent the other may extend as in walking. This is known as the crossed extension reflex. Similarly, if the head is turned to one side the limbs on that side show increased extensor tonus as if to support the weight of the body while the tonus of the opposite side decreases.

Thus we see that the central nervous system, as high up as the thalamus, is possessed of a very large degree of reflex activity which automatically promotes the interests of the animal.

Cortical Flexion.— As an animal comes out of certain anesthetics, e.g., avertin and sometimes either, it develops typical decerebrate rigidity. This, however, gives way to a flexor rigidity which is seen in the fore-limbs before the hind-limbs. It has been shown that this rigidity depends on the cerebral cortex, since it is absent if the cortex is removed (Blair and McDowall). The state is so like that present in a spinal animal that it may be suggested that it represents a group of higher protective reflexes. The phenomenon is important as it is so similar to the state of flexed fore-limbs and extended hind-limbs seen in cerebral hemorrhage in man. The so-called convulsions which occur occasionally during ether anaesthesia may be also similarly produced.

The Maintenance of Posture

The facts which have been given above show quite definitely that the maintenance of posture is purely a reflex phenomenon which does not involve the cerebrum or conscious effort. The experiments given above suggest that the muscular reflexes with which the nervous system of the elementary spinal animal is concerned are those of protection of the animal. With the greater development of locomotion are developed the anti-gravity reflexes which are exhibited by the decerebrate animal. Such extensor reflexes have arcs through the medulla and pons. They do not, however, depend, as used to be thought, on the cerebellum. Normally, however, these extensors appear to be held in check by a still higher set of reflexes involving the mid-brain. In the higher mammals this part of the brain is quite small, but in lower animals, especially those who have to maintain posture in a vertical as well as horizontal planes, e.g., birds and fishes, the so-called optic lobes of the mid-brain are more conspicuous than any other part of the brain. These are represented in the mammals by the corpora quadrigemina, which are quite small.

Muscular Co-ordination and the Maintenance of Equilibrium— Although posture and equilibrium are closely allied phenomena they are not quite identical. Equilibrium includes the maintenance of posture, but involves also maintenance of steadiness during muscular movement, such as walking. In this, the maintenance of proper co-ordination of muscular activity is essential. The reflexes concerned are very similar to those of posture, but, apparently, normally they involve to a greater extent the cerebellum and the semicircular canals.

Receptors and Reflexes Concerned in Posture and Equilibrium

The afferent impulses originates from the following four sources: skin; joints and muscles; retina; labyrinths.

In the accurate investigation of these reflexes decerebrate animals are used for the tonic postural reflexes, and thalamic animals for the righting reflexes. When one kind of receptor is being investigated it is necessary to exclude the others, e.g., by blindfolding, by removing the labyrinths, or by immobilising muscles.

1. *The Skin.*— Sherrington has shown how comparatively unimportant is the loss of tactile sensibility from the feet. A cat, in which the feet have been completely desensitised by division of nerves, can stand and walk without obvious inconvenience.

It has been shown, however, by Rademaker that certain body righting reflexes which tend to bring the body from the lateral to the normal position have their origin in the skin.

2. *The Muscles and Joints.*— We have already seen that stretching or taping of a muscle may originate nerve impulses. This occurs from the stretching or compression of the specialised nerve-endings, the tendon organs, and muscle spindles. The shortening reaction appears to depend on the tendon organs (Denny Brown) which, however, are not confined to the tendons as originally thought, while the lengthening reaction depends on the spindles. The spindles give rise to impulses by which we become aware of the movement and position of out muscles, but in this connection we are concerned with those impulses which do not reach consciousness. The fibers which carry the latter are off-shoots of the sensory fibers and reach the mid-brain and cerebellum *via* Clarke's column and the cerebellar and tecto-spinal tracts.

The reflexes which are set up are known as tonic and righting reflexes, which may arise from the muscles of the body or the neck. Some causes the body to follow the head (*neck righting reflexes*), others (*tonic neck reflexes*) cause a change in tone in certain muscles in accordance with the requirements of the head.

The difficulty experienced by quite normal persons in standing on one leg with the eyes shut is due to a reduction of the number of these impulses, for the same subjects with the eyes shut con stand quite easily on both legs; displacement of the centre of gravity, caused by standing on one leg, must however be taken into account. In many cases of tabes there is but little loss of tactile sensibility, and the condition of inco-ordination is chiefly due to the loss of impression from muscles and joints. In these cases, however, the sense of equilibrium is not lost; the man realises that he is unsteady.

3. *The Retina.*— The eyes are important sensory receptors in relation to posture and equilibrium.

They are the receptors of the *optical righting reflexes*. It can be shown that if a labyrinthectomised monkey be blindfolded and suspended in any position it makes no attempt to right itself, but does so as soon as the bandage is removed. The centres for such reflexes are in the occipital cortex.

The importance of the retina is increased when the other receptors are interfered with. This is well illustrated by the case of the tabetic who has deficient joint and muscle sense due to disease of the posterior nerve-roots; the visual postural reflexes have become educated to replace the diminished reflexes from the muscles, and directly the individual is deprived of them he becomes unsteady or even falls. This phenomenon is known as Romberg's sign. Since, however, the labyrinths are normal the subject is quite aware of his unsteadiness.

As has been indicated above, the capacity of an individual to stand on one leg depends, to a considerable extent, on impulses from the eyes. In some individuals the paralysis of accommodation by the instillation of atropine into the eyes causes interference with the maintenance of posture. This suggests that the actual focusing of objects is of special importance.

Bandaging of the eyes in animals often causes them to spin round and lose their balance. The giddiness experienced by many people on looking from a height or at moving water, or after the onset of a squint, or when objects are viewed under unusual circumstances, as in the ascent of a mountain railway, is due to the same thing. It should be understood that visual impressions in themselves are not the sole guide. It is the projection of what is seen in relation to the position of the body (ascertained by the innervation of the neck muscles and of the ocular muscles) which is the chief guide.

4. *The Labyrinth.*— An external view of the labyrinth, which is enclosed within the petrous portion of the temporal bone. The labyrinth consists of three parts— the vestibule (1), the three semicircular canals which open into the vestibule, and the tube, coiled like a snail's shell, called the cochlea. The cochlea is the part of the apparatus which is concerned in the reception of auditory impressions; it is supplied by the cochlear division of the eighth or auditory nerve. The remainder of the internal ear is concerned not in hearing but in the reception of the impressions we are now studying; it is supplied by the vestibular division of the eighth nerve. Within the vestibule are two chambers made of membrane, called the *utricle* and the *saccule*; these communicate with one another and with the canal of the cochlea (see Hearing). Within each bony canal is a membranous canal of similar shape. Each canal is filled with a watery fluid called endolymph, and separated from the bony canal by another fluid called *perilymph*. Each canal has a swelling at one end called the *ampulla*. The membranous canals open into the utricle at C, the *horizontal* canal by each of its ends; the *superior* and *posterior* vertical canals by three openings, these two canals being connected at their non-ampullary ends.

The membranous canal consists of three layers: the outer layer is fibrous and continuous with the periosteum that lines the bony canal; then comes the *tunica propria*, composed of homogeneous material, and thrown into papillae except just where the attachment of the membranous to the bony canal is closest; the innermost layer is a somewhat flattened epithelium.

At the ampulla there is a different appearance; the tunica propria is raised into a hillock called the *crista acustica*; the cells of the epithelium become columnar in shape, and to some of them fibers of the eighth nerve pass, arborising round them; these cells are provided with stiff hairs, which project into what is called the *cupula*, a mass of mucus-like material. Between the hair-cells are fiber-cells which act as supports. When the pressure of the endolymph in the interior of the canals is altered, the hairs of the hair-cells are affected, and a nervous impulse is set up in the contiguous nerve-fibers, which carry it to the central nervous system. The stimulation of the hairs is brought about by the movements of the endolymph.

The Function of the Otolithic Cavities

Since the position of the head is of such importance in maintaining posture, a special mechanism has been developed within the utricle and saccule which is affected by gravity and in which impulses are set up which are carried to the brain also by the vestibular nerve.

In each saccule and utricle is the macula, resembling the crista acusticae of the semicircular canals, but in addition there are entangled in the hairs of the hair-cells

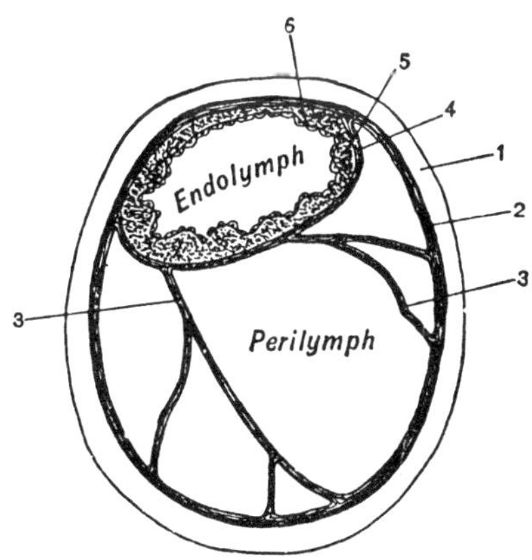

Fig. 7.8. Section of human semicircular canal. (After Rudinger.) 1, Bone; 2, periosteum; 3, 3, fibrous bands connecting the periosteum to 4, the outer fibrous coat of the membranous canal; 5, tunica propria; 6, epithelium.

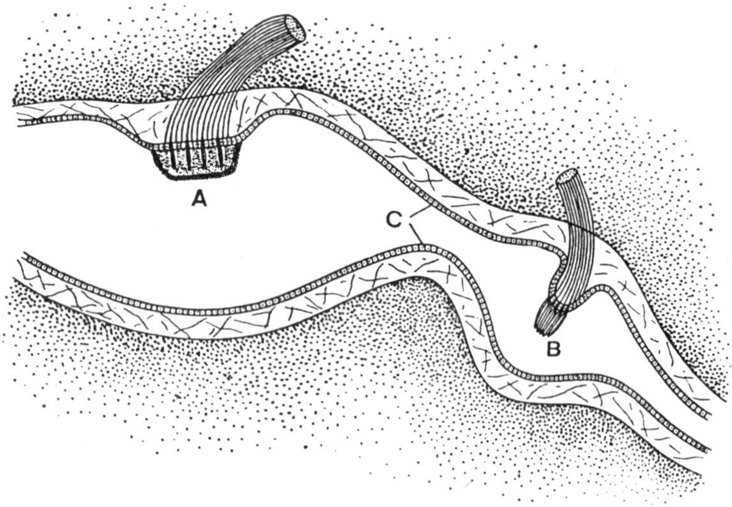

Fig. 7.9. (See text.)

calcareous bodies known as *otoliths*, which stimulate the hairs by pulling. The function of an otolithic cavity was first discovered in the crayfish, whose cavity is open to the exterior and which replaces the otoliths periodically by grains of sand; when Kreidl replaced the sand by iron filings and approached the animal with a magnet, the animal could be made to turn somersaults or to adopt any position, according to the direction of pull of the magnet. In the mammal, definite alterations in the tone of muscles are caused by change in position of the head, even when the reflexes due to stretching of the neck muscles are excluded by fixing the neck in plaster of Paris. The reflexes from the labyrinths have a longer latent period than those from the neck; the effects from neck and labyrinth are summated.

The reflexes are of two categories: (1) *tonic labyrinthine reflexes* which are shown by the decerebrate animal and which relate the position of the body and limbs to that of the head. These depend on the utricle whose otoliths lie above the horizontal maculae, and (2) *labyrinthine righting reflexes* which are shown by the thalamic animal and which are concerned with maintaining the head in the normal position in relation to the earth's surface. If the body is moved in such an animal, the head is automatically righted. The asymmetric righting reflexes depend on the saccules whose otoliths lie lateral to the vertical maculae; the symmetrical righting reflexes arise probably in both utricles and saccules.

After bilateral destruction of the labyrinth an animal soon recovers from the effect of the operation, because of its visual postural reflexes; but certain functions are never recovered. The cat, for example, never regains its proverbial power of falling on its feet if thrown from a height, and ceases to be able to rise to the surface and swim when thrown into water.

The function of the otolithic cavities only may be destroyed by centrifuging the animal, a procedure which causes it to be unable to regain its posture, but it may still respond to some extend to sudden movement of the head as the semicircular canals act normally. The otolithic cavities may then be looked upon as the organs of static equilibrium.

> The *vestibular nerve* arises from the bipolar cells of the ganglion of *Scarpa*, which is situated in the internal auditory meatus. The peripheral axons ramify among the hair-cells of the epithelium in the utricle, saccule, and semicircular canals. The central axons enter a collection of small nerve-cells between the restiform body and the descending root of the fifth; this is termed the *principal nucleus*; here they bifurcate; the descending branches run towards the lower part of the bulb, and arborise round the cells of the neighbouring grey matter (descending vestibular nucleus). The ascending branches pass upwards, some to the cerebrum, but most by the restiform body to the cerebellum; in their course they give off many collaterals which form synapses with the cells of two nuclei near the outer angle of the ventricular floor, known as the *nucleus of Deiters* and *nucleus of Bechterew*. The fibers which arise from Deiters's nucleus pass into the posterior longitudinal bundles of both sides; those which start in *Bechterew's nucleus* become longitudinal, but their destination is uncertain.

The Function of the Semicircular Canals

It will be noticed that the canals on each side are in three planes at right angles to each other, and we learn the movements of the heat with regard to the three dimensions of space by means of impressions from the ampullary endings of the vestibular nerve; these impressions are set up by the varying pressure of the endolymph in the ampullae.

Thus a sudden turning of the head from right to left will cause movement of the endolymph towards, and therefore increased pressure on, the hair-cells connected to the ampullary nerve-endings of the left horizontal canal, and diminished pressure on the corresponding apparatus of the right side. It is probable that resulting from such a movement two impulses reach the brain, one the effect of increased pressure in one ampulla, the second the effect to decreased pressure in its fellow. It may even be that increased pressure on one side of a crista is accompanied by diminished pressure on the opposite face of the same crista.

"One canal can be affected by and transmit the sensation of rotation about one axis in one direction only; and for complete perception of rotation in any direction about any axis, six canals are required in three pairs, each pair being in the same or parallel planes, and their ampullae turned opposite ways. Each pair would thus be sensitive to any rotation about a line at right angles to its plane or planes, the one canal being influenced by rotation in one direction, the other by rotation in the opposite direction."

The two horizontal canals are in the same plane; the posterior vertical of one side is in a plane parallel to that of the superior vertical of the other side.

When these canals are diseased in man, as in Menière's disease, there are disturbances of equilibrium: a feeling of giddiness, which may lead to the patient's falling down, is associated with nausea and vomiting. In animals similar results are produced by injury, and the subject has been chiefly worked out on birds by Flourens, where the canals are large and readily exposed, and in fishes by Lee.

Thus, if the horizontal canal is divided in a pigeon, the head is thrown into a series of oscillations in a horizontal plane, which are increased by section of the corresponding canal of the opposite side. After section of the vertical canals, the forced movements are in a vertical plane, and the animal tends to turn somersaults.

"When the whole of the canals are destroyed on both sides the disturbances of equilibrium are of the most pronounced character. Goltz describes a pigeon so treated

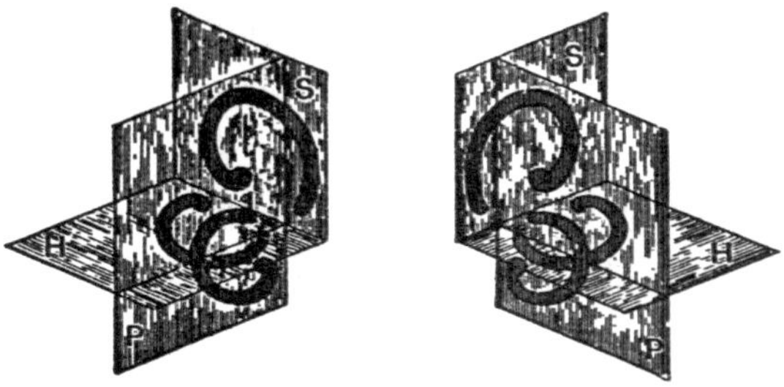

Fig. 7.10. Diagram of semicircular canals, to show their positions in three planes at right angles to each other. It will be seen that the two horizontal canals (H) lie in the same plane: and that the superior vertical of one side (S) lies in a plane parallel to that of the posterior vertical (P) of the other. (The student will understand that, though in the diagram the canals are entirely separated from one another, they are really connected.)

which always kept its head with the occiput touching the breast, the vertex directed downwards, with the right eye looking to the left and the left looking to the right, the head being incessantly swung in a pendulum-like manner. It can neither stand, nor lie still, nor fly, nor maintain any fixed attitude. It executes violent somersaults, now forwards, now backwards, rolls round and round, or springs in the air and falls back to recommence anew. It is necessary to envelop the animals in some soft covering to prevent them dashing themselves to pieces by the violence of their movements, and even then not always with success. The extreme agitation is manifest only during the first few days following the operation, and the animal may then be set free without danger; but it is still unable to stand or walk, and tumultuous movements come on from the slightest disturbance. After the lapse of a fortnight it is able to maintain its upright position. At this stage it resembles an animal painfully learning, to stand and walk. In this it relies mainly on its vision, and it is only necessary to cover the eyes with a hood to dispel all the fruits of this new education, and cause the reappearance of all the motor disorders."

It is these canals which enable the individual to know in which direction he is being moved, even though the eyes are bandaged, and the feet are not allowed to touch the ground. On being whirled round, such a person knows in which direction he is being moved, and feels that he is moving so long as the rate of rotation varies, but when the whirling stops he seems, especially if he opens his eyes, to be whirling in the opposite direction, probably owing to the rebound of the fluid in the canals. The forced movements just described in animals are due both to the absence of the normal sensations from the canals and to delusive sensations arising from the irritation, and the animal makes efforts to correct the movement which it imagines it is being subjected to.

It has been found possible by Adrian to record from the vestibular nucleus impulses set up by movement of the semicircular canals. A canal appears to be stimulated by movement in one direction only, but sometimes a resting discharge has been recorded which is abolished by movement in the other direction.

The impulses which co-ordinate reflex movements of the head, neck, and eyes are carried by the posterior longitudinal bundle which connects the nuclei of the cranial nerves with each other and the anterior horn cells of the spinal nerves.

The semicircular canals are then essentially the organs for the maintenance of dynamic equilibrium. There is some evidence that the semi-circular canals may take a greater part in maintaining static equilibrium than has hitherto been supposed, and in support of this it has been found photographically that in the standing position there is usually, if not always, a swaying movement of the head.

Lower Nervous Mechanisms Involved in Co-ordinated Movements

It will be understood that such mechanisms are not confined to the spinal cord but are concerned in the activities of those parts of the brain-stem which control the muscles of the head. A fuller description is given by Creed, Denny-Brown, Eccles, Liddell, and Sherrington, 1932.

Reciprocal Innervation of Antagonistic Muscles.— When a muscle is stimulated reflexly so as to flex a joint it is evident that the extensor muscles must at the same time become elongated. This elongation is not a passive phenomenon but is an active relaxation of the muscle which, is always in a state of tonus or partial contraction. This may be shown experimentally by separating, say, the tendons flexing and extending the knee-joint and attaching them to levers. The levers must be sufficiently weighted to stretch the muscles so that their tone may be kept up reflexly by the stretch reflex or shortening reaction. If, then, the knee is caused to be flexed by stimulating an afferent nerve of the same side it will be found that there is a lengthening of the extensor muscle. Thus there is, as first shown by Sherrington, reciprocal action between the flexors and extensors. There is, however, a very marked degree of grading between the two activities. According to Graham Brown the sum of the relaxation and the contraction is equal, the relaxation being graded to the contraction by some central mechanism.

In every voluntary act there is this reciprocal contraction and relaxation of antagonistic muscles. In some persons the relaxation of the deltoid muscle can be felt if the elbow is supported on the arm of a chair and the limb is actively pressed against the side.

Sometimes this reciprocal arrangement gets thrown out of gear. This occurs in strychnine poisoning and in lockjaw. When the unfortunate patient tries to open his mouth the stronger muscles which ought to relax contract at the same time and the jaw is fixed. Death occurs from asphyxia because the respiratory muscles go into spasm and fix the thorax as a result of the failure of the reciprocal mechanisms.

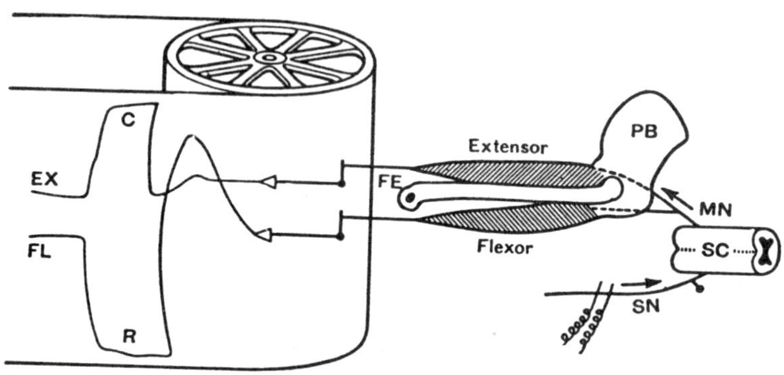

Fig. 7.11. Diagram to illustrate reciprocal innervation. The flexor and extensor muscles of the thigh are attached to levers as indicated and the femur FE and the pelvic bone PB firmly held. When a sensory nerve of the opposite side is stimulated the extensor contracts but the flexor relaxes.

It is suggested by Gasser (1937) that the inhibition is produced at certain cells by very rapidly travelling impulses which are capable of producing a subnormal phase such as occurs in peripheral nerve.

Of course by volition it is possible to contract flexors and extensors simultaneously.

The Principle of the Common Path and of Convergence.— When a muscle is made to contract reflexly the impulse which starts at the point of stimulation uses a path which can only be used by similar impulses arising from a given region of the body. It is a private path. When, however, the impulse reaches the spinal cord it uses paths used by impulses from other regions, and when it reaches the anterior horn cells through which it is finally effective it is said to use the *Final Common Path* from the motoneurone pool to the muscles concerned. This is a public path upon which all impulses intended to reach any given muscle must converge. Upon this path converge not only afferent impulses arising from the periphery but the impulses which arise in the higher parts of the brain and are concerned in voluntary activity.

It is evident that occasions must arise in which there is competition, as it were, for the final common path.

For the investigation of such a problem, the *"scratch reflex"* of the dog is one that lends itself admirably. This can best be studied in the "spinal" dog, that is in a dog in which cerebral influence is shut off by division of the spinal cord in the lower cervical region. If the skin over a large saddle-shaped area covering the shoulders and back is gently scratched or stimulated with a weak faradic current on one side, the hind leg of the same side executes scratching movements, which involve flexor muscles principally. The scratch reflex is a movement by which an animal presumably rids itself of irritating insects.

When, however, the foot is stimulated the impulses set up, if noxious, take precedence in the final common path and the scratch reflex is inhibited.

The factors which are chiefly concerned in determining predominance in the final common path are (1) strength of stimulus; (2) importance of the stimulus in relation to survival: severe pain, for example, usually dominates; (3) fatigue, however, reduces the power of dominance of a given stimulus.

The final common path is also used by a variety of reflexes, for in the language of the Oxford School "there is no reason to believe that the crossed extensor and the stretch reflex each possess a private motoneurone pool"; that is to say, the same groups of cells in the anterior horn of the spinal cord are used by a variety of stimuli arising from different sources.

Reinforcement.— Instances of reinforcing action may be found; for example, if two points of the skin of one shoulder are stimulated with a very feeble current, neither stimulus alone may be sufficient to evoke the scratch reflex, but the two together may elicit it; in order to attain this result the two points of skin must be fairly close together. Further detail is obtainable from Creed and others.

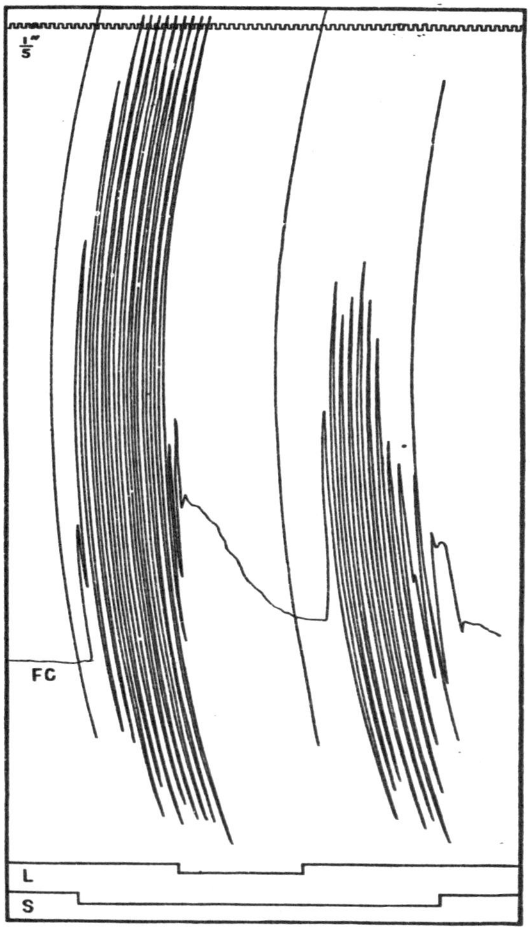

Fig. 7.12. The scratch reflex. Tracing of the flexors of left hip evoked by stimulation of the skin of the shoulder. The depression in the signal line S indicates the commencement of the stimulation, and its rise the termination. While this was going on, the left foot was stimulated, and the depression of the signal line L indicates the duration of this stimulation; during the stimulation of the foot, and for a short time afterwards, the scratch reflex is inhibited, but the scratch reflex returns soon afterwards. The time is registered in fifths of seconds. To be read from left to right.

The Phenomena of Excitation and Inhibition

The problem of excitation in the central nervous system is similar to that of the peripheral excitation of a muscle by a nerve and has already been discussed.

Present evidence suggests that an effective stimulus sets up a self-propagating action potential in a nerve which liberates acetylcholine at its ending and so stimulates the cells with which it synapses. The occurrence of what are known as central excitatory or inhibitory states suggests that an accumulation of such a chemical mediator may occur. It is possible that acetylcholine may also be responsible for inhibitory states, for minute amounts applied for some time and large amounts both produce inhibition. So also do choline and potassium, and both of these are liberated during activity. The phenomenon of inhibition is seen peripherally and centrally.

Peripheral Inhibition.—We have already noted that stimulation of the vagus produces an inhibition which is now known to be produced through the mediation of a chemical substance, acetylcholine. Inhibition of the intestine by the splanchnic nerve is similarly brought about by the production of an adrenaline-like substance. Many other drugs have inhibitory actions.

Central Inhibition.— This is seen to occur in the scratch reflex, the cross extensor reflex, the conditioned reflexes, and many others, but whether it is really similar in natural peripheral excitation and inhibition is not yet certain.

A central inhibition of the knee-jerk can also be produced, and it can be shown that it is much easier to inhibit the knee-jerk of a spinal animal than that of a decerebrate animal.

In relation to conditioned reflexes below we shall see that whatever the nature of inhibition it is an active process, while the action of strychnine, which we have noted in relation to reciprocal innervation, suggests that it is a chemical process.

The extremely rapid action of the nervous system makes it difficult to imagine that the accumulation and disappearance of chemical substances are concerned. Yet all the available evidence indicates that changes of a physico-chemical nature take place, and certainly the disappearance of acetylcholine is extremely rapid.

It can, for example, be shown that when an afferent impulse reaches the motor cell of a reflex arc a central excitatory state is set up. It is capable of summation as a result of a succession of subminimal stimuli along the same afferent nerve or of different nerves. Further, the application of one effective stimulus may reduce the central reflex time of another, and when a certain degree of excitation has accumulated it discharges. There is evidence, however, that the discharge may vary in rate, and it is suggested that muscle activity may be graded thereby. It is indeed possible to discharge the motor cell artificially by stimulating its axon and causing an impulse to pass up to cell in the wrong direction. After-discharge can thereby be prevented. The rate of discharge can be measured by recording the electrical variation of the muscle and the gradation of muscle activity (or the relative number of motor units thrown into activity) ascertained by finding the tension up by the muscle.

It may be shown that there can in the same way be a summation of a central inhibitory state. This, however, is more persistent than C.E.S. (central excitatory state), and is not discharged by "antidromic" impulses.

As already mentioned, it has been suggested by Gasser that central inhibition is due to the production of a subnormal phase in motor cells such as occurs in peripheral nerve, and this view receives considerable support from the work of Eccles who, in studying the electrical response of ganglia, has shown that the occurrence of after-potential is related to the excitatory state as in the case of nerve-fibers. Details of this difficult subject are found in a review by Eccles (see references), but it will be seen that it is very difficult to reconcile this electrical view of excitation with that of chemical transmission at the synapses.

We must assume that in the delicate co-ordinated movements of which our muscles are capable and in which, as we have seen, the cerebellum, etc., are concerned, the mechanisms of excitation and inhibition are likewise intimately concerned. For example, when we bend the elbow the inhibition of the extensors must be delicately tuned to the excitation of the flexors.

Rhythmical Activity

In many parts of the nervous system rhythmic activity is seen. The best known, perhaps, are those of the respiratory centres, the scratch reflex just described, and that of stepping. In the case of the ankle clonus we have seen that it is dependent on tension on the calf muscles being maintained. Generally, however, the phasing of rhythmic movements is not caused by afferent stimuli, although they may regulate them, for they occur if the afferent pathways are cut. The rhythmicity depends on some inherent central mechanism not yet understood.

Conditioned Reflexes

In this variety of reflex we have the participation of the cerebral cortex and apparently of consciousness in its information, and it is so called because it depends on training or conditioning for its establishment. Conditioned reflexes are not inborn, like the reflexes we have hitherto been considering, but have become acquired by the animal during its life-time. Our knowledge of these reflexes we owe largely to Pavlov, who has placed their study on an experimental basis. His classic experiment is well known. He showed that if a bell was rung each time food was given to a hungry dog, eventually the dog secreted saliva when it heard the bell although food was not presented. The showing of the food to the dog constitutes the *unconditioned stimulus*, the ringing of the bell the *conditioned stimulus*. The fact that a dog will secrete salvia when food is offered is well known, and may be looked upon as an inborn or unconditioned reflex; but it has now been shown that practically any stimulus not involving serious hurt to the animal, and provided it begins to act slightly before the normal activity, may, if it occurs simultaneously with the normal stimulus, become the conditioned stimulus. Even the cessation of a stimulus, e.g., of the ringing of a bell, may act as a stimulus. The sight of the syringe used for the injection of apomorphine is eventually sufficient to cause vomiting although no actual injection is made. Failure, however, to follow the conditioned by the unconditioned stimulus leads to weakening and eventually to *loss* or *extinction* of the reflex. Even allied reflexes are affected, a fact which indicates that the extinction is an active inhibitory process. A conditioned reflex may become established in relation to any reflex activity of the animal, even to the knee-jerk, but for the sake of simplicity most of the work has been carried out in relation to the secretion of salvia. For more accurate work the duct of a salivary gland is brought to surface, so that the saliva can be easily collected and measured.

It is evident that in the formation of a conditioned reflex two processes occur, namely, an analysis of the stimulus which takes place in the cerebrum which with the appropriate afferent nerve and nerve-ending comprises the analyser, and an association of the conditioned and unconditioned stimulus. If the appropriate part of the cortex is removed, e.g., the temporal areas in a case in which the conditioned stimulus is a sound, the reflex disappears. This experiment is important, as it indicates that the reflex does not dependent on any short-circuiting mechanism through lower centres as has been suggested.

Conditioned reflexes are of interest as they offer a method of investigation of the analysers and the power of the lower animals to differentiate between different kinds and intensities of stimuli; for example, it has been shown that a dog can differentiate between half tones on the piano. It has been possible also by their study to show that the power of localising the side from which a sound comes depends on integrity of the corpus callosum which joins the two cerebral hemispheres.

Conditioned reflexes show many of the characteristics of reflexes generally. Thus there may be *summation* from the addition of two conditioned stimuli. There may also be *spread,* but in this case it is in the area stimulated. If there is a localised conditioned stimulus from the skin, other near-by areas may subsequently give a similar response. Somewhat akin to this phenomenon is that of *linking,* in which it is found that if a reflex has become established to one sound it is much more easy to establish a second reflex from another sound.

Repetition plays a very important part in conditioned reflexes. It is not only necessary for the formation of the reflex but is essential for its maintenance, otherwise the reflex tends to *decay*. It is, however, readily reinforced by repetition of the procedure following up the conditioned by the unconditioned stimulus.

Conditioned reflexes are liable to be inhibited or stopped in certain circumstances. If, for example, an extraneous noise is heard this may cause a temporary *external inhibition* of the reflex. For this reason the animal is arranged in the special room indicated in the illustration and is observed indirectly through a system of mirrors or a periscope. If, however, the stimulus is harmful and affects the same region as the conditioned stimulus, the inhibition may be permanent. It is to be noted that the animals experimented upon are on the friendliest possible terms with the observers.

It has been found that a considerable interval may occur between the conditioned and the unconditioned stimulus, provided the former is applied first. A dog may thus be taught to secrete salvia half an hour after a bell is rung (i.e., inhibition of delay). This is known as a *trace reflex*. In the interval some definitely active inhibition must be present to prevent the stimulus from acting, since the introduction of an extraneous stimulus

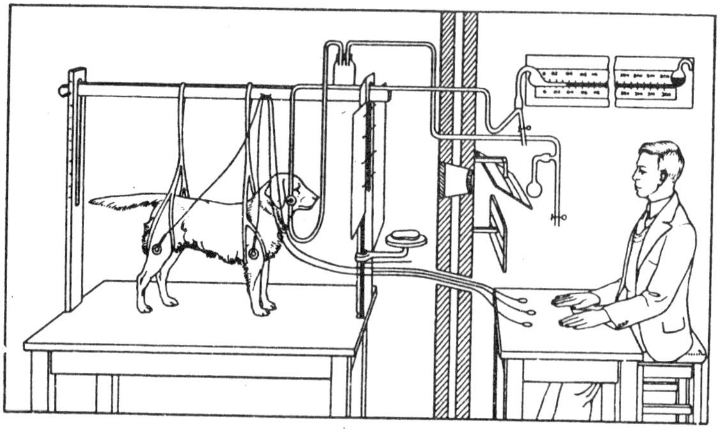

Fig. 7.13. Pavlov conditional reflex.

during the interval causes an immediate flow. If, however, in the interval, another stimulus is applied which the dog has been taught to associate with no food, it is found that an inhibition of the conditioned reflex has been produced, and that the latter cannot be elicited again for some time. This we call a *conditioned inhibition*, or if the animal has had to differentiate carefully between the positive and negative stimuli, *differential inhibition*. Conditioned leads to *extinction* of the reflex, a fact which is of considerable practical importance in relation to undesirable habits in children. When mustard is put on the fingers of a child which sucks its fingers it obtains the reverse of satisfaction from putting its fingers in its mouth and ceases to do so. All forms of inhibition other than those caused by extraneous stimuli are known as *internal inhibition*, since they involve an active inhibitory process. Evidence indicates that this inhibition occurs in the cerebral cortex. Further, it is found that if an inhibitory stimulus is repeated its after-effects may be summated, the inhibition may involve larger areas of the cerebral cortex, and other conditioned reflexes may become affected. Not only so, but the inhibition may spread more generally and the animal appears to go to sleep. Pavlov suggests that such sleep is closely related to hypnotic and normal sleep, which according to this view, is due to accumulated inhibition or the receipt of stimuli which are related to cessation of activity.

Dogs may be trained to fall asleep on a table when a dim light is switched on. This involves an enormous amount of patient work, which consists of caressing the animal, preferably when it is tired, during a period of several months when the room is lit only by the dim light. The process is akin to the singing of a lullaby to young children or rocking a cradle. In man the observance of time of night, the ceremony of preparing for bed, provide examples of similar stimuli and are of great value in promoting sleep. Experimental sleep is also very likely to occur in animals during differential inhibition, by repetition of thermal stimuli or during the interval between the application of a conditioned and its associated unconditioned stimulus as in the trace reflex. The sleep produced may be very profound and during it the animal is remarkably irresponsive to stimulation. The inhibition may involve limited areas of cortex, and an inhibition produced in one analyser may spread to another adjacent, and even the motor cortex may become involved. In man also we know that sleep may be similarly patchy, and that many activities, e.g., walking, hearing, even reasoning, may take place during sleep.

Many attempts have been made to make diagrams of possible new paths being laid down and of short-circuits formed. Such diagrams are more fanciful than useful, since the amount of exact information on such subjects in negligible. It seems indeed more probable not that new paths exist separately, but that they are merely different from the old in that the impulses pass along them at too great a rate to affect consciousness. There is now evidence, however, that it is possible to establish conditioned reflexes in dogs in which the cerebrum has been removed. In these, other parts of the brain have become the analysers, but they can only appreciate comparatively crude stimuli.

Of interest appears to be the importance of *coincidence in time* in the formation of conditioned reflexes. Since a nerve impulse is self-propagating it is reasonably possible that two impulses arising at the same time in different parts of the body may eventually meet. It may be that this hitherto little appreciated point may be of fundamental importance in relation to the formation of conditioned reflexes.

It is evident that the learning of so-called tricks by the lower animals must depend on similar mechanisms. It may be that many of the problems of memory do so also, for we can readily say that the dog "remembers" the association of the conditioned with the unconditioned stimulus.

It is but a step from the conditioned reflexes just described to the phenomenon of acquiring habits or habitual actions, such as are involved in learning to ride a bicycle or drive a motor-car. The movements are, in the first instance, acquired as a result of conscious effort, but subsequently become reflex in nature and no longer involve such effort. Until we attempt to write or use a knife and fork with the unaccustomed hands, we scarcely realise how many of our actions are reflex in character. In relation to posture, for example, we have a large number of inborn reflexes, but in addition to these we may by practice acquire a vast number of others, our total capability in relation to postural equilibrium being a combination of the inborn and the acquired. How far some of the still higher activities of the brain may be held to be a similar summation of inborn and acquired characteristics leads into the realm of psychology, which is outside our present province.

The Role of Heredity.— It is of interest to observe at this point that in spite of many experiments no evidence has been obtained that conditioned reflexes can be inherited.

In these experiments the remarkable discovery was made that puppies do not appear to have any hereditary preference for meat. That is, however, not to say that the influence of heredity may not be important in determining the ease with which certain reflexes may become established. It is well recognised that it is easier to train some horses and dogs than others, while bad traits in horses are often clearly hereditary. Some can be trained in certain duties and not in others. This is true also of humans.

Pavlov has be enable to differentiate between different kinds of nervous systems in regard to the ease with which excitatory and inhibitory states may be formed. Some are well balanced, others less so; he draws attention to similar differences which occur in human temperaments.

Some very interesting observation in this relation have been made on animals which appear to throw light on human behaviour. For example, when an animal has acquired a positive response to an object of circular form and a negative one to an ellipse, great irritability and rest-lessness are observed if an object intermediate in shape is used. The state produced is comparable to that of neurasthenia in man, or the irritability produced when one is unable "to make up one's mind."

In the ellipse experiment just mentioned, while some animals become irritable, some may fall asleep while others appear indifferent.

The Biological Function of Conditioned Reflexes

It is easy to develop a whole philosophy on the basis of conditioned reflexes, and to make out a case for the greater part of human behaviour being dependent on the development of such reflexes. This has been done by Pavlov and by Waston in what is known as the Behavourist School of Psychology; its views have, rightly, not received general acceptance, although they explain more than at first sight seems possible.

The importance of conditioned reflexes to the animal is that they constitute the basis of learning and give a greatly increased significance to sensations, and in this way give the animal a greater appreciation of its environment. Thus it may be forewarned of danger, and the acquisition of food is also facilitated.

In civilised communities the establishment of positive and negative reflexes makes community life possible through the medium of restraints and conventions of which that of language is the most important, since it makes possible the conveyance of ideas from one person to another.

8

Neurophysiology & Disorders

Autonomic Functions and Their Regulation

The autonomic nervous system continuously provides motor signals which control the functions of the visceral organs, glands, and blood vessels in such a manner that a physiologically constant internal environment is maintained throughout the lifetime of the individual. In turn this homeostasis is initiated through a vast array of sensory inputs which impinge upon the preganglionic neurons of the autonomic nerves so that the signal outputs of these neurons are stimulated to a continuous state of activity which, however, exhibits marked quantitative fluctuations with time. These fluctuations in turn depend upon the particular internal and external conditions at any given moment.

The general functions of the autonomic nervous system are revealed to some extent by artificial stimulation of particular sympathetic and parasympathetic nerves. However, the in vivo roles of many autonomic reflexes, as well as certain bodily responses which have important autonomic components, are best discussed in detail in context with the particular organ systems with which these reflexes and responses are related. Consequently the following presentation will be limited for the most part of a survey of a number of important autonomic and related effects as they occur in vivo, and thus this discussion will provide the reader with a summary of, and an introduction to, the more detailed considerations of individual autonomic reflexes and related automatic responses which follow throughout the remainder of this text.

Like the somatic nervous system, the autonomic nervous system exhibits a hierarchy of levels within the central nervous system at which vesceral functions are integrated. Thus many simple autonomic functions are integrated wholly within the spinal cord whereas particular higher brain centers are essential for the integration of the more complex autonomic responses. For example, the spinal animal exhibits a normal blood pressure at rest, and coordinated reflex contractions of the full rectum or bladder can take place in a relatively normal manner. On the other hand, the more complex visceral reflexes which regulate the pupillary responses to light as well as those underlying pupillary accommodation for distance are integrated within the midbrain.

The medulla oblongata and the hypothalamus are two particularly important regions of the central nervous system that are linked inseparably to the integration of many complex autonomic responses as well as to several complex physiologic processes that have autonomic components. Thy hypothalamus, in addition to its major role in the regulation of a number of autonomic functions, also operates together with the limbic system as a physiologic unit, a unit which provides the neurologic substrate for emotional responses as well as innate (or instinctual) behavior.

Visceral Responses and the Medulla Oblongata. The term *vital centers* is applied to those regions located within the medulla which are responsible for regulating the tone of the blood vessels (i.e., vasomotor control), the heart rate, the force of myocardial contractions, and the process of respiration. Thus damage or injury to the cardiovascular and/or respiratory centers generally is fatal.

The afferent fibers that send inputs to the vital centers of the medulla usually originate in highly specialized mechano- and chemoreceptors. Thus, for example, the receptors of the aortic and carotid sinuses as well as the aortic and carotid bodies transmit afferent signals which result in extremely delicate, precise, and graded motor adjustments insofar as heart rate and caliber of the blood vessels are concerned. Furthermore it appears that certain specialized receptor elements may be located within the medulla per se.

The medullary region of the brain stem also contains of the neural centers which integrate a number of autonomic reflexes in addition to those outlined above. Coughing, sneezing, swallowing gagging, and vomiting all are complex responses that are integrated within the medulla oblongata. It is important to note that some of these reflexes have voluntary as well as autonomic components. For example, the swallowing reflex is elicited by the voluntary propulsion of a mass of food or liquid toward the back of the pharynx, at which point this mechanical stimulation induces the fully automatic swallowing reflex proper.

Visceral Responses and the Hypothalamus. The principal hypothalamic functions range from the integration of relatively straight forward visceral reflexes to extremely complex behavioral and emotional responses. Nonetheless, in all of these processes the hypothalamus serves as the major physiologic integrative center, and in every case a clear-cut stimulus-response is evident. Stimulation of the hypothalamus under experimental conditions will evoke certain autonomic responses to be discussed below; however it also appears that many normal autonomic functions which are elicited in vivo by hypothalamic excitation are components of more complex physiologic reactions, and that the hypothalamus initiates such autonomic responses secondarily to the onset of certain emotional states, e.g., fear and rage.

Experimental stimulation of the anterior superior hypothalamic region (as well as many other areas of the hypothalamus) may induce contraction of the urinary bladder, and for this reason a so-called parasympathetic center was postulated to lie within the anterior hypothalamus. However, hypothalamic excitation produces few other clear-cut parasympathetic reactions so that the experimental evidence in favor of the existence of a hypothalamic "parasympathetic center" remains unconvincing.

On the other hand, artificial excitation of other hypothalamic areas, particularly the lateral regions, evokes pupillary dilatation, hypertension, and erection of the hairs (piloerection) among other characteristic adrenergic responses. In vivo, however, this pattern of diffuse adrenergic response does not result from afferent regulatory signals that arise within the viscera per se; rather such a response is evoked by emotional stimuli, particularly fear and rage. Such adrengergic reactions also are touched off by appropriate thermal stimulation (i.e., an extremely cold environment). and thus form part of the overall physiologic mechanism that is concerned with thermoregulation.

Dilatation of the blood vessels in skeletal muscle has been observed following stimulation of the dorsal region of the hypothalamus in the midline. This experimental finding, taken in conjunction with other evidence, tends to support the conclusion that the hypothalamus may be a component in the sympathetic vasodilator system that has its origin in the cerebral cortex, and such a cholinergic motor system has been implicated as the physiologic mechanism responsible for dilatation of the blood vessels within the skeletal muscles that takes place immediately following the onset of exercise.

When the dorsomedial and posterior hypothalamic areas are stimulated, an increased secretion of catecholamines (i.e., epinephrine and norepinephrine) takes place in the adrenal medualla. Such an enhanced adrenal meduallary secretion is a basic physiologic characteristic that accompanies the emotions of fear and rage, and this response in vivo also may be related to excitation of the sympathetic vasodilator system.

The physiologic mechanisms whereby the hypothalamus integrates the secretion of a number of endocrine substances (or hormones). The mechanism whereby secretion of the catecholamines, vasopressin, oxytocin, thyrotropin, adrenocortioctropic hormone, follicle-stimulating hormone, prolactin, and somatotropin is regulated by the hypothalamus will be discussed in context with each specific hormone.

The hypothalamus also has been implicated as a factor that is involved in the physiologic states of wakefulness and sleep. As an examination of these functional states is wholly inseparable from a consideration of the reticular activating system and other neural elements. The possible role of the hypothalamus in wakefulness and sleep will be presented as an integral part of the discussion of these functional states. Similarly, as the physiologic interactions between the hypothalamus and the limbic system are so intimate, the roles of these neuronals pools in certain behavioral states will be discussed.

The remainder of this discussion will be concerned with a consideration of the three so-called apetitive functions with which the hypothalamus is concerned directly. These functions, are thirst, hunger, and sexual behavior. Actually these fundamental drives evoke patterns of activity which involve many organ systems in addition to the hypothalamus, systems whose activation leads to complex behavioral responses on the part of the individual, which is turn lead to amelioration or satiation of the basic drive. Actually, therefore, the sensation of thirst merely provides a physiologic stimulus whereby a net deficit of water in the body is corrected and thereby homeostatic balance is restored through the ingestion of fluid. Similarly, hunger leads to food-seeking behavior and the consumption of food so that bodily energy stores are maintained.

Thirst and the Regulation of Water Balance. "Thirst" may be defined as a sensation which is referred to the mouth and pharyngeal region and is associated with a craving for liquids. Usually this sensation is associated with a desire for water. Thus a localized dryness of the oral mucosa per se is related to the sensation of thirst; therefore a certain relief from this sensation can be achieved by sucking a damp cloth or an ice cube. Experimental animals (rats) with induced lesions in the areas of the hypothalamus that control drinking behavior will ingest small quantities of water when their pharyngeal mucosa becomes dry, although a generalized tissue dehydration per se no longer is an effective stimulus to induce drinking.

The central neural mechanism that regulates water intake is located within the hypothalamus. A large tract of unmyelinated nerve fibers has its origin in neurons whose cell bodies are located within the supraoptic and paraventricular nuclei of the hypothalamus. This hypothalamohypophyseal tract courses through the median eminence and stalk of the pituitary, then terminates in the neural lobe of the hypophysis. The hypothalamohypophyseal tract has a critical physiologic role in the production and release of the hormones of the posterior pituitary. In humans, *antidiuretic hormone* (sometimes also called *vasopressin;*) is the most important endocrine substance that is elaborated by the posterior pituitary. Antidiuretic hormone stimulates the reabsorption of water into the bloodstream from the fluid that has been filtered into the tubules of the kidneys; consequently this hormone is a major factor which regulates the quantity of water which is lost from the body to the urine. Thus the volume of urine excreted per unit time is, in general, inversely proportional to the quantity of antidiuretic hormone carried in the bloodstream to the renal tubules. In turn the release of antidiuretic hormone under physiologic conditions depends upon the presence of a morphologically and functionally intact hypothalamohypophyseal tract. Pathologic or experimental damage to this system, or to the neural lobe of the pituitary itself, produces a condition known as *diabetes insipidus*. In this conditions (not to be confused with diabetes mellitus, enormous volumes (up to 20 litres per day in humans) of a dilute urine are excreted, a condition known as *polyuria*. In turn this tremendous loss of water results in an abnormally great thirst which leads to the ingestion of large volumes of water, a condition known as *polydipsia*.

In experimental animals it has been demonstrated that electric stimulation of the hypothalamohypophyseal tract by means of electrodes chronically implanted within this system would induce the secretion of enough antidiuretic hormone to inhibit the diuresis produced by the prior ingestion of a large volume of water.

In contrast to the majority of glandular tissues, such as the adrenal medulla and salivary glands in which nerve impulses induce secretory activity, the neural lobe of the pituitary is composed principally of nerve endings that are derived from the hypothalamohypophyseal tract. A few connective tissue elements also are present. These nerve terminals do not end upon secretory cells; rather they end in close proximity to the blood vessels of the neural lobe. Furthermore, not only the terminations of the nerve fibers, but also the fibers themselves, as well as the cell bodies of these neurons which lie within the supraoptic and paraventricular nuclei, all contain a high concentration of membrane-limited secretory vesicles or granules. Briefly, it appears on the basis of data obtained from histologic and physiologic studies that the entire hypothalamohypophyseal system is composed of neurosecretory cells that synthesize, transport, and release antidiuretic hormone. These hypothalamic neurosecretory cells also exhibit bioelectric properties which in all respects are similar to those found in more conventional neurons; and although it is not yet entirely clear what the precise role of this electric activity is insofar as the release of antidiuretic hormone in vivo is concerned, nevertheless it may be suggestive that electric stimulation of the hypothalamohypophyseal system causes an enhanced secretion of antidiuretic hormone.

In vivo, the excretion of water by the kidneys is dependent upon the size of the entire body pool of water. The ingestion of large volumes of water produces a relative dilution of the body fluids and a rapid decrease in the volume of water that is reabsorbed from the renal tubules with a concomitantly increased rate of urine flow or a diuresis. Conversely, a prolonged decrease in water intake results in an increased rate of water reabsorption from the renal tubules which results in the excretion of a correspondingly small volume of more concentrated urine per unit time. Homeostatic regulation of the body water content is achieved by exceedingly precise changes in the release of antidiuretic hormone, and in turn these changes in the rate of secretion of this substance are mediated through minute alterations in the osmotic and hypotonic solutions into internal carotid artery. Intracarotid injection of hypertonic saline stimulates the release of antidiuretic hormone and a decreased urine output in relation to the quantity of liquid ingested (i.e., an oliguria). On the other hand, dilution of the carotid arterial blood causes a decrease in antidiuretic hormone secretion and a diuresis ensues. Based upon experimental data such as these, it has been postulated that there are *osmoreceptors* present somewhere within the brain, and presumably these receptors lie within the supraoptic and paraventricular nuclei of the hypothalamus. Hence these osmoreceptor elements constitute a physiologic mechanism whereby the homeostatic regulation of antidiuretic hormone release, and consequently water excretion, is controlled automatically. In addition to the osmoreceptor mechanism for controlling the secretion of antidiuretic hormone that was described above, it also appears that the total volume of body water per se also may have a role in the physiologic control of antidiuretic hormone secretion. Hence the existence of volume receptors as well as osmoreceptors has been postulated. In view of the critical importance that water plays in all bodily processes, it would, de facto, be rather surprising if the quantitative regulation of the body water store were subserved by merely one homeostatic mechanism.

Presumably satiety occurs when the degree of hydration is such that is no osmotic or volume imbalance acting upon either osmo- or volume receptors, and thereby the sensation of thirst is alleviated.

In addition to playing a vital role in the control of water elimination from the body, the hypothalamus also is responsible for regulating water intake. Thus experimental lesions which are placed in suitable hypothalamic areas can decrease, or even abolish completely, water intake in experimental animals. Such alterations in drinking patterns sometimes can be obtained without changing feeding behavior. Conversely, in the dog and goat, electric stimulation of the lateral superior hypothalamic region (i.e., between the columns of the fornix and the mamillothalamic tract;) by means of chronically implanted electrodes results in a tremendous increase in water intake. In fact, the polydipsia resulting from such an experimental manipulation may result in an increase in body weight of up to nearly 50 per cent above the normal weight for the particular animal. Furthermore, the injection of minute quantities of hypertonic saline into the same areas of the hypothalamus as those subjected to electric stimulation also causes polydipsia. This finding implies that the neurons responsible for producing this effect are sensitive to alterations in osmotic pressure like those of the hypothalamohypophyseal system.

Hunger and the Regulation of Food Intake. "Hunger," or "Appetite" may be defined as the normal desire or craving for food. The sensation of hunger usually is referred in a general way to the lower chest or epigastric region. It should be mentioned here that the intermittent gnawing hunger pangs that may be experienced correlate very poorly with the actual patterns of gastric contractions which occur during the fasting state. Consequently the simplistic notion that special " hunger contractions" give rise to the subjective sensation of hunger is invalid, and it has been demonstrated conclusively in human subjects that no particular type of gastric contraction is related in a specific manner to hunger pangs. There is, incidentally, no qualitative difference between the contractions of the stomach which are observed during periods of digestion and during periods of fasting.

As in the case with thirst, the hypothalamus is related intimately to hunger and to the regulation of food intake. It has been shown experimentally that a hunger or feeding center is present in the ventrolateral hypothalamus, and that a satiety center is present in the ventromedial hypothalamus. Therefore under normal circumstances these two centers interact in such a reciprocal manner as to regulate the desire for food. Artificial stimulation of the feeding center elicits eating behavior in conscious animals, whereas destruction of this center causes a loss of appetite, or anorexia, so severe that the animal starves to death. Stimulation of the ventromedial satiety center, on the other hand, causes the animal to stop eating, but lesions induced experimentally in the same region induce a pattern of gross overeating, or *hyperphagia,* such that the animal becomes extremely obese, a condition known as *hypothalamic* obesity. When the feeding center is destroyed experimentally in rats which have bilateral lesions already present in the satiety center, anorexia results. This experiment indicates that the satiety center operates under physiologic conditions by exerting an inhibitory effect upon the feeding center. In other words, the surprisingly precise equilibrium between food intake and energy expenditure under normal circumstances that underlies the maintenance of a constant adult body weight in turn apparently results from an equally precise balance between the reciprocal. Activity of the feeding and satiety centers of the hypothalamus. According to this concept, the ventrolateral hunger center is dominant, and thus impulses from the satiety center presumably inhibit the desire to continue eating.

An important consideration is the source of the afferent inputs which provide information to the feeding and satiety centers concerning the status of the energy stores of the body. Neither radical gastrectomy nor denervation of the stomach and intestinal tract prevent the development of the hypothalamic hyperphagia that results in gross overeating and the onset of obesity following the induction of small bilateral lesions in the ventromedial nucleus whose activity underlies satiety. Therefore it is unlikely that increased afferent inputs from the gastrointestinal tract underlie the drive to increase food intake to pathologically high levels. There is, however, good experimental evidence which suggests that the activity of the feeding and satiety centers are controlled by the rate of glucose metabolism of the cells located within each of the centers; hence these cells have been called *glucostats*. A low blood glucose level, or hypoglycemia, is presumed to stimulate the feeding center and to inhibit the satiety center, whereas an elevated blood sugar level, or hyperglycemia, has the opposite effect. In support of these contentions it has been determined experimentally that hypoglycemia caused a reduction in the electric activity of the ventromedial satiety center, while that of the ventrolateral feeding center was enhanced somewhat. Hyperglycemia again produced reciprocal alterations in the electric cavity of both of the centers, but in diametrically opposite directions to the changes induced by hypoglycemia.

Stated another way, it has been suggested that when the arteriovenous difference in blood glucose concentration in the feeding center is low, the rate of glucose utilization within the glucostatic cells also is low; consequently the activity of the feeding center is uninhibited and the individual "feels hungry," the sensation being referred to the epigastric region. On the other hand, when the rate of glucose utilization is high, the feeding center is inhibited by the enhanced activity of the glucostatic cells of the satiety center and the individual no longer feels hungry.

Both of these statements of the glucostatic hypothesis for the regulation of appetite are essentially similar, and the experimental data currently available strongly supports the conclusion that the glucostatic mechanisms within the hypothalamic feeding and satiety centers are major physiologic regulatory systems insofar as feeding behavior is concerned. This hypothesis also explains the markedly increased appetite, or polyphagia, which is present in diabetes mellitus, a disease which is caused by a deficiency in the secretion of the pancreatic hormone insulin. The blood sugar level in diabetics is abnormally high, whereas the actual metabolism of glucose by most of the cells of the body is abnormally low. The lack of insulin prevents the normal transport of sugar into, and utilization by, the cells of the body. Neural tissues in general, and the brain in particular, do not require insulin to utilize glucose effectively. The ventral hypothalamic cells apparently are an exception to this general rule. Consequently the rate of glucose utilization by the hypothalamic cells is related directly to the quantity of circulating insulin like other cells of the body so that a deficiency of this hormone results in a decrease in glucose utilization, the activity of the feeding center is unrestrained, and polyphagia develops.

The rate of uptake and utilization of glucose by the cells of the ventromedial satiety center normally is quite high, as demonstrated by studies in which radioactive glucose was used as a tracer substance. If gold thioglucose, which is toxic to and produces clear-cut lesions in the ventromedial nuclei, is administered, the animals (mice) develop hypothalamic hyperphagia and subsequent obesity. The gold thioglucose performs a "chemical ablation" of the cells of the satiety center in the ventromedial nucleus so that the activity of the feeding center is manifest without inhibition.

Experimental stimulation of the mamillary and premamillary regions as well as damage to the amygdaloid nuclei of the limbic system have been demonstrated to produce enhanced feeding behavior. These neural areas also appear to be concerned in some way with the regulation of appetite, although the normal physiologic roles of these areas is obscure.

In contrast to the afferent inputs which regulate the activity of the feeding and satiety centers, not much information is available concerning the efferent pathways from these hypothalamic centers. However, it is apparent that both of these regions must give rise to tracts which innervate the motor nuclei of the brain and spinal cord which are involved in the extremely complex motor behavior involved in acquiring and ingesting food.

A number of factors are related to the control of food intake in addition to the primary regulatory mechanisms that are located in the hypothalamus. For example, a warm environment depresses whereas a cold environment enhances the appetite, and both of these responses are related directly to the net metabolic rate, hence, overall energy consumption by the body. Similarly the quantity of physical work (or exercise) performed is an important factor is regulating appetite through the quantity of energy consumed. In humans, cultural and environmental factors are extremely important determinants of food intake, as are prior conditioning experiences related to the sight, odor, and taste of food. At times the physical availability of food alone is the major factor in determining intake.

The net effect of the operation of the several physiologic and other mechanisms which govern hunger is that in normal adult animals and humans the caloric intake balances the energy expenditure of the body over long periods of time so that the body weight is maintained within close tolerances.

Sexual Behavior and the Hypothalamus. Like thirst and hunger, the basic sexual drive results in the development of extremely complex behavioral patterns for its amelioration, and behind this activity lies a number of equally complex physiologic mechanisms. Thus many endocrine and neural factors operating together in a smoothly coordinated fashion are indispensable to normal mating behavior. The following discussion will emphasize the role of neural processes in mating with particular stress being placed upon the role of the hypothalamus in these processes.

Sexual behavior is integrated at all levels of the nervous system. Hence penile erection and ejaculation can be evoked in humans and animals following complete transaction of the spinal cord, although such sexual activity is fragmentary in that it represents only a small and isolated part of an entire behavior pattern that is present normally. It is impossible to evoke complete and normal patterns of sexual behavior in either paraplegics or in spinal animals, despite the fact that certain fundamental sexual reflexes are integrated within the cord. When the brainstem and greater part of the midbrain are intact, stimulation of the vagina will elicit some of the postural adaptations necessary for mating, but again this behavior is only a small part of the entire pattern necessary for successful copulation.

Thus copulation per se merely consists of a number of reflexes that are integrated in spinal and lower brain centers. However, the behavioral patterns that attend this activity, the sexual drive itself which leads to copulation, and the highly coordinated sequence of physiologic mechanisms in both male and female that lead ultimately to pregnancy are controlled in large measure by the hypothalamus acting in conjunction with the limbic system.

There is an inverse relationship between the phylogenetic status of a particular species of animal and the direct importance of hormones in the initiation of mating behavior. The hormones involved are testosterone in the male and ovarian hormones, i.e., estrogens and progesterone, in the female. Thus in rats mating behavior is dependent strictly upon the availability of a sexually receptive female (i.e., a female in estrus or heat) to a sexually mature male, and in both sexes of this species mating behavior is determined entirely by sex hormones. Copulation in rats which have had no prior sexual contact or experience proceeds quite normally at the first attempt; learning does not appear to play a role in mating in this species. Such behavior is innate (or instinctual) and is triggered solely by the presence of certain chemical substances.

On the other hand, conditioning or learning plays an extremely important role in the development of mating behavior of primates, including man. In humans, sexual functions are closely related to the high degree of encephalization present in this species and hence are conditioned to a large extent by social as well as by psychic influences.

The hypothalamus is essential to ovulation and to the development of estrus, or heat, in lower mammals.* Estrus in turn leads to mating behavior in the majority of mammals, and this effect as well as ovulation is mediated by way of hypothalamohypophyseal pathways. Therefore if suitably placed lesions are made in the anterior hypothalamus, the animal fails to come into estrus and mate, whereas ovulation per se may be normal. These facts indicate that these biologic mechanisms are regulated independently by separate hypothalamic regions. Furthermore the injection of estrogenic (female) hormones into such operated experimental animals does not cause the reappearance of estrus, a fact which suggests strongly that the hormones normally responsible for the production of estrus exert their functions upon a particular hypothalamic region, and that this region also is crucial to the development of an entire somatic behavior pattern which results in mating.

When lesions are introduced in the hypothalamus between the ventromedial nucleus and the mamillary body, ovarian atrophy and a cessation of estrus ensue. Presumably these effects are caused by injury resulting from the operative procedure upon the release of pituitary gonadotropins. Conversely, artificial stimulation of the ventromedial nucleus also can induce ovulation.

The sexual behavior of male animals also is affected by the hypothalamus and other regions of the brain. Artificial stimulation of the tuberal region causes ejaculation

* *The term "estrus" signifies the restricted period of sexual receptivity which occurs in a cyclic fashion in female mammals (other than primates). Periods of estrus are marked by an intense sexual drive. The sexual cycle of the human female as well as a few other primates of reproductive age is called the menstrual cycle.*

in rats, whereas stimulation of the medial forebrain bundle and adjacent hypothalamic areas induces penile erection coupled with marked emotional displays in monkeys. In castrated rats, which have a greatly diminished, or completely absent, sex drive, the implantation of pellets of testosterone into the hypothalamus restores the normal pattern of sexual behavior. In normal rats, suitably located anterior hypothalamic lesions will abolish completely all interest in sexual matters, whereas lesions situated in the mamillary region may cause enhanced sexual activity in male rats.

Generally complete extirpation of the neocortex will inhibit sexual activity in male experimental animals, whereas subtotal cortical ablation can produce a partial inhibition of such activity. The extent to which sexual behavior is decreased by such a procedure is not related to the degree to which motor defects are induced concomitantly by the surgical manipulation. The diminution of sexual behavior following subtotal cortical ablation is most evident when the frontal lobes are involved.

In marked contrast to the decrease in sexual behavior noted above which follows cortical injury, when bilateral lesions are placed in the pyriform cortex of the limbic system overlying the basal amygdalar nucleus the animal usually develops a pronounced hypersexuality. Thus cats and monkeys subjected to this operative procedure not only copulate with adult females of their own species, but also attempt copulation with immature females, other males, animals of other species, and even with inanimate objects. Such indiscriminate and misdirected sexual behavior clearly lies beyond the normal range for the particular species involved. This excessive sexual activity was found to decrease somewhat following castration but was not itself induced by a greater secretion of testosterone following the initial operative procedure upon the pyriform cortex.

In most mammals the sexual activity of the male is relatively continuous,* whereas that of the female occurs in a cyclic manner called the *estrous cycle* which is dependent upon oscillations in the blood estrogen level. During the periods of heat, or estrus, the increase in the circulation estrogen level which occurs at this point in the estrous cycle causes an alteration in the behavior of the female such that the company as well as the sexual advances of the male no longer are rejected. Rather, during estrus the female actively seeks out the male and attempts to mate. The females of certain species, particularly the rabbit and ferret, come into estrus and remain so until pregnancy intervenes. In such species, ovulation per se is due to a neuroendocrine reflex which operates through the hypothalamus. Direct stimulation of the genitalia and other sensory areas at the time of copulation excites the hypothalamus; in turn the signals from this region of the brain are transmitted directly to the pituitary and cause the release of gonadotropic hormones which then are carried by the bloodstream to the ovaries where they induce rupture of the ovarian follicles and liberation of the ova. In many other species, including humans, the ova are liberated spontaneously and in a cyclic fashion. In lower mammals this release of the female germ cells coincides with estrus. In humans, this event takes place at the approximate midpoint of the menstrual or sexual cycle as discussed.

---

* *Notable exceptions to this statement are found in the male rhinoceros and elephant, which species enter a state of rut at intervals that coincide with peaks of greatest sexual excitation.*

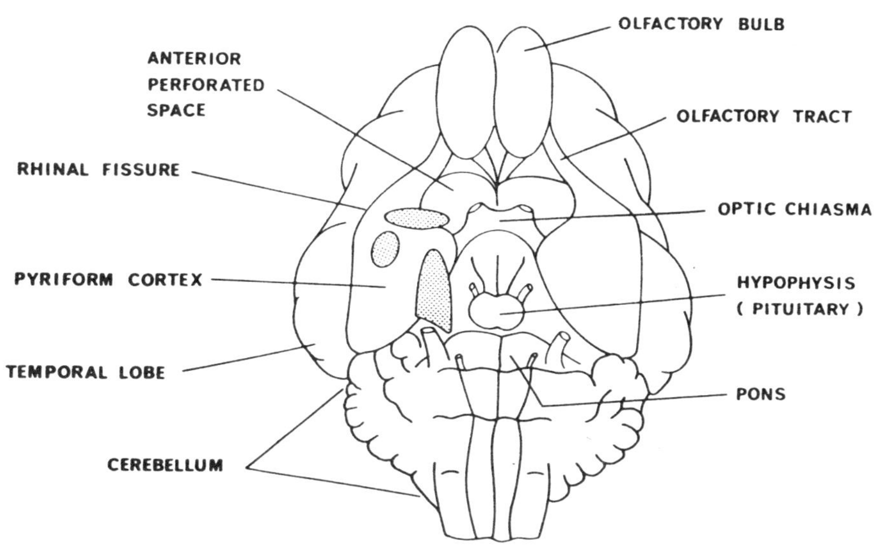

Fig. 8.1. Ventral surface of cat brain showing areas (shaded) where lesions placed in the pyriform cortex over the amygdaloid nucleus cause hypersexuality.

In female experimental animals, extirpation of the neocortex and/or the limbic cortex completely eliminates the male-seeking behavior by the female during estrus. However, the other aspects of this physiologic process remain unchanged, including the slight rise in body temperature that occurs. Induced lesions of the pyriform and amygdaloid regions do not produce hypersexuality in the female as they do in the male, although discrete lesions placed in the anterior hypothalamus do abolish the behavioral effects of estrus but without altering the normal pituitary-ovarian cycle of hormonal changes.

The implantation of tiny pellets of estrogens into the anterior hypothalamus will induce estrus in ovarectomized rats; however implantation of the hormone into other parts of the brain as well as into regions that are located outside of the brain produces no such response. Consequently it would appear that some hypothalamic structure is responsive to the circulating estrogen level and is activated by a high circulating estrogen level so that the sexual behavior typical of the estrous state is induced.

Voluntary Regulation of "Involuntary" Functions. Generally the functional activities of the autonomic nervous system are carried out at wholly subconscious levels and furthermore these activities cannot be regulated ordinarily through a conscious effort of the will. Although several investigators have studied the physiologic effects of meditation (Yoga and Zen Buddhism) on a number of readily measured functional parameters, the results often were conflicting, perhaps because of the differences in technique employed by the subjects to induce the meditative state itself. Recently, however, several controlled investigations have been carried out upon normal human subjects all trained in the same technique of meditation. During this state, called "transcendental meditation, " the subject achieves an extremely relaxed physical condition while remaining fully conscious and alert. In general the specific functional alterations observed in subjects during transcendental mediation were consistent with several of those alterations which were observed earlier in yogas and practitioners of Zen meditation. These data are summarized in this section, as it now is clear that a number of supposedly involuntary processes are indeed subject to modification through the application of conscious mental effort on the part of the subject. The potential clinical significance of some of these findings will be indicated in context. In the studies to be cited, each subject served as his own control.

During periods of transcendental mediation, the rates of both oxygen consumption and carbon dioxide production declined sharply, but the ratio of carbon dioxide excretion to oxygen consumption (volume/volume) remained unchanged for all practical purposes when compared to the nonmeditation control values. The respiratory rate decreased slightly as did the minute volume of air respired (i.e., the volume of air breathed per minute measured in litres;). These facts suggest strongly that the overall metabolic rate of the subject declines during periods of meditation. Furthermore, the rate of decrease in oxygen consumption that is seen during meditation is quite different from that observed during sleep.

The mean arterial blood pressure remained at fairly low and constant values during periods of meditation. However, it is interesting to note that this blood pressure was achieved during the quiet interval which preceded meditation, and that the blood pressure did not change appreciably following the meditation. The heart rate was observed to decline very slightly during meditation, on an average of three contractions per minute.

The partial pressures of oxygen and carbon dioxide in the arterial blood (Po_2, Pco_2) remained practically unaltered during mediation, but the blood pH declined very slightly, a fact that was indicative of negligible metabolic acidosis.

The electric resistance of the skin increases sharply (up to four times the control value) during meditation. Supposedly this factor is related to the "degree of relaxation"; that is, the greater the resistance, the more at ease the subject is.

The blood lactic acid concentration is a direct indicator of anaerobic metabolism. During transcendental mediation, the blood lactate concentration was found to decline at a rate which was up to four times as rapid as that measured in the nonmeditating

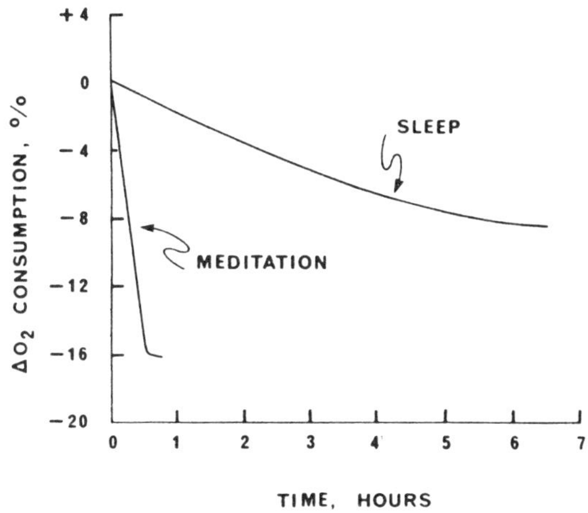

Fig. 8.2. Comparison of the effects of transcendental meditation and sleep on the rate of oxygen consumption. Hypnosis per se causes no alteration in the rate of oxygen consumption (see also text).

subject who was merely resting in a supine position, and the lactate concentration remained low even at the end of the postmeditation interval. The explanation for this effect appears to lie in the fact that during mediation blood flow through the skeletal muscles increases significantly, as indicated by flow measurements in the forearm. This factor would increase the rate of delivery of oxygen to the muscles during meditation, and thus anaerobic production of lactic acid would be minimized as the principal source of this compound in vivo is within the skeletal muscles.

As noted above, the blood pressure and heart rate remain at essentially constant levels during meditation; therefore under such circumstances alterations in blood flow are affected principally by changes in the caliber of the vessels. Consequently it appears that during meditations the vascular bed in the skeletal muscles undergoes vasodilatation, and it has been suggested that the cholinergic sympathetic vasodilator nerves may be responsible for this effect. It also has been suggested that patients having anxiety neuroses, as well as patients suffering from essential or renal hypertension might benefit markedly from transcendental meditation and the concomitant sharp reduction in blood lactate that accompanies this state. It is known, of course, that such neurotic patients tend to develop a marked hyperlacticacidema when under stress, and it has been demonstrated experimentally that injections of lactic acid into such patients (or even normal persons) can precipitate anxiety attacks. Furthermore, both classes of hypertensive noted above exhibit higher-than-normal blood lactate levels in the resting state than do nonhypertensive subjects. It is tempting to speculate upon the possible physiologic role of the low blood lactate concentration found in meditating subject insofar as the etiology of this state is concerned. Furthermore, the potential clinical value of meditation to the hypertensive or anxiety neurotic is such as to warrant further investigation in this area.

In addition to the physiologic and biochemical alterations discussed above, electroncephalographic recordings obtained from meditating subjects revealed that a pronounced increase in the alpha-wave activity of the cortex takes place in all subjects, and in some individuals a concomitant development of theta-wave activity was observed in the frontal area of the brain. Suffice it to say at this point that from a physiologic standpoint the state induced by transcendental meditation in no way resembles that evoked by sleep, hypnosis, autosuggestive techniques, or operant conditioning.

The overall functional pattern that is evoked voluntarily by meditation in trained subjects appears to resemble an integrated reflex that includes a number of autonomic responses that are coordinated by the central nervous system, and in contrast to the sympathetic "fight or flight" reaction that involves activation of the entire sympathetic nervous system, it would appear that transcendental meditation exerts quite the opposite effects with the net result that the individual is extremely relaxed, though in full possession of his mental faculties.

Other studies have demonstrated clearly that suitable conditioning techniques can be employed to train a person or an experimental animal to control certain individual visceral functions at will. These studies, which contrast somewhat with the more widespread physiologic responses evoked by transcendental meditation, will be discussed in context together with the phenomenon of learning.

Neurophysiology of Behavior: Motivation and Emotion

The term "behavior" can be defined as any activity which is performed by a particular organism, especially activity which can be observed externally and measured in quantitative terms regardless of whether the activity is induced by internal or external stimulation. Thus in broadest terms, behavior is anything or everything that an organism does in response to various stimuli.

Behavioral responses in toto are not the result of the activity of mutually exclusive regions of the nervous system. Rather, behavior is a function of the entire nervous system acting as a coordinated unit. This statement also should be construed to mean, however, that certain types of behavior can be (and are) dominated by the activity of certain regions of the nervous system that may act in concert with other organ systems of the body.

In this section the physiologic mechanisms which underlie motivation and emotion will be discussed. The problems encountered in studies of motivation tend to overlap those encountered in studies on emotion. The reader must realize that the topics presented under each of the following two subheadings have been separated arbitrarily. Thus the material concerned with intracranial autostimulation has been considered under the heading of motivation, although it could have been considered just as readily under emotion.

Motivation. The term "motivation" can be defined as any of the forces which regulate the behavior of an organism such that this behavior is directed toward the satisfaction of certain basic needs or the achievement of certain goals. Motivation can be considered to be made up of two aspects, one of which guides the *direction* in which the motivation is channeled and is chiefly a product of learning, whereas the other is concerned with the intensity or *drive* which underlies the behavior. In this section, emphasis will be placed upon the physiologic mechanisms that underlie the drive aspect of motivation.

From an experimental standpoint, the drive component of motivation can be studied quantitatively by observing the measurable alteration in one aspect of behavior after altering the intensity of some stimulus. The stimulus which is varied can be either external or internal with respect to the organism. For example, food or water deprivation can be varied quantitatively to give variable internal stimuli, whereas alterations in the intensity of applied sound, light, or electric shocks all will provide similarly variable external stimuli. In turn, the effects induced by the application of such interceptive or exteroceptive stimuli can be estimated by measuring any of several behavioral changes, including, for example, gross motor activity, alterations in autonomic responses, latent period of a learned response, choice made between two or more different stimuli, and the intensity (or force) of a response to a given stimulus. It should be borne in mind, however, that the relationship between motivation and learning is exceedingly complex, so that even under the best of experimental conditions the quantitative measurements of motivation per se as derived from studies on either human or animal subjects are only refined approximations, and not absolute certainties.

When the observed drive (or intensity) of a particular behavior pattern changes, it is tacitly inferred that the activity of the central nervous system has changed, although direct proof of this contention may be lacking. Nevertheless, several well-known classes of stimuli can alter markedly the behavioral patterns of humans as well as experimental animals; these factors and their physiologic roles in behavior may be summarized briefly.

Afferent Input Stimuli. The afferent inputs that influence motivated behavior can be divided into exteroceptive and interoceptive stimuli.

Exteroceptive Stimuli. Generally speaking, and sensory input can alter the drive aspect of motivated behavior, provided that the magnitude (or intensity) of the stimulus is sufficiently great. For example, extremes of temperature, very loud sounds, and strong illumination all can motivate avoidance behavior under certain circumstances. It appears that those sensory inputs having a marked affect upon the subject either in a pleasant or unpleasant (painful) direction exert the most pronounced motivational effect.

In humans, it also has been found that sensory deprivation can be deleterious to the subject as an abnormally strong sensory input. Thus a pronounced deterioration of higher mental faculties including the ability to reason and memory, followed a prolonged (6-month) interval of isolation in one subject. Furthermore, hallucinations (i.e., false sensory impressions) commonly develop in subjects undergoing extended periods of sensory deprivation, and the ability to perform even simple motor tasks also declines appreciably. Most important to the present discussion, however, is the fact that isolation can produce an extreme state of apathy or lassitude in the subject.

Interoceptive Stimuli. Sensory inputs to the central nervous system that arise within the body per se, in particular the viscera, are an important source of afferent signals that underlie motivated behavior. Thus alterations in the caliber of blood vessels and mechanical displacement or stretching of internal organs may evoke afferent impulses that in turn stimulate extremely complex behavioral patterns to alleviate the condition. The sensation of pain is the major example of a visceral sensation that induces such behavior patterns.

Humoral Stimuli. The chemical agents which are included under the heading of humoral substances consist of a variety of hormones, metabolities, nutrients, and drugs, all of which are carried by the bloodstream to the blood-brain barrier. After crossing this barrier, these humoral agents can exert their effects directly upon particular groups of nerve cells within the brain and thereby alter motivated behavior accordingly. In addition, the temperature as well as the osmotic pressure of the blood per se also can exert direct influences upon certain behavioral patterns.

Hormones. Two examples of the direct effects of endocrine substances upon particular areas of the central nervous system that are involved in behavior may be cited. First, it has been shown experimentally that sex hormones can lower the response threshold of the reticular formation to electric stimulation. Second, epinephrine has been demonstrated to facilitate the transmission of impulses in the ascending reticular activating system.

Metabolites and Nutrients. Certain metabolites have been considered to have a role in the onset of fatigue, which in turn motivates one toward entering the sleep phase of the diurnal wakefulness-sleep cycle. Although lactic acid has been implicated in this motivational process, the relationship between the two has not been established unequivocally.

During the course of normal metabolism, the concentration of some constituents of the blood decreases whereas the concentration of other blood constituents may increase. In turn, these alteration in the concentrations of blood nutrients may appear across the blood-brain barrier so that an altered function of the nervous themselves develops. For example, a relative deficiency of glucose in the brain that is caused by the presence of an excessively high insulin level may bring about marked behavioral changes that can range from symptoms resembling those of alcoholic intoxication to outright convulsions.

Thermal Stimuli. The temperature of the blood itself provides an extremely potent physical stimulus to the activation of complex motivated behavioral patterns that are involved in the maintenance of body temperature. It should be mentioned here that the maintenance of body temperature within very narrow limits is exceedingly important to survival. Mammals (as well as birds) have evolved a very complex and precise thermoregulatory system that involves certain automatic components which underlie the bodily mechanisms that balance heat production against heat loss. In addition to the automatic thermoregulatory mechanisms of the body, motivated behavioral responses also are invoked by thermal stresses in either direction, and these behavioral patterns tend to balance discrepancies between heat load and heat loss in the body. For example, an animal may seek shelter or curl up in a ball (thereby diminishing the surface exposed to heat loss) in order to conserve body heat in a cold environment. A human being, on the other hand, may alter the amount of clothing being worn or adjust the thermostat in a building in order to achieve the same goal.

In addition to the motivated behavior patterns discussed above that the potentially mediated by alterations in blood temperature per se, it should be mentioned that any marked alteration in blood or body temperature undoubtedly will influence behavior directly, merely because of the effects of temperature changes upon the rate of all chemical reactions in the body, including those taking place in brain and peripheral nervous tissues.

Osmotic Pressure. It was noted earlier that the injection of a hypertonic saline solution into the carotid arteries will induce highly motivated drinking behavior. Consequently it would appear that alterations in the tonicity of the plasma itself can affect the irritability of certain nerve cells in such a manner as to influence markedly certain behavior patterns concerned with thirst.

Inherent Neural Stimuli: Circadian Rhythms. Practically all plants and animals exhibit regular cyclic variations in many of their functions. The duration of particular functional cycles can vary markedly (e.g., the menstrual cycle lasts for about 28 days), however among the most evident are those whose duration is approximately 24 hours in length, and these cycles are called *diurnal* or *circadian rhythms*. In man as well as in lower mammals the daily oscillations in body temperature, sodium and potassium excretion, white blood cell (leucocyte) count, adrenocortical function, urine volume, and wakefulness and sleep are the best-studied cycles, although many other diurnal fluctuations in particular functions are known.

As discussed above, afferent inputs and humoral influences are the most readily detectable means whereby the activity of the central nervous system; hence behavioral intensity, is altered, however many changes in behavior cannot be ascribed to these sources. Certain of the circadian rhythms enumerated above thus have been ascribed to the operation of a so-called biologic clock mechanism. Thus rhythmic processes taking place either in the environment external to the organism, or within the organism itself but outside of its central nervous system, then affect either the afferent or humoral mechanisms which in turn alter the activity of the central nervous system and thereby alter behavior indirectly and in a cyclic fashion. On the other hand, some rhythmic physiologic alterations in the activities of various organisms indicate that the central nervous system per se exhibits cyclic fluctuations in its activity that are independent of extraneural cyclic events. It would appear that the central nervous system has inherent mechanisms which can operate in a cyclic ('clocklike") manner, and thus modify behavior even though an external stimulus is absent.

In certain lower organisms (insects, fish, birds) the morphologic patterns of organization within the nervous system are so arranged that appropriate stimuli can evoke stereotyped, often complex and highly motivated, but unlearned, behavioral patterns called *instincts*. In mammals, however, it is difficult to ascertain the actual role of instincts in behavior, because such innate behavior as may be present is dominated by the far greater capacity for learning that is present. Hence instinctual behavior is governed to a great extent by learned behavior patterns so that the two merge and become, de facto, indistinguishable.

From a neuroanatomic standpoint, it appears that the mechanisms which control some of the diurnal rhythms are located within the limbic system. For example, damage to the fornix alters the adrenocortical rhythm, whereas more generalized lesions of the limbic system provoke abnormal sleep-wakefulness and the body temperature cycles without interfering with thermoregulation per se.

Affect and Motivated Behavior: Neural Centers *Which Underlie Approach and Avoidance Responses*. Within the past 20 years, it has been determined experimentally that a number of hypothalamic and closely related structures are concerned intimately with the affective component of sensory experience. Thus if an animal is confined to a cage having a lever that can be pressed, eventually the animal depresses this lever by accident. Now if electrodes are implanted in the brain of the animal, and the lever is arranged as a switch which can be manipulated by the animal to deliver an electric stimulus to the brain each time the lever is pressed, the affective properties of the stimulus can be deduced from the behavior of the animal. Thus when the electrode tip is located in certain regions of the brain (e.g., the tegmentum, posteromedial hypothalamus, and septal nuclei) the animal will stimulate itself repeatedly for long periods of time, even to the point of exhaustion, whereas if the electrode tip is situated in other brain areas (e.g., the posterolateral hypothalamus, dorsal midbrain, entorhinal cortex) the stimulus causes the animal to avoid pressing the bar at all following the initial excitation.

The areas of the brain in which implantation of the electrodes causes repetitive voluntary stimulation are far larger than those from which an avoidance reaction can be evoked. However each of these regions is distinct from the other, even though the two areas may be closely situated within the brain.

Experiments such as those described above have given rise to the concept that the hypothalamus and related structures contain two general affective sensory regions which variously are termed "reward" and "punishment," "approach" and "avoidance," or "pleasure" and "pain" centers, depending upon the positive or negative behavior patterns that are elicited by autostimulation of particular brain areas.

It is clearly impossible for an investigator to ascertain or to sense precisely what an experimental animal feels or perceives when the reward (or approach) system is stimulated electrically through its own efforts, but clearly the evoked sensation is such that repetition of the stimulation is in order, and this repetitive behavior has been interpreted as arising from a pleasurable affective response. Alternatively, however, it is just as reasonable to suppose that the presence of the electrode tip in the so-called reward center actually provides an extremely strong irritation of some type and the animal quickly learns that rapidly repeated lever pressing will ameliorate this situation for as long as the mechanical behavior continues (death of the animal may intervene, but satiation, insofar as lever pressing is concerned has not been observed).* In this view, the repeated lever pressing by an experimental animal is somewhat analogous to the behavior of a confirmed heroin addict who seeks the drug no longer as a pleasurable and temporary escape from reality, but rather to avoid the intrinsic misery of withdrawal symptoms.

Similarly it is impossible for an investigator to appreciate what actually is felt by an experimental animal when the avoidance system of the brain is stimulated.

Regardless of the interpretation given to the experiments on stimulation of the approach system of the brain, it is clear that from a physiologic standpoint much normal human, as well as animal, behavior is motivated by primary stimuli which gives rise to a pleasant affect as well as by other stimuli which give rise to an unpleasant, or even painful, affect.

Emotion. The term "emotion" can be defined as a physiologic departure from a condition of homeostasis during which a state of strong mental excitement (or depression) is present. The respiratory, cardiovascular, neuromuscular, endocrine, gastrointestinal, cutaneous, and other physiologic changes which are accompaniments of emotion prepare the individual for overt behavioral responses or acts which may or may not be carried out. Thus normal emotion is a temporary functional imbalance that is characterized by profound autonomic (visceral) and somatic as well as phychic alterations; and as noted earlier, emotion cannot be initiated or terminated voluntarily, the latter owing to the prolonged after-discharge of the limbic system whose functions are linked inseparably with those of the hypothalamus to the physiologic manifestations of the emotional state.

Emotions involve several distinct parameters, including cognition, conation, and affect as well as the specific physical changes summarized above. Cognition signifies an operation of the mind whereby one becomes aware of objects of thought or perception; this term also signifies an awareness of a sensation, and frequently its cause. *Conation* indicates that components of emotion (and other mental states) in which a positive and conscious tendency to act is involved; often conation is referred to in the vernacular as "will power." *Affect* is, of course, the subjective component of any sensation. In emotional states the affective component is either "pleasant" or "unpleasant," but never "neutral."

The common words employed to describe or indicate various emotions clearly indicate their affective (or subjective) content, insofar as human experience is concerned; i.e., learning plays an important role in the expression of emotion. For example, the

---

* *Verbal reports given by patients (i.e., schizophrenics and epileptics) in whose brains electrodes were implanted chronically indicate that the sensations evoked by autostimulation generally were "pleasurable," and caused "relief of tension." Intervestingly, certain subjects who exhibited the highest lever-pressing rates could not describe why they performed this activity at all. Conversely, if the electrodes were placed in areas of the brain in which autostimulation normally was avoided, stimulation of these areas evoked sensations ranging from a slight uneasiness or fear to outright terror.*

terms love, desire, joy, elation, surprise, anger (or rage), fear, gloom, hate, anxiety, and disgust all may have somewhat different connotations, but in general all of these words signify either a pleasant or an unpleasant affect when used in a particular context.

In brief, therefore, emotion is a state of mind as well as a behavioral response, a state which is accompanied by motivation either toward or away from an object or event.

The following discussion is limited primarily to the neurophysiologic aspects of emotion as studied by neuroanatomic, neurosurgical, electro-physiologic, and observational techniques. Electroencephalography is a particularly useful technique for detecting objective signs of excitement and alerting in experimental animals as well as human subjects.

Functional Manifestations of Emotions. When studied under controlled laboratory conditions in human subjects, emotional responses have been found to have parasympathetic as well as sympathetic components. That is, both divisions of the autonomic nervous system can participate simultaneously in the altered physical signs present during emotional states, and these signs may include erection of the hairs, tachycardia, hypertension, papillary dilatation, inhibition or stimulation of the gastrointestinal tract and urinary bladder, and so forth.

Emotions can be accompanied by marked excitement or depression. In the former instance the mental processes are accelerated, whereas in the latter they become dull, retarded, or sluggish.

Neuroanatomic Basis of Emotion: The Hypothalamus and Limbic System. The vascular, glandular, and visceral alterations that take place during emotional states are regulated by the autonomic nervous system, which in turn is controlled in large measure by the hypothalamus. This structure also is the neural center which underlies the genesis of certain emotional states including rage as well as elaborate patterns of sexual behavior, but many other structures are involved in these responses in addition to the hypothalamus.

When small lesions are induced within the ventromedial nuclei of the hypothalamic region, the experimental animal develops a state of rage and makes accurately directed and ferocious attacks upon anyone in the vicinity. When artificial stimulation by means of electrodes chronically implanted within the hypothalamus is employed, it is possible to localize rather accurately the hypothalamic regions that are responsible for evoking two general behavioral states. First, a pattern similar to rage (or fight) behavior can be evoked in which the animal (e.g., cat) growls, hisses, extends his claws, flattens the ears, arches the back, erects the hairs (piloerection) develops pupillary dilatation, and exhibits other sympathetic responses. Second, a pattern similar to fear (or flight) can also be evoked, and this response includes pupillary dilatation, glancing back and forth, turning the head back and forth laterally as though seeking an avenue of escape, and ultimately flight. These experimentally evoked behavioral patterns are complete and they involve highly integrated somatic and visceral reactions of the entire body, not merely isolated parts. In brief, the responses elicited by stimulation of appropriate hypothalamic areas resemble those exhibited normally upon presentation of a suitable stimulus to a cat, e.g., a dog.

It appears that the fight (or defense) reaction is localized within the dorsal portion of the central thalamus which surrounds the descending part of the fornix; this "center" then extends rostrally into the preoptic and ventral septal area as well as caudally into the posterior hypothalamus within which region the tissue dilates into the central gray matter of the midbrain. Consequently the part of the brain from which the fight or defense reaction can be elicited consists of a narrow (1 to 1.5 mm) band or lamina of tissue which traverses the entire hypothalamus. According to certain workers, the flight reactions are evoked by stimulation of the external portion of this lamina, whereas fright (or flight) reactions are elicited by stimulation of the central part of the lamina. Other investigators feel that the neural mechanisms which subserve the flight reaction merely are located somewhat rostrally to those which underlie the escape reaction.

Similar fight or flight reactions can be evoked by stimulation of the amygdalar portion of the limbic system.

Despite the lack of unanimous agreement as to the precise areas of the brain wherein the rage and fear responses are localized, nevertheless it is apparent that an area which starts in the telencephalon, traverses the hypothalamus, and extends into the midbrain is the neural region wherein aggressive motor behavior as well as escape reactions, together with their autonomic components, are integrated. Furthermore, it has been demonstrated that excitation of other hypothalamic areas than those discussed above, as well as the cerebral cortex and hippocampus, does not evoke emotional responses. However, it has been shown that a fiber system which involves the ventromedial hypothalamic nuclei apparently is involved as a check upon emotional activity, since destruction of these regions results in unrestrained aggressive behavior.

The other neural system which plays an intimate role in the genesis of emotional states is the limbic system. It must not be inferred that the limbic system operates independently of the hypothalamus merely because the functions of these two parts of the brain in the development of emotional responses have perforce been discussed separately. Quite the contrary; these two parts of the brain are inseparable from a functional standpoint.

The olfactory function of the limbic system is discussed in relation to the sense of smell. It is clear, however, that only a small portion of this system is activated by olfactory stimuli, and the functions of the nonolfactory structures of the limbic system are related intimately to emotional states.

The major anatomic components of the limbic system may be reviewed briefly. The principal structures that comprise the limbic system are two rings of limbic cortex and a number of related subcortical nuclei, including the amygdala, the septal nuclei, and the anterior thalamic nuclei.

Experiments performed by stimulation or ablation of specific regions within the limbic system indicate that this part of the brain not only is concerned with olfactor, but also with feeding behavior (i.e., sniffing, salivation, chewing, licking, swallowing, retching, and gagging). Acting in concert with the hypothalamus, the limbic system also is involved in the control of certain autonomic functions, biologic rhythms, sexual behavior, and in motivated behavior, as well as in the emotions of rage and fear.

Stimulation of the limbic system causes a number of autonomic responses, in particular alterations in heart rate, blood pressure, and respiratory rate. Since these responses are evoked by stimulation of many limbic structures, there do not appear to be any localized centers for the integration of these responses. Consequently it would appear that the autonomic effects which are mediated by the limbic system are parts of more complex behavioral patterns including emotional responses. Stimulation of the amygdaloid nuclei, on the other hand, evokes the complex motor responses noted above that are related directly to feeding behavior (eg, chewing, licking, and so forth). Lesions in the amygdala occasionally cause some hyperphagia.

The defense responses evoked by stimulation of the amygdala are like those produced by stimulation of the hypothalamus and midbrain. However, these reactions are produced with greater facility when the amygdala is stimulated directly, but it is clear that this structure exerts its effects indirectly and through excitation of hypothalamus and midbrain, although the specific pathway by which these effects are transmitted is unclear.

When the amygdala is stimulated simultaneously with a hypothalamic region known to produce and aggressive behavior pattern, sometimes the effects of the dual stimulation are facilitory. More frequently, however, the aggressive behavior is moderated by such dual stimulation, and these two responses have been obtained by stimulation of two entirely discrete areas within the amygdala. These data support the contention that the amygdala is located at a higher neural level than the hypothalamus insofar as the integration of emotional behavior is concerned.

When the septal region of the limbic system is extirpated, in experimental animals such as rats, the responses to a situation which normally would produce extreme anxiety or fear in the animals are decreased considerably. On the other hand, such operated animals become quite vicious, and will attack each other or the experimenter readily.

Following bilateral ablation of the anterior temporal lobes in monkeys, portions of the limbic system, in particular the amygdala, generally are damaged. Following such a procedure, the animals suffer a number of profound behavioral and other disturbances including psychic blindness (i.e., visual agnosia), and a marked impulsive exploratory behavior develops, together with loss of normal aggressive tendencies. The animals concomitantly become quite docile, passive, and unresponsive, and their dietary habits become deranged. That is, a herbivore may be converted into a carnivore. Collectively these postoperative symptoms are known as the Klüver-Bucy syndrome.

In contrast to the loss of aggressive behavior which accompanies the Klüver-Busy syndrome, other kinds of emotional response, in particular sexual activity, become increased markedly. The experimental subjects (monkeys) became hyper-sexual, and the normal sex drive of the male often becomes channelled into clearly abnormal directions.

Some years ago it was proposed that the limbic cortex and related structures together with certain thalamic and hypothalamic regions formed a neuroanatomic unit that functionally was responsible for the genesis of emotions. It has been demonstrated that the emotional changes which are observed to take place in the Klüver-Busy syndrome are caused by loss of the pyriform cortex and the subjacent amygdalar nuclei. The docility which also develops following amygdalectomy is specific, but such a placid animal sometimes can be made fierce and subject to bouts of rage by placing lesions is the ventromedial hypothalamic nucleus. On the other hand, amygdalectomized animals, which have become docile following the operation, occasionally can be rendered savage by subsequently placing lesions in the septal region.

The hippocampus has anatomically well-defined neural connections to the hypothalamus by way of the fornix, and with the anterior cingulate gyrus by way of the mamillary bodies and the anterior thalamic nuclei. Nevertheless, the significance of these pathways in the genesis and integration of emotions has not been established clearly. Furthermore it has been proven experimentally that the hippocampal formation does not underlie any demonstrably obvious type of emotional behavior.

It has been proposed that the Papez circuit mediates the cognitive as well as other subjective features of emotion, and the hippocampal formation in particular seems to have been implicated to some extend in the subjective aspects of emotions. Beyond these rather nebulous statements, nothing more edifying on the relationships between the neuroanatomic and neurophysiologic aspects of emotion can be presented with certainty at present.

Drugs and Behavior Modifications. For basic scientific as well as clinical reasons, considerable interest has developed in the action of a number of drugs that alter human behavioral patterns. Pharmacologic agents that produce such effects on behavior include tranquilizers, such as reserpine, which decrease anxiety; *psychotomimetics,* such as mescaline or lysergic acid diethylamide (LSD), which produce hallucinations and other psychotic symptoms; and *psychic energizers,* such as amphetamines, which are antidepressant agents that increase drive and interest as well as serve to elevate the mood. The action of many psychoactive drugs appears to be through modification of synaptic transmission in various regions of the brain, consequently the discovery of such chemical agents has led to considerable research on the biochemistry and functional characteristics of various neurotransmitter agents.

Electroencephalography

All living cells exhibit characteristic bioelectric properties, as emphasized repeatedly throughout earlier chapters of this book. In particular, the tissue of the cerebral cortex consists of a vast, highly organized array of neuronal and glial elements that is characterized by a continuous rhythmic oscillation of electric potential (the *spontaneous rhythm*) in addition to a number of larger-voltage responses that occur locally and as the result of excitation of specific receptors (the *evoked potentials*).

It has been known for about a century that spontaneous, rhythmic variations in voltage can be recorded from the brain of an unanesthetized animal. However, systematic analysis of these "brain waves" resulted from the pioneering efforts of Berger, who introduced the term *electroencephalogram* (EEG) to denote the recording made of the alterations in electric potential that can be obtained from various parts of the brain by means of electrodes placed upon the skull of an intact human or animal subject. The EEG also can be obtained by placing the electrodes directly upon the pial surface of the cerebral cortex after the skull has been opened, in which case the recording sometimes is called an *electrocorticogram.*

An EEG recording may be bipolar; in this instance, the potential difference or voltage generated by the brain is measured between two active electrodes placed upon the skull or cortex. Alternatively, a monopolar recording of the EEG indicates the changes in potential at a single active lead, which are compared with a "stable" or "indifferent" electrode that is located on the body at some distance from the cortical electrode. In practice, establishing a valid reference electrode for recording monopolar EEGs is extremely difficult, consequently bipolar recording of EEGs is the method of choice. Although only two leads are shown, in practice many more leads actually are employed, and the records obtained may be subjected to computer analysis.

EEGs yield information that is of interest to the clinician as an index to the functions of the brain in health and disease. In addition, EEGs provide objective data concerning certain functions of the brain during various functional or behavioral activities, for example during the waking and sleeping states. The spontaneous wave patterns encountered in the EEGs obtained from normal humans now will be discussed together with the evoked cortical potentials that can be recorded following stimulation of particular sensory receptors. The latter technique also has proven to be of major importance in mapping the pathways from specific peripheral sensory receptors to their final terminations within particular regions of the cerebral cortex.

Spontaneous Cortical Rhythms. When suitable leads are placed upon the head of a normal human subject, extremely small and irregular potentials can be recorded from the frontal, parietal, temporal, and occipital regions. The actual voltages recorded are in the range of microvolts (μ v), and the maximum peak-to-peak voltage recorded from normal human subjects is about 50 μv.

Characteristic differences are present between EEGs obtained from different regions of the brain, the specific patterns that is recorded being dependent upon the physiologic conditions prevailing at the time of recording as well as upon the technique used for making the EEG (i.e., a bipolar or unipolar arrangement of the electrodes).

The normal EEG is composed of a large number of waves having irregular amplitudes as well as frequencies. However, during any particular physiologic state one frequency usually dominates, and this property is far more significant than in the amplitude of the individual waves in the interpretation of EEGs. Thus the frequency of the dominant EEG wave in any recording is the basis upon which EEG patterns are named, and these frequencies are denoted by Greek letters as follows.

If the predominant wave frequency of an EEG lies between 8 and 14 per second, an *alpha rhythm* is present. This pattern characteristically is recorded with electrodes which are placed upon the scalp of an adult human sitting with the eyes closed and the mind at rest. The amplitude of the alpha waves thus recorded is about 50 µv. A *beta rhythm* is present when the frequency of the dominant rhythm is 14 to 60 waves per second. A *theta rhythm* is indicated by a frequency of 4 to 8 cycles per second, whereas a *delta rhythm* is manifest by fewer than 4 waves per second. A number of other minor rhythms are recognized in addition to those defined above, but in all instances the amplitude of the waves is related inversely to the characteristic frequency of the particular wave pattern. Furthermore, it is a convention of electroencephalographic terminology that high-frequency waves (of short duration) are called fast activity, whereas low-frequency waves (of long duration) are termed *slow activity*.

Factors that Modify Spontaneous Cortical Rhythms. The pattern of frequency of the EEG is quite labile, and thus is modified by a host of factors. In humans the frequency of the dominant rhythm varies with age. At birth the principal rhythm are 0.5 to 2.0 waves per second and 20 to 50 per second, the latter resembling a fast adult beta pattern. During childhood, theta rhythms are most evident. The delta rhythm of infancy as well

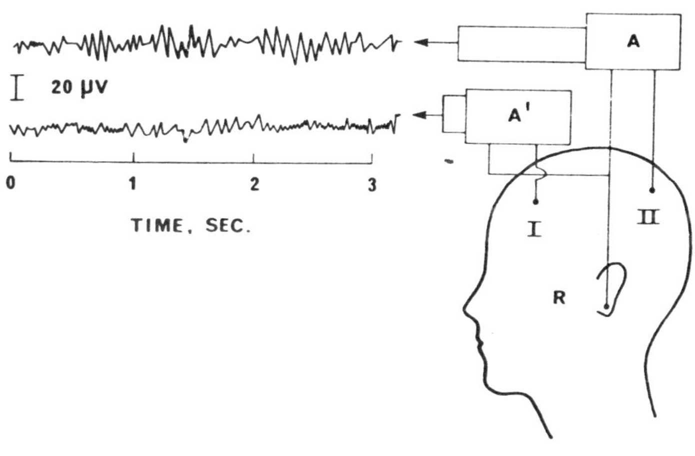

Fig. 8.3. Technique used for recording electroencephalograms (EEGs). A, A' = amplifiers; I = frontal lead; II = occipital lead; R = reference lead. Note the low amplitude, fast wave activity recorded between I and R compared to the higher amplitude, slower activity recorded between lead II and R.

as the theta rhythm of childhood are seen most clearly when recorded over the occipital and temporal areas of the brain. Gradually, however, these characteristic EEG patterns of immaturity change to the alpha rhythm of the adult so that between the ages of 14 and 19 years the adult EEG pattern is developed.

The particular EEG pattern that becomes established during maturation is a specific characteristic of the individual (like the fingerprints), and this functional property remains unaltered, assuming that no injury of disease or the brain occurs subsequently.

The frequencies of EEG's that are recorded from the frontal and parietal areas generally are higher than those recorded from the occipital region.

The alpha frequency of the adult EEG pattern can be decreased markedly by a reduction in the blood sugar level, a low body temperature, a high arterial partial pressure

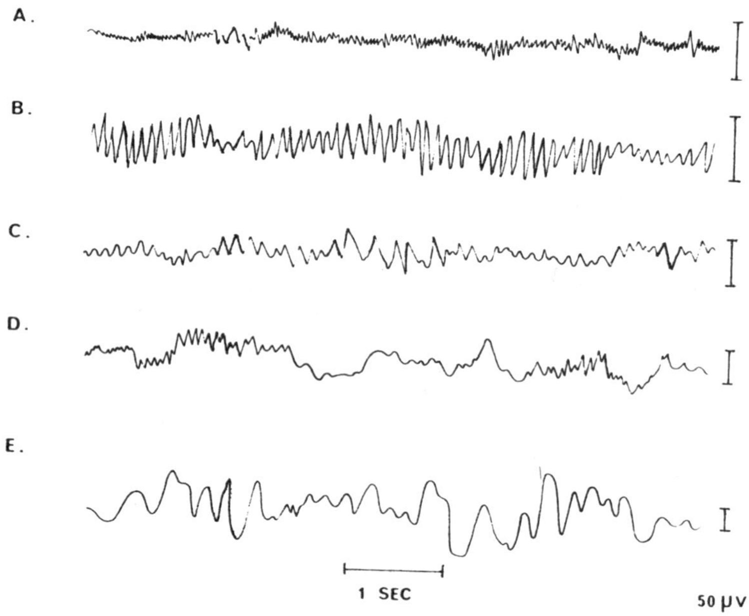

Fig. 8.4. Tracings of electroencephalographic patterns recorded from human subject during various states. A. During excitement, i.e., the attentive, alert state. The activity is of low amplitude, fast, generally irregular, and "desynchronized" in that no consistent rhythmic wave patterns are present B. Subject relaxed with eyes closed. Note regular alpha rhythm. C. Subject drowsy. D. Subject asleep. Note two groups of regular waves with a frequency of about 14/sec, the so-called sleep spindles. E. Deep sleep, irregular slow waves of high amplitude.

of carbon dioxide, or a decline in the blood concentration of adrenal glucocorticoid hormones. In general, therefore, those factors which reduce metabolism simultaneously tend to decrease the rate of alpha discharge in the brain. Conversely, a high blood glucose level, an elevated body temperature, a low arterial Pco_2, or an increase in the circulating adrenal glucocorticoid level all accelerate the alpha wave frequency (i.e., the fast-activity component of the EEG increases). Hyperventilation, or forced respiration, sometimes is employed clinically in order to reveal latent abnormalities in the EEG, as this procedure markedly lowers the arterial Pco_2 in the brain, and thus enhances fast activity in the EEG.

The alpha rhythm of the adult cortex normally predominates during the waking state, and this pattern is recorded when the subject is relaxed, the mind is wandering, and the eyes are closed. If, however, the eyes are opened so that a strong visual stimulus is presented suddenly and the attention is thereby fixed, the alpha waves are replaced by a high-frequency, irregular rhythm having a low voltage, but which has no dominant rhythmic pattern. This phenomenon, which is called *alpha blocking*, also is caused by any type of sensory excitation or mental concentration. Alpha blocking also is called *desynchronization*, because it indicates that the coordinated, or synchronized, activity of the neural elements which underlie production of the alpha wave pattern is interrupted by the sensory stimulus. Since desynchronization is induced by sensory excitation, and is correlated with the aroused (or alert) state, this phenomenon also is called the *arousal* or *alerting* response. Once the sensory stimulus no longer engages the subject's attention, the slower alpha rhythm appears.

Another factor that exerts a considerable influence upon the dominant pattern of the EEG is the state of arousal of the individual; sleep per se exerts a profound effect upon the EEG pattern. Sleep will be discussed subsequently in relation to the waking state and to the participation of the reticular activating system in these processes. It should be mentioned at this juncture, however, that there is an interesting direct relationship between the predominant frequency of the EEG and the evident state of arousal of the subject.

Physiologic Mechanisms that Under-Lie the Electric Activity of the Cortex. The alpha and slow-wave sleep patterns of the EEG exhibit rhythmic waves; it would appear that neural elements are firing in a regular and repetitive manner to produce these recorded electric oscillations. Actually, there is considerable evidence which indicates that the EEG depends upon the electric characteristics of the cortical cells themselves. In particular, the outermost two cell layers of this structure (i.e., the molecular or plexiform layer and the external granular layer, have been shown to be responsible for generating the largest portion of the primary evoked response of the cortex, to be discussed below.

The appearance of rhythmic waves in the EEG suggests that neural elements are firing in a synchronous rather than in a random fashion, and that such activity could be explained, at least partially, by simultaneous and coordinated oscillatory or reverberatory activity in a large number of closed neuronal circuits. Alternatively, certain neurons could exhibit autorhythmicity, and thus drive adjacent groups of neurons to rhythmic activity.

The best evidence that is available at this time indicates that the rhythmic changes recorded in the cortical EEG apparently are caused by current flow in the oscillating dipoles that are produced upon the dendrites of the cortical cells and their cell bodies by fluctuating afferent inputs. The superficial layers of the cortical gray matter contain relatively few cells; however the abundant dendrites in this region form an exceedingly dense mass of interdigitating fibers. Since dendrites usually do not transmit all-or-none action potentials, local (or nonpropagated) hyperpolarizing and hypopolarizing potentials are produced on the dendritic processes by excitatory (facilitory) or inhibitory endings on the dendrites. In turn, activity in these presynaptic endings produces a localized current flow into (and out of) the postsynaptic nerve cell body as well as its dendritic processes. Consequently the functional interrelationship between the nerve cell body and its dendrites becomes an ever-changing dipole, and the current flow in this dipole would induce detectable oscillations in a volume conductor (e.g., the interstitial fluid). If the net sum of the dendritic activity is positive with respect to the cell body, the cell is hyperpolarized and consequently less excitable. Conversely, when the net sum of the electric activity on the dendrites is negative relative to the cell body then the cell is hypopolarized, hence nearer to threshold, and thus hyperexcitable. In other words, the net dendritic potentials fluctuate rhythmically and thereby the excitability of the entire never cell membrane will be influenced by the electrotonic spread of such current fluctuations. Therefore the electric characteristics, hence the irritability, of a large number of nerve cells in a particular area of the cortex can change simultaneously, provided that no afferent (i.e., desynchronizing) inputs are received which would disturb this regular process and when the electric activity of large groups of nerve cells fluctuates in synchrony, rhythmic electric waves are detectable in the EEG.

There are two factors which lead to the synchronous electric activity of large groups of cortical dendrites such that rhythmic waves appear in the EEG. First, afferent impulses transmitted from the thalamus and other subcortical areas can induce synchronous cortical activity. A shallow, circular cut made in the cortex does not desynchronize the alpha rhythm, provided that the circulation is undamaged; therefore a lateral spread of impulses in the cortex is not essential to synchrony. However, the rhythmic wave pattern

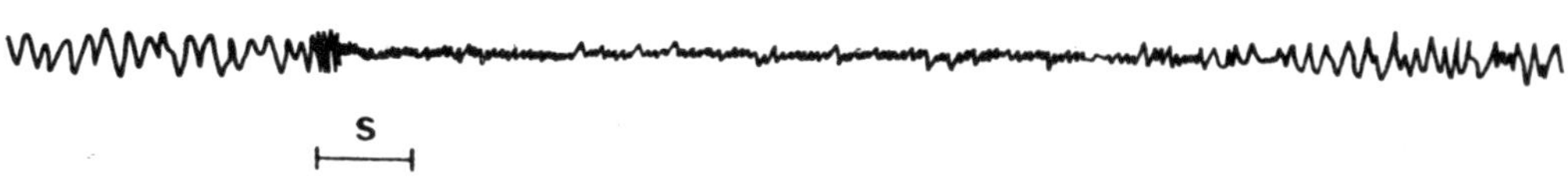

Fig. 8.5. Desynchronization of the EEG in the rabbit induced by an olfactory stimulus (S). Note the sudden appearance of irregular, high frequency, low amplitude waves upon application of the stimulus.

becomes much deranged if the deep-lying connections beneath the cortical area within the circular cut are severed.

The second type of synchrony takes place between adjacent and parallel dendritic processes. When two (or more) nerve fibers are in lateral contact with each other in a volume conductor, and one fiber is stimulated, the electric properties of the second fiber are modified appreciably even though the second fiber may not discharge an all-or-none impulse. The excitability of the second fiber is altered by passage of the impulse down the first fiber as follows. Flow of current into the depolarized region on the active fiber hypopolarizes the adjacent region of the second fiber, but hyperpolarizes the second fiber at two other points, and thus areas which are more positively charged with respect to other regions of the nerve develop at loci where inhibitory (i.e., hyperpolarizing)

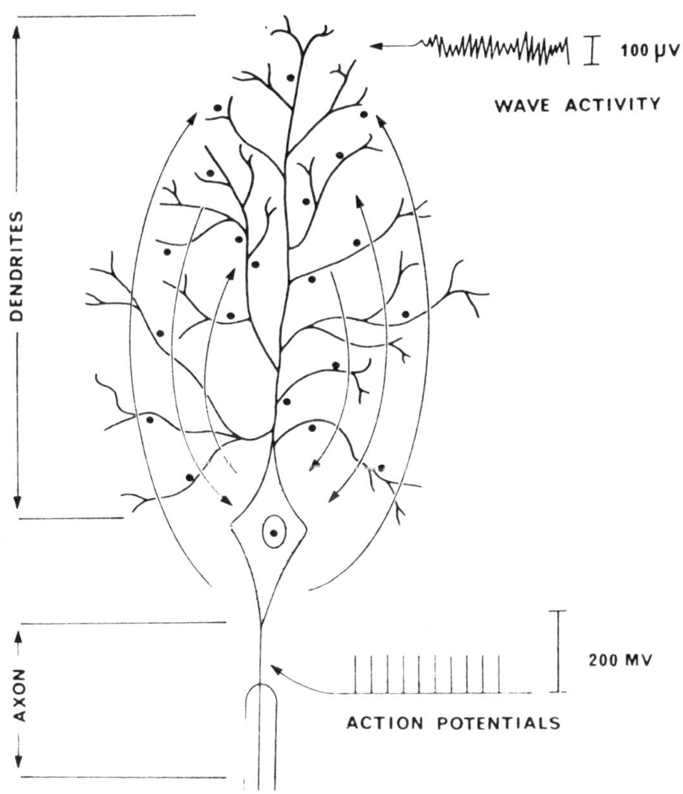

Fig. 8.6. The electric activity as recorded from the dendrites compared to that recorded from an axon. The ebb and flow of current on the active presynaptic terminations on the dendrites (black dots) causes potential fluctuations that are recorded as wave activity. In contrast to these localized potential alteration, all-or-none action potentials are transmitted along the axon.

nerve terminals are active. This purely electric transmission of impulses, or of electric effects, from the membrane of one nerve fiber to that of another fiber in lateral contact with it is called *ephaptic conduction*, and such physical junctions are called *ephapses*. This physical and functional arrangement is in marked contrast to conventional synapses, and it will be apparent to the reader that since no transmitter substance is involved, ephaptic conduction is entirely an electric effect which can take place in either direction.

Since the outermost layers of the cerebral cortex are composed essentially of extremely dense networks of neural processes that are oriented in similar planes with respect to each other, then the generation of current sinks and sources in adjacent fibers tends to synchronize current flow by the process of ephaptic conduction.

The cortex of the cerebellum as well as that of the hippocampus are both quite similar morphologically to the cerebral cortex, insofar as having complex patterns of parallel subpial dendritic processes overlying a layer of neurons is concerned. Therefore, both the cerebellum and hippocampus generate rhythmic oscillations in surface potential that are like those recorded in EEGs made from the cerebral cortex.

In contrast to the synchronizing mechanisms discussed above, it was noted earlier that desynchrony of the alpha wave pattern occurs when specific sensory inputs to the cortex are increased, and the rhythmic pattern of the EEG is altered so that an irregular low-voltage activity develops. Stimulation of the specific sensory nuclei and pathways up to, but not above, the level of the midbrain causes desynchronization. However, stimulation of the specific sensory relay nuclei of the thalamus or the primary cortical sensory areas does not produce desynchronization. In contrast to these responses, high rates of stimulation applied to the reticular formation in the tegmentum of the midbrain as well as to the nonspecific thalamic projection nuclei produces desynchronization of the EEG and will awaken a sleeping animal. When massive lesions are placed in the midbrain such as to interrupt the medial lemnisci in addition to other specific ascending sensory pathways, desynchronization still occurs following appropriate sensory stimulation. However, lesions induced in the tegmentum of the midbrain which interrupt the reticular activating system, but without disturbing the specific sensory systems, are accompanied by a synchronized EEG pattern which is not modified by sensory stimulation. Experimental animals which have the midbrain lesions described above are conscious, whereas animals having tegmental lesions remain comatose for extended intervals. Consequently it would seem that the afferent inputs to the cortex which are responsible for producing the desynchronization which follows stimulation of particular sensory endorgans are transmitted up the specific sensory systems to the midbrain. Thence the signals enter the reticular activating system by way of collateral fibers; subsequently the signals pass to the thalamus and ultimately reach the cerebral cortex via the nonspecific thalamic projection system.

Evoked Cortical Potentials. The cerebral cortex not only manifests continuous electric activity as described in the previous sections, but also a number of specific types of electric response can be evoked in the cortex by stimulation of peripheral sensory receptors or loci along the pathways that ascend from the receptors to the cerebral cortex. Careful study of such evoked potentials has revealed that two fiber systems functionally (as well

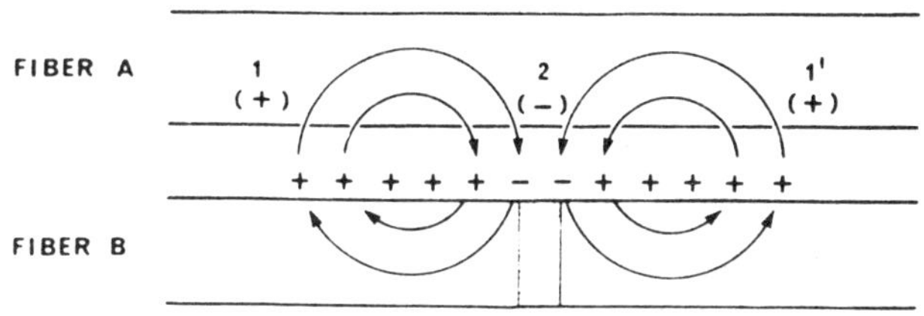

Fig. 8.7. The electric properties of two adjacent nerve fibers. Current flows into the depolarized (stippled) area of active fiber B from the surrounding membrane as an impulse passes along the nerve. At points 1 and 1' on the membrane of the inactive fiber A, positive charges build up (+), thus the membrane becomes slightly hyperpolarized in these two regions. At point 2 of fiber A, on the other hand, positive charges are "removed" so that the membrane undergoes a slight depolarization at this point.

as morphologically) connect the receptor endorgans to the cortex. The first of these fiber systems transmit impulses from the sense organ directly to specific cortical areas via a chain of three or four interneurons, and this system exhibits an extremely high degree of spatial orientation of its component fibers; hence the signals transmitted by this system are oriented similarly, so that a high degree of sensory localization results. The second fiber system branches from the direct pathway outlined above at the levels of the medulla and midbrain, and thus afferent signals are transmitted to the cortex indirectly via the reticular formation of the brain stem and diencephalon. The terminations of this second fiber system within the cortex thus are quite diffuse, in contrast to those of the direct afferent pathway. Another component of the diffuse fiber system diverges at the thalamic level.

The functional characteristics of each of these two afferent fiber systems are understood chiefly from the potentials which they produce in the cerebral cortex as well as by the manner in which these systems induce or alter spontaneously rhythmic cortical activities.

From a technical standpoint, the electric events which occur following excitation of a sense organ can be recorded by an exploring electrode placed upon the cortex, an indifferent electrode being located some distance away upon or within the body. The exploring electrode can be placed either intra- or extracellularly; however, in the latter instance the net electric activity of a much greater number of neurons may be sampled than with an intracellular electrode (cf., microelectrode studies of individual cerebellar neurons).

Following excitation of a particular sensory endorgan, two general types of potential are generated and can be recorded from the cerebral cortex. First, a sudden potential change called the unit spike can develop, and this activity persists for only one or two milliseconds. Second, the other type of potential develops relatively slowly, is of long duration, and is called the primary evoked response (or primary evoked potential).

The *unit spike* is related to the electric field in the immediate proximity of a single active cortical neuron, hence is recorded by microelectrodes whose tip diameter is relatively small (i.e., on the other of 2 μ) in order to prevent damage to the cell (or group of cells) under study. Recordings of unit spike activity have provided important data concerning the specificity of individual neurons and their pathways insofar as receptive fields are concerned.

Primary evoked potentials are detected by placing a large electrode on the cortical surface; hence the recordings reflect the summated activity of a large number of neurons which are located beneath the electrode. Subsequent excitation of a sense organ, a peripheral sensory nerve, or a thalamic relay nucleus produces a diphasic potential having a magnitude up to 1 mv, the potential being localized specifically in the sensory receptive areas of the cortex. In fact, the ultimate cortical locus where the primary evoked potential can be recorded from stimulation of a particular sense organ is so specific that the evoked potential has been used to map the specific primary sensory areas in the postcentral gyrus of the cortex. This technique has been used to map the projections of the cutaneous, retinal, and cochlear receptors upon the cortical sensory areas. Such a neurophysiology procedure is valid for determining the spatial orientation of peripheral as well as central endings because the electric activity in the direct, rapid-conducting sensory pathways not only is synchronous, but also because these pathways have an exquisite spatial orientation of their component neurons and their fiber processes.

The actual configuration of the primary evoked potential depends upon the position of the recording electrode. Thus when this electrode is placed upon the cortical surface, the initial deflection usually is positive, and this phase is followed by a more prolonged negative phase. On the other hand, when the exploring electrode is inserted "deep" (i.e., 0.2 to 0.3 mm) into the cortex, this pattern is inverted; i.e., the initial deflection is negative, and this phase is followed by a positive deflection.

Apparently the external granular layers of the cortex are related to the genesis of the evoked cortical potentials, however these bioelectric phenomena cannot be ascribed to any one neural source. The primary evoked potential commences as electric activity ascends from below into the terminal ramifications of the thalamocortical afferents, and then continues for an interval of 20 to 30 milliseconds. It has been demonstrated that individual cortical neurons may discharge spikes one or more times while the primary evoked potential is present.

If the experimental animal is anesthetized lightly, the primary evoked potential may be followed by a short volley of low-frequency positive waves (i.e., about 10 per

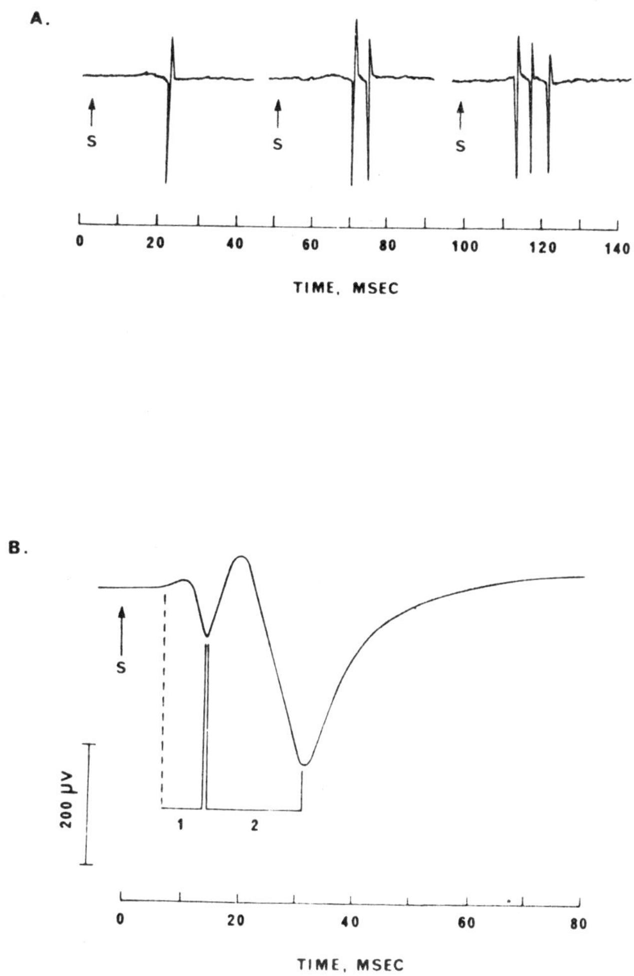

Fig. 8.8. Unit spikes recorded extracellularly from a single neuron of the postcentral gyrus (monkey) at different times following delivery of a single stimulus (S). Note that the cortical neuron can fire one or more times in response to a single stimulus. The latency of response also is subject to spontaneous variation. B. Evoked electric response recorded from the cat sensory cortex following contralateral sciatic nerve stimulation (S). 1 = primary evoked response; 2 = secondary response.

second). These repetitive waves are produced in the thalamus by the initial afferent volley of impulses and have been considered to be an after-discharge that is caused by oscillatory activity between the cortex and the thalamus.

If, on the other hand, the animal is anesthetized deeply, the specific primary evoked potential frequently is succeeded by a second positive-negative change. This secondary *evoked discharge* (or *response*), in contrast to the highly localized primary evoked response discussed above, is quite diffuse and it appears simultaneously over most of the cortex and other parts of the brain after a rather consistent latency of between 30 and 80 milliseconds the initial stimulus.

The diffuse secondary response is not altered by a circular cut through the gray matter which isolates a "button" of tissue containing the locus of the primary evoked potential from all lateral connections. This fact, together with the consistent latent period that elapses before the appearance of the secondary evoked response, argues in favor of the conclusion that this electric activity must arise from subcortical regions. Apparently the diffuse or nonspecific thalamic projection system is involved in the genesis of the secondary evoked discharge.

Furthermore, within the primary sensory receptive areas of the cortex the neurons which fire during the course of the primary evoked discharge do not fire while the secondary discharge is taking place. Consequently a different group of neurons must be involved during the secondary process. Lastly, the secondary evoked discharge is not similar everywhere throughout the cortex. Thus the secondary activity that is elicited in the association areas is different from that which takes place simultaneously within the visual cortex, both of which were evoked by one stimulus, i.e., primary visual stimulation.

The secondary evoked response is related intimately to another bioelectric phenomenon. When an experimental animal is anesthetized rather deeply, and obvious sensory inputs are absent, trains or bursts of almost synchronous waves having a frequency that ranges between 8 and 12 per second can be recorded from large areas of each cerebral hemisphere. These spontaneously occurring *cortical burst waves,* like the alpha waves and sleep spindles tend to wax and wane. Although such spontaneous bursts of cortical waves are not true evoked potentials, a similar bioelectric phenomenon can be evoked by stimulation of the reticular system of the thalamus.

The primary evoked potential is unaltered by the presence of spontaneous bursts of cortical activity; however such activity does prevent the appearance of the diffuse secondary evoked response. This burst activity apparently is indicative, but not a cause, of the spontaneous physiologic changes in the irritability of the central nervous system, as evoked cortical responses generally are greater during periods of burst activity, but depressed during the intervals between bursts.

Spontaneous cortical bursts are produced through activation of a diffuse (nonspecific) thalamic projection system, in contrast to the repetitive waves which are generated in the specific thalamic projection nuclei.

The secondary evoked potential also is related to another bioelectric phenomenon called the recruiting response. Thus a series of electric stimuli applied to the intralaminar thalamic nuclei causes the appearance of a train of negative-then-positive diphasic potential waves to appear in both cerebral hemispheres following a lag period of 15 to 60 milliseconds. If the frequency of the applied stimulation lies between 5 and 15 per second, then the amplitude of the evoked potentials gradually increases at first. Subsequently, the trains of evoked potentials rhythmically increase and decrease in amplitude, their frequency ranging between 8 and 12 per second. The configuration and frequency of the potentials evoked by the recruiting response are like those of the spontaneous cortical bursts. Furthermore, the spatial distribution of the recruiting response in the cortex is identical with that observed when spontaneous burst activity occurs.

The functional classification of the thalamic nuclei has been developed as the consequence of studies done on the cortical potentials which are evoked following stimulation of the thalamic nuclei. Thus extremely localized stimulation of the relay and association nuclei produces a similarly localized focal activity in the cerebral cortex following a latent period of 1 to 5 milliseconds; hence these structures are called *specific thalamic nuclei*. Excitation of the other thalamic nuclei produces diffuse, bilateral, cortical potentials which are indicative of a recruiting responses; these structures are called the *nonspecific thalamic nuclei*. The latter nuclei discharge the cortical nuclei which in turn generate the continuous electric activity of the brain that is recorded as the EEG.

Wakefulness and Sleep

The normal diurnal wakefulness-sleep cycle is one of the most obvious circadian rhythms that can be experienced as well as observed, and the mental and physical benefits which accrue to the individual from alternating periods of wakefulness and sleep are equally evident. From a strict physiologic standpoint, however, the specific benefits that are derived from intermittent periods of sleep are far less clear. It is plain that sleep directly affects the performance of the entire nervous system, as prolonged bouts of sleeplessness (pervigilium) result in a progressive deterioration of one's mental and behavioral characteristics. Apathy, listlessness, and mental dullness or irritability may be the accompaniment of extended periods of wakefulness. In turn, the irritability may yield to outright psychotic manifestations, provided that the lack of sleep is extended for a sufficiently long interval. In fact, such neurologic symptoms can appear following deprivation of one component of normal sleep, namely the rapid eye movement (REM) phase of this state.,

The particular functional effects of sleep upon the various somatic and visceral structures of the body are even more nebulous than those seen to occur in the nervous system, and there is even some evidence which indicates that no impairment of such functions occurs even though these structures are not subjected to a regular wakefulness-sleep cycle.

During periods of wakefulness, the nervous system exerts certain general influences upon somatic and visceral functions. Thus tone of the skeletal muscles is increased and net sympathetic discharge likewise is augmented during the waking state. Conversely, during periods of sleep, impulse transmission to the somatic musculature may fall so low that tonus of the skeletal muscles becomes practically nil. Concomitantly, the discharge of the sympathetic nervous system also decreases markedly, whereas parasympathetic nervous activity may (or may not) be enhanced. A number of additional physiologic changes accompany the altered patterns of neural activity seen during the sleep state. For example the body temperature declines somewhat leading to a fall in the metabolic rate to basal levels. The heart rate declines and the vessels of the cutaneous vascular bed dilate; consequently the arterial blood pressure falls. The excretory function of the kidneys declines, whereas the activity of the gastrointestinal tract may increase somewhat

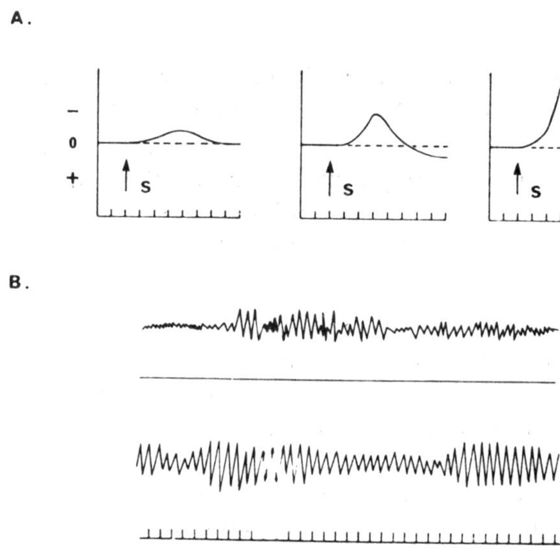

Fig. 8.9. A. Recruiting response to three successive stimuli of constant intensity which were delivered singly to the intralaminar (nonspecific) region of the thalamus. The polarity is indicated on the left. Note that the amplitude of the evoked response recorded from the cortex increases progressively. B. Electric responses of cortex to rhythmic electric stimulation of the intralaminar portion of the thalamus. Upper trace, "spontaneous" burst of activity; lower trace, waxing and waning response.

depending upon whether or not the functional state of the parasympathetic nervous system is augmented.

For the purpose of the following discussion, the waking, aroused, or alert state can be defined as that condition in which a person or animal is capable of responding to various sensory stimuli and of having subjective experiences. Conversely, normal or physiologic sleep can be considered to be reversible state of mental as well as physical rest during which volition and consciousness are partially or completely absent. Sleep also may be defined as a reversible behavioral state during which a characteristic and immobile posture is assumed, and the individual is relatively insensitive to external or internal stimuli.

It must not be inferred that wakefulness and sleep are sharply distinct and mutually exclusive phenomena. Rather there is a smooth and graded continuum from keen alertness through drowsiness to light sleep and thence to deep sleep. Furthermore, depending upon internal and external conditions, an individual may fluctuate back and forth, both readily and rapidly, between any of these states. Therefore, wakefulness and sleep actually consist of many degrees of intensity, and these may shade either perceptibly or imperceptibly into each other.

The neuroanatomic and neurophysiologic substrates upon which the waking and the sleeping states are based now will be considered, and this material will be followed by a discussion of the particular physiologic aspects of the various sleep states.

Roles of the Hypothalamus and Thalamus in Wakefulness and Sleep. When lesions are placed in the posterior hypothalamus of experimental animals a state of prolonged and comatose sleep ensues. Similarly, artificial stimulation of the dorsal hypothalamus of conscious animals induces sleep. Experimental observations such as these have led to the postulate that "wakefulness" and "sleep" centers are present in the hypothalamus. However, more recent experimental studies performed upon the reticular activating system as well as the nonspecific thalamic projection nuclei have indicated that the role of the hypothalamus, if any, in producing or regulating sleep is neither direct nor specific. Thus it is important to mention that the posterior hypothalamic lesions that produce a sleeplike comatose state in experimental animals also damage RAS fibers as they course to the thalamus and cortex. Consequently, the effects of such posterior hypothalamic lesions doubtless can be explained on the basis of destruction of a part of the RAS that is involved in producing wakefulness, rather than due to destruction of a presumed hypothalamic center that performs this function.

Similarly, the interpretation of experiments in which stimulation of dorsal hypothalamic areas produces sleep in conscious animals also can be criticized. Thus the dorsal hypothalamic areas which appear to induce sleep when stimulated lie extremely close to the nonspecific thalamic projection nuclei. Sleep is induced when the frequency of stimulation is at a rate of about 8 per second. However, this frequency of stimulation is the same as that required to produce sleep when applied to the nonspecific thalamic projection nuclei, the orbital surface of the frontal lobe, and certain regions of the brain stem. Consequently it would appear that the effects of hypothalamic excitation are caused by stimulation of a nonspecific and diffuse neural system whose stimulation produces sleep, and thus the hypothalamus is not involved directly in the mechanism responsible for inducing this state.

Insofar as the thalamic component of a possible "sleep center" is concerned, it has been shown that electric stimulation of the lateral and ventral portions of the massa intermedia by chronically implanted electrodes will induce sleep in conscious animals. In contrast to the effects of hypothalamic stimulation described above, thalamic stimulation produces an organized behavioral pattern leading to sleep. A definite sequence of sleep-related activities is evoked by thalamic stimulation, including yawning, seeking an appropriate sleeping site, lying down, closing the eyes, somatic relaxation, and ultimately sleep.

Role of the Reticular Activating Systems (RAS) in Wakefulness and Sleep. Although the actual source of an individual's capacity to perform intellectual as well as volitional motor functions, to learn, and to perceive as well as to localize particular sensations lies within the cerebral cortex, the cortex itself cannot perform these functions unless it is "turned on" or "awake" so that a conscious or alert state is present. The principal neuroanatomic structure which is critical to production of a conscious state in the cortex of a sleeping person or animal is the *reticular formation*. This phylogenetically ancient core of the medulla oblongata and midbrain also has a number of other functions, including centers which participate in the regulation of respiration, cardiac rate, blood pressure, somatic movements, and the secretion of certain endocrine glands. The reticular formation also has been shown to participate in the modulation or control of sensory inputs to the brain.

About 25 years ago it was discovered that stimulation of the reticular formation of a sleeping or drowsy cat by means of a chronically implanted electrode would awaken the animal as peacefully as though it awakened naturally. This experiment provided direct evidence that excitation of the reticular formation was responsible for producing arousal or alerting of the cortex. Subsequently, the reticular formation of the brain stem and midbrain was named the reticular activating system (RAS) because of its ability to induce the waking state when stimulated.

As noted earlier, all of the major sensory pathways of the body emit enormous numbers of collaterals which enter the reticular formation. Thereby somatic, visceral, auditory, visual, and other sensory signals from practically all regions of the body not only are transmitted directly to the cortex via the appropriate thalamic nuclei, but also are shunted into the reticular formation. Thus various sensory inputs can excite the reticular formation so that this structure in turn transmits signals to the cortex producing arousal (or wakening) of the cortex. The aroused or awakened cortex then is able to interpret directly the sensory signals which are being received.

The function of the RAS in producing arousal is nonspecific in that it responds identically to any sensory input. Hence the response of the RAS to any sensory stimulus is to arouse or alert the brain and not to relay any particular information concerning the input signal per se. The signals that are relayed from the RAS are not focused upon any one particular cortical area as are those transmitted by the specific sensory systems. Rather the cortical inputs from the RAS are diffuse.

The RAS apparently is able to learn to discriminate among various sensory inputs. Thus a stimulus which would awaken one individual instantly is completely ineffective when applied to another person. For example, a person who has lived for a along period near a railroad depot would sleep undisturbed throughout the in evitable racket caused by the operations of the depot, whereas a newcomer to the area would be disturbed and awakened constantly by the barrage of auditory (and perhaps olfactory) stimuli. On the other hand, the individual who was conditioned to living near the sounds of the depot might awaken instantly at the relatively slight noise produced by a door opening in his home in the middle of the night, and this selectivity to different stimulus intensities also appears to reside within the RAS.

The RAS also plays a role in focusing the attention selectively on particular sensory inputs during the waking state.

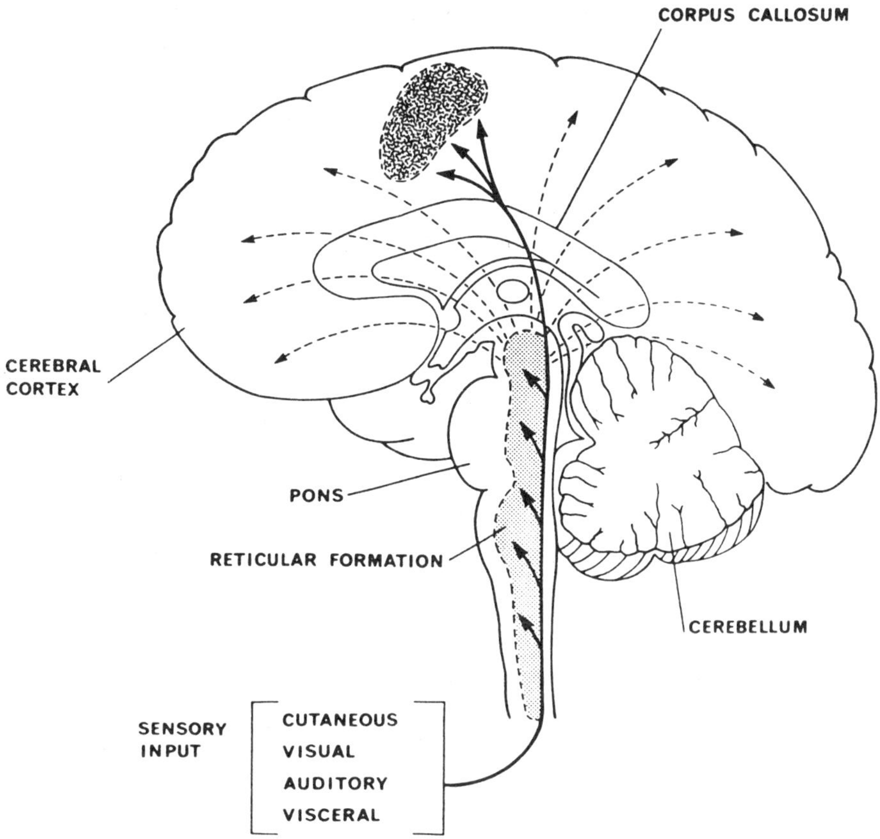

Fig. 8.10. The reticular formation of the human brain. Various sensory inputs send nonspecific impulses into the reticular formation via collaterals as well as to specific sensory areas of the cerebral cortex (shaded). In turn, the reticular formation sends nonspecific impulses throughout the cortex (curved dashed lines) to "awaken" the entire brain.

The RAS not only is responsible for producing cortical arousal, but also it is necessary or maintaining the individual in a conscious state once aroused. Therefore if a person has suffered permanent injury to, or pathologic destruction of, the RAS, an irreversible coma ensues which only can terminate in death. When the RAS is uninjured, however, it can maintain a state of wakefulness (but not of consciousness) even when the cortex is absent. For example, in a normal newborn infant whose cortical functions are nil, periods of wakefulness are present throughout the day. Similarly, anencephalic monsters (i.e., infants born with a congenital absence of the cerebral hemispheres) may live several years with proper care, but such creatures never have any true understanding of, or communication with, their environment. Nevertheless, in both instances cited above intervals of wakefulness are present during which feeding, swallowing, digestion, and other basic physiologic activities are carried out. The conclusion is inevitable that a rudimentary form of wakefulness can be present even in the complete absence of the cerebral cortex provided that the RAS can function adequately. For long periods of normal wakefulness to be maintained, however, the presence of the cerebral cortex is essential, and the alert state appears to be sustained through a reciprocal feedback of signals between the cortex and the RAS. Consequently the RAS is stimulated by impulses from some areas of the cortex as well as by impulses that originate in the sensory receptors that are located throughout the body. This fact can be demonstrated, for example, by electrically stimulating the orbital surface of the frontal lobe or the superior temporal gyrus in monkeys. This localized cortical stimulation will arouse a sleeping monkey and cause augmented reticular activity in such an animal. However, if the stimulation is applied to these cortical areas while the monkey is awake, the animal may immediately cease whatever prior activity in which it was engaged, and look about intently, if not to say questioningly, for want of a better term to describe the evoked response. Consequently it appears that the cerebral cortex, acting in concert with the RAS via diffuse systems of corticofugal fibers, has an important role in focusing attention during the waking state as well as providing a pathway whereby intracortical processes can initiate and sustain arousal of the individual. For example, direct fiber pathways pass into the RAS from nearly all areas of the cortex. However, the sensorimotor cortex (i.e., the precentral and postcentral gyri), the frontal cortex, the cingulate gyrus, the hippocampus and other limbic structures, as well as the basal ganglia give rise to especially prominent corticofugal pathways that course into the reticular formation. Furthermore, such corticoreticular fiber systems conceivably might underlie the alerting responses which accompany emotional states and which can take place in the absence of any clearly demonstrable external stimulus.

There is some experimental evidence which indicates that the various functions carried out by the RAS are localized and it has been postulated that the caudal portion of the reticular formation underlies the wakefulness-sleep patterns. On the other hand, the thalamic portions of the reticular system are believed to be responsible for regulating the localized arousal patterns which constantly shift or scan from one area of the cortex to another with time as the normally active person is confronted with a broad range of specific sensory stimuli that change rapidly.

Impulses that ascend in the RAS desynchronize preexisting synchronized patterns of cortical activity; however, the mechanism that underlies this effect is obscure. Furthermore, experimental stimulation of the RAS inhibits spontaneous cortical burst activity and the recruiting response.

Since stimulation of the RAS causes arousal and alerting of experimental animals, it might be anticipated that such excitation would produce an elevated rather than a depressed irritability of the cortical neurons. It is known, however, that certain neurons located in the sensory cortical projection areas discharge at random during sleep but during the waking state the same neurons discharge only in response to particular sensory inputs. Consequently it seems as though the activity of the RAS eliminates the random firing that occurs during sleep by inhibiting cortical activity to some extent, and thereby the affected neurons are unhampered by extraneous impulses so that they now are able to respond solely to specific sensory inputs. In other words, the input signal is tuned more sharply even though the overall sensitivity of the entire system to excitation (i.e., the net irritability) is decreased somewhat.

Certain pharmacologic agents initiate (or mimic) the physiologic action of the sympathetic nervous system on the RAS. Thus the catecholamines (epinephrine and norepinephrine) as well as amphetamine all cause behavioral alerting as well as electroencephalographic arousal patterns. This effect is brought about through a reduction in the threshold to firing of the reticular neurons located within the brain stem. Under physiologically stressful conditions, the adrenal medulla normally secretes quantities of catecholamines directly into the bloodstream. One major effect of the generalized adrenergic discharge that occurs during emergencies is an intensification of the alert state that in turn is essential to effectual response to the emergency state per se.

The reinforcement of the alerting response to the secretion of catecholamines during periods of physiologic stress is mediated indirectly. That is, the epinephrine and norepinephrine liberated from the adrenal medulla do not act directly upon the excitability of the reticular neurons. Rather, these agents increase the blood pressure (i.e., they exert a pressor effect) and it has been demonstrated that an increase in blood pressure alone, from whatever cause, will concomitantly increase the irritability of the neurons that comprise the reticular formation; that is, these neurons apparently possess a mechanoreceptor function.

In conclusion, what physiologic mechanisms appear to underlie the normal wakefulness-sleep cycle?

It is clear that awakening or arousal from the sleeping state is produced when sensory (or afferent) input signals to the cerebral cortex via the RAS reach a sufficient intensity to "turn on" or "activate" the cortex in a general fashion. The particular sensory receptors that provide these input signals are irrelevant, as the cortical arousal produced by the RAS is nonspecific and crude. It is far from clear, however, how these sensory inputs to the RAS become quantitatively adequate to trigger normal awakening following a night's sleep. One clue is available which perhaps may be relevant insofar as this process is concerned. A number of investigators have demonstrated experimentally the presence of as yet unidentified biochemical factors in cerebrospinal fluid as well as blood plasma of well-rested animals which can induce wakefulness when injected or transfused into recipient animals. Consequently it is tempting to speculate upon the possibility that under physiologic conditions one (or more) specific humoral substances can reach a sufficiently high level in the body fluids that the irritability of the RAS increases markedly. Thus any minor sensory input to the RAS would be adequate to produce cortical arousal.

Alternatively it could be suggested that normal arousal following a period of sleep is triggered by the depressed activity of a sleep center (or system) whose function when fully active is to inhibit the activity of the RAS and/or the cortex either directly or via certain humoral agents. Reciprocal activity between a "Wakefulness System" (the RAS) and a "Sleeping System" (several structures, particularly the thalamus?) would result in the normal wakefulness-sleep cycle.

In any event, once the waking state of the cortex is achieved, the alert or aroused condition normally is maintained for a number of hours by a continuous bombardment of the RAS by sensory inputs that arise in somatic as well as visceral structures, and in turn these inputs, in particular those from the muscle spindles, serve to maintain cortical arousal via the RAS. In addition, the cerebral cortex, once aroused, transmits impulses back to the RAS, and these signals automatically tend to enhance RAS activity. In other words, a positive feedback loop is established functionally between the cortex and the RAS during periods of wakefulness. Lastly, any sympathetic neural activity that is present in the waking state would tend, a priori, to enhance the activity of the RAS, although the quantitative significance of this factor under physiologic conditions is unknown.

As the waking state becomes prolonged, the familiar symptoms of "drowsiness" or "fatigue" develop. Undoubtedly many factors contribute to these symptoms, including not only marked physical activity which induces neuromuscular fatigue, but also monotony and boredom. The latter two factors, of course would contribute to drowsiness by decreasing sensory inputs to the RAS, hence the degree of cortical arousal would decline automatically. In addition, it has been shown experimentally that humoral agents are present in the plasma of fatigued subjects which can produce sleep in rested animals. Presumably such chemical agents have a role in the physiologic onset of sleep through their depressant action on certain areas of the nervous system (e.g., the RAS and/or cortex), and possibly their stimulant action on a "sleep center" or "system" of which thalamic areas probably are a component. According to this view, therefore, normal arousal following an adequate period of sleep could be due to the elimination and/or metabolic in activation of the humoral agent (or agents) responsible for producing sleep, so that the depressed excitability of the RAS neurons caused by the humoral agent returned to "normal" or "physiologically active" levels. The circumstantial evidence in support of this contention will be presented in the next section.

In this regard, it is of interest that the ability of general anesthetics to produce the unconscious state depends (at least partially) upon their ability to inhibit or depress conduction within the RAS.

Alternatively, the subjective feelings of drowsiness or fatigue which lead to sleep on a more or less regular daily basis also could be induced, in part at least, by a depletion of neurotransmitter substances in the neuronal pools which comprise the arousal system. This view is all the more attractive since the RAS is composed of enormous numbers of polysynaptic neural circuits; therefore depletion of transmitter substances conceivably would occur more readily here than in more direct pathways having fewer synapses. In any event, and regardless of the specific neural and biochemical mechanisms that may be involved, when the signal output of the RAS to the cerebral cortex decreases below a certain level, sleep ensues. There also is a strong implication that excitation of certain thalamic structures may participate actively in the behavioral patterns that lead to the sleeping state.

Physiologic Correlates of Sleep States. The EEG has been used extensively to gain some objective insight into the neurophysiologic alterations that occur during sleep. Some of the changes in the EEG that are recorded from normal human and animal subjects can be related directly to the depth of sleep. In addition to EEGs, eye movements, body temperature, reaction time, stimulus intensity for arousal, sequence in which various sleep patterns appear, electro-myographs, heart as well as respiratory rates, and the fluctuations in blood levels of certain hormones all have been studied and correlated with one another in normal subjects during periods of natural sleep.

It has been recognized since ancient times that there are two clearly different levels of sleep. However, only within the past half century has use of the electroencephalograph enabled investigators to demonstrate conclusively that there are fundamentally two sleep patterns that alternate with each other throughout a period of normal repose. Thus, a period of light sleep accompanied by slow brain waves of large amplitude characteristically is followed by a period of deep sleep in which the bioelectric activity of the cortex is accelerated markedly. Each of these two distinct sleep states may now be considered individually.

Light Sleep. Immediately following the onset of the sleep state in a relaxed and drowsy human or animal subject, the alpha rhythm of the EEG is replaced by a series of low-frequency waves having a large amplitude than those seen during the alert state. The subject can be awakened readily from this state of *light sleep*. As the period of light sleep progresses, groups of alphalike synchronized waves called *spindles* appear in the EEG, and some muscular tone still is present. Occasional gross body movements occur, but any eye movements that take place during light sleep are slow and of rare occurrence. The respiratory cycle is regular and deep, the heart rate is rhythmic and slow compared to the waking state, and the blood pressure also is somewhat below making levels. In the male, penile erections do not occur during light sleep. Such mentation as occurs is repetitive and thoughtlike.

Light sleep also is called *synchronized sleep, slow sleep*, or *spindle sleep*, because of the characteristic EEG patterns that may be recorded. Light sleep also is called *non-rapid* eye movement (or *non-REM*) sleep because of the absence of conjugate eye movements during this state.

Deep Sleep. The light sleep state described above gives way after variable intervals throughout the entire sleep period to an entire spectrum of physiologic changes that mark the onset of periods of *deep sleep*. The high-amplitude slow waves seen in the EEG during light sleep generally are replaced in deep sleep by low-voltage, high-frequency, irregular (desychronized) waves that are far more characteristic of the alert than the sleeping state, although regular theta waves occur consistently at the hippocampal level, Hence deep sleep is also called *desynchronized sleep*. Despite this high level of cortical activity during deep sleep, arousal from this state is difficult, and complete muscular atony also is present. These observable facts present a distinct physiologic paradox; hence deep sleep also is called *paradoxical sleep*.

During periods of deep sleep, rapid lateral or back-and-forth (occasionally up-and-down) eye movements take place in a conjugate fashion, and these eye movements have been demonstrated to be associated with periods of dreaming. Consequently deep sleep is also called *rapid eye movement* (REM) *sleep* or *dreaming sleep.*

REM sleep is accompanied by involuntary twitches of the somatic musculature at irregular intervals, rhythmic contractions of the stapedius and tensor tympani muscles of the middle ear, a shallow respiration of variable rate, and a rapid heart rate. The blood pressure also may vary somewhat during REM sleep. Penile erections occur frequently in males during REM sleep, and in those individuals who exhibit bruxism (spasmodic or rhythmic grinding of the teeth not related to mastication), this condition is manifest during intervals of deep sleep.

Periods of light sleep alternate with periods of deep sleep throughout the night, REM sleep intervals superseding light sleep about every 60 to 90 minutes. Typically, periods of REM sleep become longer toward morning, and in young adults approximately 20 per cent of an average night's sleep is spent in the state of paradoxical sleep. In fact, studies in humans have indicated that there is an inverse relationship between the percentage of the total sleep period spent in REM sleep and age. Thus, infants a few days old spend approximately 50 per cent of their sleep time in REM sleep, despite the fact that dreaming is unlikely because of their limited cortical experience. At the other end of the scale, persons in their seventh decade spend only 15 per cent of their total sleep time in REM sleep. During the intervening years, between infancy and old age, proportionate declines in REM sleep also are seen with age.

Possible Mechanisms of Light and Deep Sleep. If humans or animals are awakened every time an interval of REM sleep commences so that a net deficit of REM sleep is produced, the subjects may (or may not!) become irritable and "anxious." Subsequently, when allowed to sleep undisturbed, REM-deficient human and animal subjects spend a considerably greater proportion of their total sleep time in REM sleep than otherwise would be the case. These studies, among others, have led some investigators to the conclusion that a deficiency of paradoxical sleep causes a buildup of some biochemical factor, possibly an amine, which normally would be eliminated during periods of REM sleep. Although the present evidence for this statement is not wholly conclusive, nevertheless it is convincing.

Insofar as the neuroanatomic-biochemical system involved in the production of light sleep is concerned (in the cat, at least) it has been demonstrated that the nuclei of the median raphe of the brain stem are the chief source of serotonin in the brain. Subtotal destruction of these nuclei induces a state of relative sleeplessness (i.e., the total per cent of each day spent in sleep declines appreciably); consequently it would appear that this neurochemical system may play a role in the cyclic inactivation of the RAS leading to light sleep, as the decrease in net serotonin concentration caused by subtotal brain stem injury causes an increased wakefulness.

On the other hand, the neurochemical elements responsible for causing REM or paradoxical sleep appear to reside in the dorsal pons, specifically in an area known as the *locus caeruleus.* If the brain stem of a cat is sectioned at the upper level of the pons, a rhythmic cyclic variation between the states of wakefulness and paradoxical sleep develops. The latter state can be detected readily, of course, by rapid eye movements as well as atony of the skeletal muscles, in particular those of the neck. If, however, the brain stem is sectioned at the caudal level of the pons and immediately rostral to the medulla, paradoxical sleep no longer is seen. Therefore, the area of the brain stem responsible for inducing paradoxical sleep lies in the middle of the pons, and further investigations have indicated that this region is the locus caeruleus, whose cells contain an abundance of norepinephrine. It appears that this neurochemical system plays a role in the etiology of REM (or paradoxical) sleep like that of serotonin in the genesis of light sleep.

Insofar as the mechanisms related to the development of atony in the skeletal muscles during paradoxical sleep are concerned, it appears that the source of this inhibition lies principally within the spinal cord.

The physiologic roles of REM sleep and dreaming are quite obscure, and from a phylogenetic standpoint this type of sleep occurs only in mammals and birds. The latter animals only exhibit very brief intervals of REM sleep (i.e., up to 15 seconds); consequently only 0.5 per cent of the total sleeping time is occupied with paradoxical sleep. Mammals, on the other hand, spend a considerably greater proportion of their total sleeping time in REM, up to 20 to 30 per cent in higher mammals such as apes and man.

In conclusion, it is evident that the "sleeping state" actually represents two distinct and individual physiologic conditions which alternate normally and "spontaneously" throughout the normal period of respose. Furthermore, it is evident that each of these two states of sleep represents a highly complex physiologic state, and neither is accomplished simply by "turning off" the cortex via decreasing afferent inputs from the RAS, as other neurochemical systems undoubtedly are active participants in the process.

A Comparison of Physiologic Alterations During Sleep and Transcendental Meditation. Certain physiologic changes that are observed during transcendental mediation were discussed earlier, and at that time it was noted that these changes have little in common with those observed during normal sleep. For example, oxygen consumption declines rapidly within a few minutes after a subject commences a period of transcendental meditation, hypnosis causes no appreciable change in this parameter, and during sleep several hours must elapse before oxygen consumption decreases significantly.

The blood concentration of carbon dioxide rises significantly during sleep, a fact which indicates a decrease in respiration. Concomitantly there is a negligible decrease in the pH of the blood (i.e., it becomes more acid), and this factor can be related to the decrease in pulmonary ventilation that accompanies sleep, and not to metabolic changes like those which accompany transcendental meditation.

The increase in skin resistance which accompanies sleep takes place at a much slower rate, and is of a significantly lower magnitude, than that which is measured during transcendental meditation.

The EEG patterns characteristic of the sleeping state are composed primarily of low-frequency waves (roughly 12 to 14 cycles per second) which have a relatively high amplitude (i.e., voltage), together with a heterogeneous collection of lower-amplitude waves having a number of frequencies. This typical sleep pattern is not seen during transcendental meditation.

In marked contrast to either the sleeping state or to periods of transcendental meditation, during hypnosis the EEG assumes the pattern that typically is found in the mental state which has been suggested to the subject. Similarly, the alterations in heart rate, blood pressure, respiration, and skin resistance all follow patterns like those of the suggested state in a hypnotized subject.

The Modulation of Sensory Inputs: Attention. If any higher organism, particularly a mammal such as man, were forced to give equal attention to, as well as act upon, all of the sensory stimuli to which it is exposed constantly in the course of everyday life, the total mass of this sensory information converted into signals within the nervous system would be such as to overwhelm the circuits responsible for producing orderly and effective response patterns by the organism. As such affective responses are critical to survival not only of the individual but also of the species, it would appear a priori that certain brain mechanisms must have evolved which function to protect the individual from sensory overload and to direct his attention selectively to those particular stimuli which require action most urgently. In the case of the human species, interest as well as mere biologic urgency plays a considerable role in the priority given by the individual to particular stimuli. Consequently attention and the neurophysiologic mechanisms which underlie and direct this process are an important aspect of the waking state. The term "attention" per se means a selective awareness of a part or an aspect of the environment, as well as a selective responsiveness to one type of stimulus. Obviously, therefore, experience (i.e., learning) plays a critical role in determining which factors warrant attention by any particular species.

The remainder of this section will present a brief summary of several experimental findings which indicate that the brain contains specific mechanisms which are able to regulate the generation of sensory impulses, as well as to control their transmission in specific sensory systems.

Stimulation of the reticular formation in the medulla inhibits transmission of sensory impulses at the first synapse in the lemniscal and spinothalamic systems as well as in the trigeminal nuclei.

Sensory transmission in the cochlear nucleus of the auditory system can also be inhibited by excitation of the cochlear nerve, although some investigators feel that this effect is caused in part by contraction of the stapedius and tensor tympani muscles. Nevertheless, the cochlear nerve contains efferent fibers which pass to (and terminate within) the cochlea, and whose stimulation directly inhibits the generation of impulses within the organ of Corti. Similarly, the optic nerve also contains efferent fibers, and when these fibers are stimulated, retinal activity is either increased or decreased.

The foregoing observations clearly indicate that the central nervous system contains neural mechanisms which are able to enhance or diminish the afferent signal input traffic to the brain, and these mechanisms may operate through their effects upon the specific sensory pathways or upon the sense organs themselves. Some of these mechanisms which regulate the sensory input traffic volume are found in the reticular formation of the brain stem and diencephalon, whereas others are not. For example, stimulation of the sensory cortex can produce inhibition at presynaptic terminals which are located within the cuneate and gracile nuclei. Similarly, other inhibitory mechanisms are located in the dorsal horns of the spinal cord and the specific thalamic nuclei as well as in the cerebral cortex. All of these mechanisms share one common function, and that is to modulate (or regulate) the volume of sensory inputs to the central nervous system.

Another effect upon sensory input which is altered by stimulation of the brain can be mentioned. When physiologic excitation of central nervous structures causes a generalized release of epinephrine, the threshold to firing of the cutaneous receptors is decreased considerably. This response serves to increase markedly the excitability of the peripheral receptors in emergency states during which an overall adrenergic response occurs, and signal output from the receptors is enhanced greatly.

When a human or animal subject focuses his attention upon a particular object, the bioelectric activity of some of the mechanisms which modulate sensory input can be evoked and recorded. For example, electrodes can be implanted chronically within the cochlear nucleus of a cat to record the electric activity of this structure. Following recovery, each time a sharp noise (e.g., a click) is produced, a spike potential can be recorded from the cochlear nucleus. However, when the animal's attention is focused upon a particular stimulus such as a mouse or the odor of fish, no potential can be evoked by the clicking sound. However, when either the mouse or fish odor stimulus is removed, a cochlear potential is generated once again by the sound. It is apparent that when the attention is confined to a particular and narrow area or object in the external environment, at least part of this attention-focusing effect is caused functionally by a decrease in afferent input signals generated in the peripheral receptors themselves. Hence afferent signal transmission to the cerebral cortex may be reduced in the periphery, rather than centrally, during periods of focused attention.

The regulatory effect of central nervous structures upon the sensitivity of the muscle spindles provides another example of central regulation of sensory input. Hence the net activity of the gamma efferent neurons that pass to the spindles is controlled not only by facilitory but also inhibitory effects through descending tracts which are located in the lateral funiculi of the spinal cord; and as discussed earlier, stimulation of one portion of the reticular formation of the brain stem facilitates gamma efferent discharge whereas stimulation of other persons of the reticular formation inhibits this process. In turn, the net gamma efferent discharge at any particular moment regulates the tension of the intrafusal fibers, hence the sensitivity of the spindles per se. Similar to the reticular formation, the cerebellum, the basal ganglia, and the motor areas of the cerebral cortex all contain inhibitory centers which modulate sensory inputs in relation to the control of somatic motor activities.

Higher Cortical Functions; Learning and Memory

The higher mental faculties of the human species, collectively termed the "mind" or "intellect," have their principal neuroanatomic origin within the cortical neurons of the cerebral hemispheres. The term "mind" can be defined as those functions of the brain whereby an individual becomes aware of his surroundings and of their arrangement is space as well as in time, and by which he experiences (or perceives) feelings, emotions, and desires. Additional functional attributes of the mind enable the individual to remember, reason, attend to (or concentrate upon) either general or specific matters (stimuli), either of external or internal origin, to decide (or judge), and to associate ideas. In short, the mind enables one to feel, to think, to reason, and to synthesize ideas. In turn, an "idea" or "thought" can be defined, to paraphrase Darwin, as an abstract secretion of the neural elements of the brain.

It is patently ridiculous to assign the source of the mind to any transcendental, supersensible (i.e., metaphysical), or vitalistic origin which lies beyond the limits of human experience. For example, in support of this statement, one merely has to reflect for a moment upon the complete lack of mental capacities in a congenital anencephalic monster or upon the derangement of mental (as well as physical) abilities which can follow necrosis of neural tissue in certain regions of the brain subsequent to a cerebrovascular accident in a previously normal individual. The studies to be discussed below, which were performed upon "split-brain" humans and animals further substantiate the concept that the "mind" is a product of some billions of neurons which are linked together both morphologically and functionally in fantastically complex patterns. Although these patterns and their workings are at present obscure to a large extent, the mind is nevertheless amenable to ultimate understanding, but only insofar as this understanding is grounded upon sound and rational physicochemical principles.

There are five basic techniques whereby some of the phenomena associated with higher mental processes as well as learning and memory can be studied in human and animal subjects. First, clinical observations made in humans can be correlated with the locus as well as the magnitude of brain damage seen at autopsy. Second, the information obtained from clinical studies can be extended by stimulation of specific cortical regions during neurosurgical operations that are carried out under local anesthesia. Third, subcortical structures may be stimulated by means of chronically implanted electrodes in patients suffering from, for example, Parkinson's disease or epilepsy. Fourth, the study of conditioned reflexes in humans and animals has shed some light upon the processes of learning and memory. Fifth, the alterations in psychic functions that develop subsequent to the performance of specific surgical procedures can be studied. Of particular interest to the present discussion are observations made upon patients following complete section of the corpus callosum, so that each cerebral hemisphere functions as an independent unit.

General Psychic Functions of the Cerebral Hemispheres (Neocortex). The properties of learning and memory are not functions which reside within any circumscribed region of the brain in either humans or animals; however, the centers which underlie the so-called higher functions of the nervous system, in particular those related to language (i.e., speech and reading), appear to be localized to some extent in the neocortex, and area of the brain which achieves its highest level of development in the human species.

From the standpoint of comparative anatomy, humans exhibit the greatest ratio between brain weight and body weight of any animal, and the most obvious gross anatomic features of the human brain is the enormous and disproportionately great development of the three principal association areas of this structure. The *frontal association area* lies rostral to the motor cortex; the *temporal association area* lies between the superior temporal gyrus and the limbic cortex; and the *parieto-occipital association area* is found between the somesthetic cortex and the visual cortex.

To recapitulate briefly, these association areas are a portion of the six-layered mantle of neocortical gray matter which invests the surfaces (cortices) of the cerebral hemispheres. In turn, the slight histologic differences which Brodmann used to classify various cortical areas usually, but not invariably, can be correlated with functional differences.

The interconnections among the individual neurons of the neocortex form an exceedingly complex network. Thus the descending axons of the larger elements of the pyramidal cell layer emit collateral fibers which feed back via interneurons to the dendrites of the cells from which they originate. Consequently, highly complex oscillatory (or reverberatory) mechanisms can develop. Such recurrent collateral fibers can also be related functionally to adjacent neurons of the same layer, whereas some of these fibers can also terminate upon inhibitory interneurons which then end upon the original neuron so that negative feedback loops are formed.

On the other hand, the large and complex dendritic processes of the neurons lying deep within the neocortex can receive ascending nonspecific thalamic projection fibers, reticular afferent fibers, and intracortical association fibers which can terminate within all layers of the neocortex. In addition, the deep-lying neocortical cells can receive specific thalamic afferent fibers that terminate in layer IV of the cortex (i.e., the internal granular layer). From a functional standpoint, the role of the intracortical association fibers is unclear, as these elements can be sectioned without producing any obvious effects. From a physiologic standpoint, use of the term "association area," although convenient, is not entirely valid, as these areas of the neocortex must have far more complex and subtle functions than a mere interlining of different regions of the brain.

It has been clearly established from an anatomic as well as a functional standpoint that the cerebral hemispheres of normal humans are asymmetric. For example, in one study it was demonstrated that a greater anatomic development in the left auditory area was present in 65 per cent of the brains examined whereas 11 per cent of these organs exhibited a more pronounced development in the same region of the right cerebral hemisphere. The remaining 24 per cent of the brains studied in this series had an equal development of the auditory area in each hemisphere. Other investigations have established the fact that human language functions, including the analysis of spoken words, are localized to a somewhat greater extent in one cerebral hemisphere than in the other as discussed below, whereas the analysis of music occurs in the contralateral hemisphere.

The hemisphere which is concerned with the understanding of symbols (such as words) and the classification (or categorization) of ideas often has been referred to as the *dominant hemisphere* and its opposite member as the *nondominant hemisphere*; however now it is apparent that the second hemisphere is just as specialized in other functional areas than is the dominant hemisphere. Perception of temporal and spatial relationships either in the real or in the abstract sense takes place in the nondominant hemisphere. Hence the nondominant hemisphere is responsible for performing such mental functions as the identification of objects through their shape, and the recognition of faces as well as themes in music. Because of these facts, the concept of a "dominant" and "nondominant" cerebral hemisphere appears to be outmoded and less accurate than a concept in which each hemisphere is considered to be specialized functionally in a mutually complementary manner to its contralateral partner. One cerebral hemisphere is specialized to subserve the functions involved in language and is called the *categorical hemisphere*, whereas the other is specialized for the perception of temporal and spatial relationships and is called the *representational hemisphere*.

Damage to the categorical hemisphere causes aphasias, whereas extensive lesions in the representational hemisphere do not produce such a defect, because the language functions are localized roughly within the neocortex of the categorical hemisphere. An understanding of printed as well as spoken words and the expression of ideas in writing and in speech may be defective when an aphasia is present, even though vision, hearing, and motor functions may remain normal.

When lesions are present in the representational rather than in the categorical hemisphere, *astereognosis* results so that the individual is unable to recognize common objects merely by handling them. The term "agnosia" signifies a general inability to recognize particular objects through the use of a specific sensory modality, even though the functions of that sensory modality are normal. Parietal lobe damage usually is associated with agnosias.

The complementary specialization of hemispheric functions is related to left- and right-handedness. Thus the left hemisphere is the categorical hemisphere in right-handed individuals. In left-handed persons, on the other hand, the right cerebral hemisphere is the categorical hemisphere in only about 30 per cent of such individuals. In the remaining 70 per cent of left-handed persons, the left hemisphere is the categorical hemisphere.

Damage produced in either the categorical or the representational hemisphere in an adult induces the characteristic defects associated with these regions, and these defects persist for long periods of time. Children who must undergo hemispherectomy (e.g., for brain tumors) usually regain the functions subserved by the missing hemisphere quite rapidly, and regardless of which hemisphere was extirpated.

When the neocortex of the *frontal lobes* is dissected out of a primate, at first the animal exhibits apathy. This interval is followed by the development of an abnormally great motor activity (hyperactivity) so that the animal walks or paces constantly. The overall "intelligence" appears to be unaltered in general, and the responses to tests which require a prompt reaction to an environmental stimulus are unimpaired, whereas those responses which requires the use of information that was learned earlier are abnormal. In human patients, frontal lobectomy causes defects in the recognition of events in their normally occurring temporal sequence. A lobectomized human may be unable to recall how long ago he was a specific picture used as a stimulus. Right frontal lobectomy causes a major defect in the ability to recognize visual stimuli, whereas following left frontal lobectomy the principal defect is seen in tests that involve words as stimuli.

A mental patient can suffer from incapacitating tensions caused by delusions, phobias, and compulsions as well as by real (or imaginary) failure to perform adequately. If the white matter of the frontal lobes is severed from the rest of the brain by an operation called a *frontal* (or *prefrontal*) *lobotomy*, the tension is blocked despite the fact that the delusions, phobias, and other symptoms still are present. In other words, the patient becomes indifferent to the symptoms. Similarly an indifference to extreme and intractable pain develops after frontal lobotomy. From a practical standpoint, however, frontal lobotomy can be followed by a number of additional psychic and behavioral alterations which can be quite dissimilar among different patients depending upon the preoperative experience, personality, and environment, the quantity and site of the brain damage produced by the surgery, and so forth. For example, a given patient may become irresponsible, highly profane, vacillating, stubborn, indifferent to others and to the usual social amenities following lobotomy. Nowadays, tranquilizers and other psychotherapeutic drugs rather than lobotomy are the methods of choice for the treatment of mental disease. Nevertheless the clinical studies that have been performed on lobotomized patients have yielded some insight regarding the general functions of the frontal regions of the neocortex in humans.

Similarly, bilateral ablation of the temporal lobes in monkeys resulting in development of the Klüver-Bucy syndrome has yielded some information concerning this part of the brain. The effects of this experimental operation were discussed earlier in relation to the neurophysiology of behavior, but may be reviewed briefly. Monkeys become docile, hyperphagic, and the males become hypersexual following bilateral temporal lobectomy. All of these effects can be ascribed to removal of components of the limbic system. The operated monkeys also exhibit visual agnosia as well as an abnormally great increase in oral activity as manifest by a continual and repeated mouthing, licking, and biting of all movable objects in their environment. It has been postulated that this behavior pattern could be induced by an inability to identify objects and/or to a memory loss caused by extirpation of the hippocampus. Such Klüver-Bucy animals are distracted readily, every stimulus, minor or not, being explored regardless of its relevancy.

In humans, bilateral hippocampal lesions produce an impairment of memory for recent events. Some patients who have suffered bilateral injury to the amygdaloid nuclei and pyriform cortex may develop hypersexuality. In other words, certain aspects of the Klüver-Bucy syndrome are seen in humans suffering from lesions in particular neuroanatomic loci. However, the abnormalities which are observed following temporal lobe lesions in particular, as well as those caused by neocortical lesions in general, do not lend themselves well to the synthesis of any coherent and overall hypothesis of intellectual functions at this time.

On the other hand, a number of extremely important observations concerning motor as well as psychic functions of the individual cerebral hemispheres have been made in animals as well as humans who have undergone a total surgical section of the corpus callosum, the enormous transverse band of white fibers which functionally interconnects the two cerebral hemispheres.

About 25 years ago it was found that cutting through the corpus callosum as well as the optic chiasm of the cat resulted in a preparation in which each cerebral hemisphere not only functioned independently of the other, but also whose visual input from each eye went only to the ipsilateral hemisphere. When the animal was faced with a problem to solve, and only one eye was exposed, the visual information could pass only to the ipsilateral cortex. The animal could learn to perform a certain action, or solve a problem, based upon the information supplied solely to one eye. However, when the "informed" eye was covered, and the other "uninformed" eye was exposed to the same problem, the animal was unable to recognize the situation as the same problem, and necessarily was forced to learn the solution over from the beginning by use of the other half of the brain. This experiment indicates conclusively that the mammalian brain is indeed a dual organ, and this fact has been confirmed repeatedly by more recent studies.

To date a number of human patients have undergone section of the corpus callosum for therapeutic reasons, i.e., for the treatment of uncontrollable epilepsy. Since this operation did not appear to impair the mental faculties of experimental animals, it was hoped that the procedure would confine the epileptic seizures to one of the hemispheres. Actually, callosal section eliminated practically all epileptic attacks, even those occurring unilaterally. Thus it would appear, at least superficially, as though the corpus callosum served to facilitate the epileptic attacks, presumably is some type of feedback mechanism.

The remainder of this discussion will present the results of a number of studies performed upon "split-brain" human and animal subjects.

Callosal section causes no apparent change in the personality, general intelligence, or temperament of the patient, although some alterations in daily behavior are evident. For example, the patients tended to favor the right side of the body insofar as their response to sensory stimuli was concerned. The right side usually is controlled, of course, by the left hemisphere (categorical hemisphere). For an extended period of time following the surgery, the patients rarely performed spontaneous movements with the left side of the body, and likewise tended to ignore.

Tests were employed to examine the responses to visual stimulation presented in such a way that both left and right halves of the visual field were scanned individually, and as lights were flashed in a horizontal sequence the patients were requested to describe what they saw. Every patient stated that lights were flashed in the right half of the visual field, but when lights were flashed only in the left half of the visual field, the patients reported that no lights were seen. The patients were no blind in the left field, however, because when they were asked to point to, not describe verbally, the flashing lights, their responses were almost entirely accurate. It was demonstrated that the right cerebral hemisphere is almost the same as the left insofar as visual perception is concerned. But since the speech centers of the brain are localized in the left (the categorical) hemisphere in most individuals, then it was not surprising that the patients were unable to state visual perception in the right hemisphere verbally, although perception of the stimulus per se was unimpaired as indicated by the ability to respond correctly when manual signals were used.

Stereognostic tests in which the patients were requested to describe and name various objects merely by touch resulted in findings that were similar to those obtained by visual stimulation. That is, if an object was held in the right hand, sensory signals were transmitted to the left hemisphere and the subjects were able not only to name, but to describe, the test object verbally. But when the object was placed in the left hand, whence sensory information is transmitted principally to the right hemisphere, the subjects could not describe the object verbally, although nonverbal matching tests whereby the test object was compared to a similar object at random revealed that stereognosis was unimpaired. Interestingly, it was also found that each cerebral hemisphere receives some sensory input from the ipsilateral side of the body as well as from the contralateral side. The latter input, of course, is the principal source of sensory information normally, and the ipsilateral sensory input to each hemisphere was found to provide relatively crude information such as where the stimulus is located upon the body surface as well as whether or not a stimulus is present at all. However, the ipsilateral input cannot ordinarily relay signals that convey information about the qualitative aspects of the stimulus or test object.

When tests of motor control were applied to patients following callosal section, it was found that the left cerebral hemisphere exerted normal control over the right hand. However, the left hemisphere exerted less precise control over the left hand. The same results were obtained insofar as the right hemisphere was concerned. That is, the right hemisphere exerts full control over movements of the left, but not the right, hand. When the two individual hemispheres were in conflict insofar as initiating completely different movements in the same hand were concerned, the hemisphere on the side contralateral to the hand usually became dominant and the movement was carried out in accordance with signals emanating from the hemisphere on the opposite side of the body.

The results obtained on the intellectual capacities of split-brain human patients now may be summarized. A number of visual as well as tactile tests were employed in these studies, and these tests were administered in such a way that the test information was transmitted to only one hemisphere at a time. It was found that when visual or tactile stimuli were presented only to the categorical left hemisphere, the subjects were able to describe the stimulus (e.g., a picture) accurately and normally not only orally, but also in writing. Conversely, when similar stimuli were directed to the right hemisphere, no accurate oral or written responses were evoked, and only random guesses as to the nature of the stimulus were offered, assuming that the subject made any attempt to verbalize a response at all. When nonverbal identification of visual and tactile stimuli was substituted for verbal answers, it became clearly evident that the right hemisphere possessed a considerable ability to perform accurately. But even when the subject held an unseen object in his left hand, he still was unable to describe it verbally, a fact which suggests that the left hemisphere was isolated completely from the right hemisphere, insofar as perception and knowledge are concerned. Additional tests did reveal that the right hemisphere had a certain capacity to comprehend language, although this ability was limited to mere recognition of common words by association of these words with the object they described and vice versa. But verbalization of the names of the objects was impossible when only the right hemisphere was involved.

Auditory inputs to one ear are transmitted equally to both sides of the brain. Tests were devised to investigate the ability of the right hemisphere alone to answer questions put to the subject orally. This was accomplished by having the subject use his left hand to retrieve various common objects from a bag hidden from his sight. Even abstract statements concerning the nature of the objects were followed by correct retrievals, but even when the correct test object was being held in the left hand, the subject was unable to name or to describe the object verbally. Hence it was clear that tactile information was being transmitted exclusively to the right hemisphere.

The capacity to perform specific feats with language differs considerably between the left and right hemispheres among individual patients who have undergone callosal section. However, it has been demonstrated quite clearly that the right (or representational) hemisphere was greatly inferior to the left (or categorical) hemisphere in the particular subjects which have been studied. Interestingly, the right hemisphere may respond accurately in tests to a concrete noun, whereas verbs are understood rather poorly. The grammar function is also poorly developed in the right hemisphere as indicated, for example, by the inability of this hemisphere to form plurals.

A number of different neurologic observations point to the conclusion that up to the age of about four years, a child has an approximately equal capacity and skill for language functions in each cerebral hemisphere. Beyond this age, however, a functional separation develops between the hemispheres insofar as proficiency with language is concerned. This separation of functions ultimately results in the presence of a categorical (usually the left) and a representational (usually the right) hemisphere in the adult, as discussed earlier. The reason for this functional dichotomy between the hemispheres with advancing years is completely unknown.

Although language functions are highly developed in the categorical hemisphere, regardless of which side of the brain it happens to be on in any particular individual, the representational hemisphere does have some extremely important and specialized functions. For example, it has been demonstrated in patients following callosal section that the left hand (i.e., the right hemisphere) was able to perform quite accurately mechanical operations such as piling blocks or making drawings that involved spatial, or three-dimensional, information provided by a visual pattern. Conversely, the right hand under instructions from the left (categorical) hemisphere was unable to perform the same operations.

Insofar as emotional expression is concerned, it appears that each hemisphere functions to an equal extent in the generation of an emotional response.

Collectively the studies performed upon human patients as well as animals following section of the corpus callosum indicate that two functionally independent brains are present within one individual, and that each brain is capable of performing highly sophisticated mental functions independently of the other. Furthermore, there is abundant evidence to substantiate the conclusion that each cerebral hemisphere of the normal adult is specialized to perform certain functions well and others poorly, and that these functions tend to supplement each other. Interestingly, there is direct evidence which indicates that following callosal section monkeys are able to handle twice as much visual information as they could prior to the surgery. This fact raises an interesting question regarding the possibility that a split-brain individual could learn twice as much information per unit time, or learn to perform twice the number of manual tasks in the same time span. One thing is evident, however, from all of the studies cited above. Section of the corpus callosum to that each cerebral hemisphere can function independently of the other produces an individual having "two independent spheres of consciousness within the same cranium." Therefore the psychic properties of consciousness, awareness, and perception are divisible in the literal sense of the word!

In conclusion, what may be said regarding the normal function of the corpus callosum? Some experimental evidence indicates that signals related to complex visual indicates that signals related to complex visual patterns are transmitted from one hemisphere to the other across the corpus callosum. It also appears that nerve impulses related to learning and memory are encoded, and these complex signals then are transmitted across the corpus callosum so that both hemispheres presumably are able to learn (and to recall?) the information simultaneously. However, the foregoing statement must be regarded as tentative rather than conclusive, and far more detailed factual information must be obtained before the physiologic role of the corpus callosum can be stated accurately.

Neurophysiology of Learning. The ability to learn is a fundamental characteristic of man as well as of many other organism, and as consequences of the learning process, habit patterns, skills, and behavior are modified by experience. The capacity for learning (as well as that for memory) lies wholly within the nervous system and may be considered to reside in a sort of "functional plasticity" of this complex system whereby physicochemical modifications can occur as the result of experience. Although the mechanisms which underlie neural plasticity remain obscure for the most part, it is quite clear that the activities of the nervous system can be formed (or molded) by experience in such a way that responses to various stimuli can be altered considerably. Furthermore, as a result of this plasticity the nervous system is also able to store and to retrieve information through its memory functions (which actually are inseparable from the learning process), and can even recover functionally in some instances even though irreversible neural damage has been incurred in certain areas of the brain.

One particularly enigmatic feature that is shared in common by the memory as well as the learning process is the temporal scale upon which these events take place. Thus the majority of neurophysiologic processes have a duration lasting for a few milliseconds or perhaps a few seconds. Learned information may (or may not!) take considerably longer to "store," and once committed to memory the information may be retained for many years. These generalizations imply strongly that the fundamental mechanisms which underlie the learning process are quantitatively as well as qualitative different from those underlying simple reflexes.

The remainder of this section will deal principally with experimental studies concerned with learning, and in particular with certain overall behavioral modifications which are brought about by experience. The discussion of memory in the next section will consider several modifications that have been demonstrated to take place in the nervous system at the ultramicroscopic and molecular levels following a period of learning.

Some General Aspects of Learning. Frequently, and erroneously, it is assumed that the learning process is an exclusive function of the cerebral hemispheres. However, primitive forms of "learning" can be demonstrated readily to take place in many species including, for example, insects and worms. The octopus, a particularly interesting marine mollusc, has a demonstrably remarkable capacity for discrimination learning. In fact, this species can even exhibit a rudimentary form of intelligence, provided that one is content to define this term as a "comprehension" of, as well as an ability to respond appropriately to, peculiar environmental situations.

Furthermore, "learning" phenomena have been demonstrated to occur in mammals at subcortical as well as spinal levels in the central nervous system. For example, posttetanic potentiation, which is the facilitation observed to take place in a synaptic pathway after repeated stimulation, is an excellent example of this kind of subcortical learning phenomenon.

The pigeon provides another example of a submammalian organism which is able to learn quite rapidly a number of highly complex and sophisticated visual discriminations.

Despite the facts summarized above, the more highly advanced learning processes that take place in man require the participation of the cerebral cortex even though the brain stem is also involved. The structural changes that have been observed to take place subsequent to a period of learning.

Learning Processes. Fundamentally two principal types of learning process are recognized, depending upon whether or not the subject plays a passive or an active role. During *classic* (or *Pavlovian*) *conditioning*, as well as during *habituation*, the subject plays a relatively involuntary or passive role; hence this type of learning is considered to represent a relatively "primitive", "simple", or "generalized", learning process. On the other hand, during *operant conditioning* (also called *instrumental conditioning* or *trial-and-error learning*) the subject exerts a considerable degree of voluntary control over the learning process so that this type of conditioning is considered to represent learning at a much "higher" level than either classic conditioning or habituation.

The principal features of each of these learning processes now may be discussed individually, but it should be stressed that each of these processes is extremely important to the individual organism insofar as net learned information is concerned.

Classic Conditioning. Classic conditioning results in the formation of learned responses called *conditioned reflexes.* A conditioned reflex in turn is an automatic (or reflex) response to a stimulus which previously did not evoke the response. This effect is produced by repeatedly pairing the stimulus which normally does not produce the response (the conditioned stimulus, CS with a second stimulus which normally produces a specific and innate response (the *unconditioned stimulus,* US). When the unconditioned and conditioned stimuli are applied in the correct temporal sequence and for a sufficient number of times, then ultimately presentation of the conditioned stimulus alone will evoke the response which originally could be elicited only by the unconditioned stimulus.

Among the classic experiments performed by Pavlov, salivation was induced in the dog in response to placing meat in the mouth (the unconditioned stimulus). If a bell was rung immediately before the meat was placed in the mouth, and this process was repeated a number of times, then eventually ringing the bell (i.e., the conditioned stimulus) alone was sufficient to evoke salivation.

In order for conditioning of this type to take place at all, the conditioned stimulus *must* precede the unconditioned stimulus. If the conditioned stimulus is applied after the unconditioned stimulus no conditioned reflex develops. The conditioned response follows the conditioned stimulus by a time interval which is practically identical to that which separated the conditioned stimulus and the unconditioned stimulus during the training period. This delay between stimulus and response may range from a second or so up to 1.5 minutes, and when a considerable time such as this elapses between the application of the conditioned stimulus and the development of the conditioned response, the latter is called a *delayed conditioned reflex.*

When first developed, a conditioned reflex can be elicited not only by the conditioned stimulus but also by similar stimuli, e.g., by ringing bells having slightly different tones to evoke salivation in the example cited above. If only one particular conditioned stimulus (i.e., a bell having one specific tone) is reinforced by repetition, whereas the similar stimuli are not repeated, when an animal can learn to discriminate between the different stimuli with amazing accuracy, and this process is called discriminative conditioning. The phenomenon whereby the response to stimuli other than the conditioned stimulus is eliminated exemplifies the effect of internal inhibition, as discussed below. Discriminative conditioning is an exceedingly useful tool for studying color vision and pitch discrimination, among other sensory modalities, in various subhuman species.

Once a conditioned reflex becomes established, if the conditioned stimulus is applied a sufficient number of times in the absence of the unconditioned stimulus, eventually the conditioned response disappears. The process whereby this effect takes place is called *internal inhibition* (or *extinction*). On the other hand, if the animal is distracted or disturbed by an external stimulus which is presented immediately following the conditioned stimulus, the conditioned reflex may not take place, and this effect is called *external inhibition.* If, however, the conditioned reflex is reinforced occasionally by pairing the unconditioned and conditioned stimuli, the conditioned response will remain unaltered for extremely long periods of time.

An enormous number of specific and visceral effects can be evoked as conditional responses following application of suitable conditioning stimuli to humans as well as to animals. Insofar as the visceral responses are concerned, it has been demonstrated clearly that these supposedly automatic functions can be altered readily by appropriate discriminative conditioning regimes in a manner quite similar to those used to produce somatic conditioned reflexes; i.e., a person can learn to alter his visceral functions in response to appropriate stimuli. for example, heart rate, blood pressure, intestinal contractions, rate of urine formation, and the caliber of the blood vessels all can be increased or decreased by the use of appropriate discriminative conditioning techniques. In this regard, it must be noted that conditioned reflexes are particularly difficult to form if the unconditioned stimulus evokes a purely motor response. Furthermore, the signals evoked by excitation of the sensory endings in the muscle spindles cannot be used as afferent inputs to form a conditioned reflex, whereas afferent signals from the skin, eyes, or ears readily participate in such a function. On the other hand a conditioned response can be formed with relative facility, provided that the unconditioned stimulus is coupled to either a pleasant or unpleasant affect. Thus stimulation of the "pleasure" or reward system in the brain provides strong *positive reinforcement* for such learned visceral responses as were outlined above, whereas stimulation of the "pain" or avoidance system of the brain (as well as a painful cutaneous stimulation) provides an equally strong *negative reinforcement* for such conditioned responses.

One fact is obvious concerning the neurophysiologic mechanism that underlies learning by classic conditioning techniques. That is, during this process a new functional connection (or connections) must be formed within the nervous system. For example, in the classic study by Pavlov concerned with salivation in response to ringing a bell it is obvious that a functional pathway is developed during the conditioning period between the auditory pathway and the autonomic centers in the brain that control salivation.

Although decortication can depress the formation of many conditioned reflexes, it is also known that the new functional connections present after a conditioned reflex has become established may or may not involve the cortex. For example, if a complex sensory pathway (such as is involved in vision or hearing) is necessary in order to transmit the conditioned stimulus, then the cortical sensory area that underlies perception of the particular sensory modality involved also must be intact, otherwise no conditioned response can develop. The remainder of the cortex, however, is unnecessary so that conditioned reflexes which do not involve discrimination and which are formed in response to simple sensory stimulation can develop when the entire cortex is absent. Under circumstances such as these, of course, subcortical structures obviously provide the neural substrate within which new functional pathways and connections are produced during conditioning.

Habituation. When a human or animal is exposed to a new (or novel) sensory stimulus, the subject becomes alert, and actively pays keen attention to the stimulus. The EEG exhibits a diffuse arousal (i.e., desynchronized) pattern, and evoked secondary electric responses become clearly evident in many parts of the brain. The behavioral response described above has been called "What is it?" reflex, but more commonly the response is known as the orienting reflex (Pavlov).

When the stimulus is "neutral," that is, it evokes neither a pleasant nor an unpleasant affect, repetition produces progressively less and less response in the subject. Ultimately the arousal changes in the EEG are not observed following habituation, and the subject learns to ignore the stimulus completely. The gradual diminution in the behavioral response which is produced by the repeated application of a stimulus without reinforcement is known as habituation.

Habituation generally develops after the stimulus has been applied only a few times and it occurs in many species; therefore it has been used experimentally as a model of plasticity in the nervous system.

If a stimulus used to produce habituation in an animal now is paired with a second stimulus which elicits arousal (as evidenced by the EEG pattern), typical classic conditioning takes place. Thus after a few applications of the paired stimuli, the neutral stimulus to which the subject exhibited habituation now produces arousal (i.e., desynchronization of the EEG) when administered alone. This type of conditioned response to a neutral stimulus is called *electrocortical conditioning* (or the *alpha block conditioned reflex*). If such electrocortical conditioning is not reinforced, extinction takes place rapidly; and concomitantly with this effect, the EEG develops quite regular, high-amplitude waves in the cortical area which was associated with the formation of the reflex in the first place. Experimental data such as these suggest that extinction (or unlearning) is similar to learning in that an active neural process is involved. Therefore extinction is not merely a passive subsidence of a previously active mechanism in the nervous system.

The functional connections produced during electrocortical conditioning appear to be formed at (or beneath) the thalamic level of the brain. Thus such conditioning is not altered by severing the lateral connections of the sensory areas of the cortex; however, this response does not develop following placement of lesions in the nonspecific thalamic projection nuclei.

The general arousal response to any particular stimulus can evolve into a behavioral reaction in which the attention is focused sharply and selectively; and when this state is present then extraneous sensory inputs are inhibited. At a behavioral level, habituation and conditioning to the arousal value of various stimuli are common and everyday human experiences. For example, one can become habituated very rapidly to commercial advertisements which are presented visually and/or orally, and unless such stimuli produce a particular affect they will be ignored totally. On the other hand, a person becomes so conditioned to the sound of his own name that a specific arousal response is evoked immediately when that particular name is spoken. The adaptive value of such habituation and arousal responses are obvious.

Operant Conditioning. During classic (or Pavlovian) conditioning the subject has a passive role in the learning process so that the paired stimuli that elicit this type of learning always are presented in a stereotyped temporal pattern irrespective of the behavioral response that is evoked. In marked contrast to classic condition in, operant conditioning results in the animal being taught (i.e., learning) to make a response voluntarily, and this voluntary in turn determines whether or not the conditioning is *reinforced*. In other words, the subject must perform a task or "operate on the environment", hence the name "operant conditioning" (Skinner). Affect is an important aspect of operant conditioning, hence the unconditioned stimulus may be either a pleasant or an unpleasant event (e.g., food or an electric shock), whereas the conditioned stimulus is a signal (e.g., a light flash or a sound) which alerts the subject to perform the task. Motor responses which are conditioned in such a way that they enable an animal to avoid a noxious stimulus are called *conditioned avoidance* (or *escape*) *reflexes*. On the other hand, the subject may be taught to perform a task following which a reward is given (e.g., food), and this reward tends to reinforce the learned behavioral response.

In practice, operant conditioning involves an apparatus wherein an animal, such as a monkey or rat, can perform specific motor responses which then can be observed and/or recorded readily and quantitatively. In other words, the apparatus is an instrument upon which the subject performs a task, hence this type of learning also is called *instrumental learning* or *instrumental conditioning*.

A large number of problem boxes, discrimination apparatuses, and mazes have been constructed with which various aspects of instrumental conditioning can be investigated in many species. Only one such apparatus will be discussed here, the so-called Skinner box. In this type of apparatus, which can take a great variety of specific forms depending upon the species and problem under study, an animal such as a rat can be trained to press a lever each time a light flashes and thereby receive a food pellet. This exceedingly simple type of stimulus-response pattern clearly illustrates the principal feature of instrumental learning, namely that the animal must participate (or respond) actively in order to be reinforced. In practice, instrumental response can be *shaped* or *patterned* according to *schedules of reinforcement* so that the animal might receive a food pellet only after each third press on the lever or after a particular time interval. In such a way the ultimate behavioral response that the investigator wishes to achieve is not produced at random but by gradual and deliberate shaping by successive reinforcements.

Animals can be taught, for example, to displace distinctively shaped or colored blocks, as well as to respond only to specific tones, light intensities, and colors following the administration of specific cues. In this way studies on cortical learning as well as localization and specificity of sensory functions can be carried out on normal as well as on experimentally altered animals with considerable accuracy following periods of so-called *discrimination learning*. For example, the conditioned avoidance response, mentioned above, often is used in practical pharmacologic tests of psychoactive drugs, such as the tranquilizers, which modify behavior. For example, an animal can learn to avoid an electric shock delivered through a grid in the cage floor by pressing a bar, and this behavior can be recorded against time. Following administration of a specific dose of a particular drug, the quantitative alteration in the bar pressing over a period of time can be taken as an index of the effects of the drug on that particular behavioral response in the animal under study. However extrapolation of such data to human behavior may (or may not) be valid.

In conclusion to this discussion, the term *reinforcement* now may be defined as it applies both to classic and to instrumental learning. During classic conditioning, reinforcement merely refers to the pairing of the conditioned and unconditioned stimuli in time, and as noted earlier, the former always must precede the latter in order for conditioning to occur at all. In instrumental learning, on the other hand, the term reinforcement signifies the pairing of a *response* on the part of the subject to some specific consequence of the original stimulus, for example, food, or the avoidance of a shock.

Interhemispheric Transfer of Learning. Classic as well as instrumental conditioning techniques have played vital roles in establishing to some extent the functional roles of the brain structures which underlie the interhemispheric transfer of learned information, and as noted earlier, the corpus callosum plays a key role in this process. Two particularly relevant studies on this area of the brain were performed about 50 years ago in Pavlov's laboratory. If a normal dog is conditioned by the classic technique to salivate in response to tactile stimulation of one particular locus on the body surface, stimulation of the same point on the opposite side of the body evokes the same response. If, however, the corpus callosum was sectioned prior to the conditioning, the salivatory response was limited to cutaneous stimulation on only one side of the body. If the corpus callosum was sectioned prior to conditioning, then individual conditioned responses could be produced in each hemisphere. More recently it has been demonstrated unequivocally that not only the corpus callosum, but also the optic chiasm as well as the anterior and posterior commissures all play essential roles in the transfer and sharing of visual as well as other types of sensory information between the two cerebral hemisphere. It has been demonstrated experimentally in monkeys that signals transmitted via the corpus callosum are able to trigger memory traces that are stored in the contra-lateral hemisphere, but this structure does not underlie the transfer of *memory traces*, or *engrams*, between one hemisphere and the other. On the other hand, engrams actually can be transmitted from one hemisphere to the other by encoded signals that are carried in the anterior commissure. Stated in the language of the computer scientist, the corpus callosum only can command a memory "read-out," whereas the anterior commissure can induce interhemispheric memory storage or "write-in".

Memory and Related Mechanisms

Types of Memory. Even as learning causes alterations in response that are based upon prior experience, so memory enables an organism to store learned information for retrieval at a later time. Hence memory is that mental faculty whereby particular sensations, impressions, and ideas are stored for recall.

Fundamentally it appears that three interlocking mechanisms are operative in causing memories, because there are basically three types of memory, each of which in turn is classified by its temporal characteristics. First there is a *short-term memory* which underlies the immediate recall of events that occur on a moment-to-moment basis. This type of memory, enables an individual to process hundreds of sensory impressions for a second or so or until the most important of these impressions can be acted upon; the overwhelming majority of these impressions, however, rapidly become extinct (or are forgotten). Second, *intermediate memory* of sensations and events lasts somewhat longer, and recall is on the order of from minutes to hours. This type of memory, for example, enables one to remember an address until the destination is reached. Third, *long-term memory* represents the highest level of information storage. This type of memory consists of sensory and other impressions that are gathered throughout a lifetime; and, once acquired, such memories are indelible. Learning at this memory level usually requires several hours to become complete, but once the information is stored, or consolidated, it remains stable for the lifetime of the individual.

Long-term memory is remarkably persistent, even when severe brain damage is present, and this fact contrasts sharply with the severe impairment or total loss of memory for recent events that may occur in persons suffering from various neurologic diseases or lesions.

Neuroanatomic Substrates of Memory. What can be said to the specific areas of the brain which are involved in the storage of memories? As is the case with the learning process itself, no one specific area of the central nervous system can be invoked as the primary area for all types of memory storage. However, the temporal lobe appears to be intimately concerned with storage of experiences that occurred in the distant past, at least in patients suffering from epilepsy in this region of the brain. Studies have been performed on such patients in that various regions of the temporal lobe, exposed by local anesthesia, were stimulated artificially. The result was that exceedingly detailed and complete patterns of visual and/or auditory memories, which frequently could not be recalled voluntarily, were evoked by the stimulation of particular loci on the temporal cortex. The memories produced by such temporal lobe stimulation are "replayed" accurately with a time sequence similar to that of the original event, but only for as long as the stimulation is continued. Frequently the patient felt as though he were an "outsider" viewing the memory replay as a detached observer. The evoked memories were complete, even to subjective impressions of the environmental situation surrounding the recalled events; however it is quite interesting that no reports of olfactory sensations were reported (or recorded) in connection with the recollections evoked by electric stimulation of the temporal cortex.

The facts described above differ markedly from the specific visual, auditory, and other sensory responses evoked by similar artificial stimulation of particular cortical sensory areas, again in conscious patients. For example, direct stimulation of the visual cortex evokes bright luminous objects (e.g., stars or streaks) or dark forms. On the other hand, a veritable kaleidoscope of colors may be perceived. These evoked visual images may either move or remain stationary, but in no way do they resemble anything seen in the environment despite the fact that they exhibit form and color.

Direct stimulation of the auditory area can elicit ringing, buzzing, or knocking sounds; but no words or auditory memories having regular patterns are evoked.

Stimulation of the somesthetic cortex can produce a sensation of numbness, tingling, or a sense of actual movement. Perception of an unpleasant odor may follow stimulation of the cortical olfactory area, and a strong taste similarly may follow excitation of the gustatory area.

It is apparent from these facts that excitation of particular cortical sensory receptive areas follows generalized and innate (or inherited) patterns, whereas responses evoked by stimulation of the memory areas of the temporal lobe are quite different, and thus represent as well as reflect the specific experiences of that particular individual. In other words, the memories evoked by temporal lobe stimulation are a "hallucination of recollection."

The memory traces (or engrams) themselves do not appear to be stored within the temporal lobes. Rather it appears that excitation of the temporal lobes merely fires or "cues" an associative circuit thereby releasing impressions that are stored elsewhere in the brain so that an earlier impression or perception reaches the conscious level.

Occasionally a patient may alter his interpretation of his immediate environment following stimulation of different areas of the temporal lobes other than those which are involved in producing memories. Thus application of the stimulus may cause the patient to feel that an event which is currently in progress has occurred previously, or he may feel strange in familiar surroundings or vice versa. Such an untimely sense of familiarity with new events (or surroundings) is called the *déjà vu phenomenon*. Occasionally this occurs in normal individuals, although more frequently such a phenomenon is seen in an epileptic as an *aura*, the sensation which occurs just before a seizure develops.

In an experimental animal, the retrieval of a learned response is nullified completely if the brain is subjected to an electric shock (or the entire animal is chilled sharply) within five minutes of the training session. If, however, the animal is subjected to such treatment several hours after the training period, no failure of learning occurs, as indicated by the ability of the subject to perform adequately. Experiments such as these indicate that a definite period of time is necessary in order that long-term memory engrams be *consolidated* or *encode* in the brain, and that the memory trace is labile (or unstable) for a period of time after exposure to the stimulus which produces the learning.

The hippocampus and its interconnections are known to be concerned intimately with the consolidation of learned information. For example, when human suffer bilateral destruction of the ventral hippocampus, or when the same region of the brain is damaged in experimental animals, the memory for recent events becomes seriously deranged. Human patients who have suffered such hippocampal destruction still possess normal long-term memory, and such persons are able to cope adequately with everyday activities, but only so long as they pay close attention (i.e., concentrate) on what they are doing at all times. If such patients are distracted from any task for even a very short period of time, however, all recollection of what was being done is lost, together with any plans that were present for undertaking new activities. Consequently, patients suffering from bilateral ventral hippocampal lesions are unable to form new intermediate and long-term memories in a normal manner.

Further evidence for an important role of the hippocampus in the formation of memories is obtained from human patients who have electrodes chronically implanted in this region of the brain. Thus stimulation of the hippocampus through these electrodes so as to cause disruption of the normal pattern of repetitive bioelectric activity in the hippocampal neurons produces a loss of memory for events that took place in the recent past. Furthermore, certain drugs which alter or impair the recall of recent events also can induce abnormal electric discharge patterns in the hippocampus.

Sometimes alcoholics suffering from brain damage concomitantly exhibit a pronounced loss of memory for recent events, and it appears that there is a good correlation between this derangement and the consistent finding of pathologic alterations in the mammillary bodies of such patients. Therefore it would seem that these structures play some role, albeit obscure at present, in the genesis of memory storage, i.e., engram formation.

Physicochemical Mechanisms Involved in Learning and Memory. Any general hypotheses that are advanced to explain the learning and memory functions of the nervous system must be able to account satisfactory for the mechanisms that underlie and characterize short-term, intermediate, and long-term (or stable) memory.

The process of learning as well as that of memory may involve merely the functional creation of new circuits within the nervous system in response to experience (i.e., appropriate stimuli), whereas the basic and enormously complex neuronal patterns that underlie the morphologic aspects of these functions of the brain are developed highly and almost completely during prenatal life so that by the time the individual is born such patterns are clearly established. In turn, this complex neuroanatomic circuitry is determined during embryonic life by the genetic constitution of the particular organism, and furthermore it appears that the pathways formed in the brain during this stage develop in part because of specific chemical interactions between the membranes of particular neurons; i.e., *cell recognition*, a common phenomenon in biologic systems, plays an important role in this process. In addition, the individual neurons, which in toto comprise the nervous system, do not undergo mitosis in postembryonic life, a fact which undoubtedly confers a certain measure of long-term anatomic stability on functional circuits, once these circuits have become established through learning processes. Furthermore, such long-term neuroanatomic stability doubtless plays some role in the stability, hence the retention, of long-term memory engrams.

An important distinction exists between the *formation of an engram* during the learning process and the *storage of an engram* as a part of the past experience of the individual. Thus it has been suggested that the acquisition and long-term storage of memories occurs in two stages. According to this view, during the learning process an immediate, unstable, and short-term memory trace (or engram) is formed and stored temporarily. Subsequently, this short-term memory engram may be "consolidated" into a long-term (or permanent) memory engram, and presumably the short-term engrams serves as a "template" which facilitates his consolidation process.

The physical mechanisms which have been postulated to underlie the three types of memory belong to two general categories. In the first, a bioelectric process is involved, whereas in the second, morphologic changes in the neurons, synapses, and/or biochemical changes within the neurons themselves are deemed responsible for producing the memory engrams.

Mechanisms Involved in Short-Term and Intermediate Memory. It has been postulated that the memory traces for recent events are produced by the activation of reverberatory (or oscillatory) circuits within the brain. Information is stored as memory engrams by closed circuits of neurons whose components reactive each other in a cyclic fashion.

As noted earlier, electrically induced convulsions, deep anesthesia, and certain neuropathologic situations tend to abolish memory for recent events, whereas such treatment does not interfere with long-term memory patterns. These facts would tend to indicate that reverberatory mechanisms are not involved in all learning and memory processes. However, there is some evidence that reverberatory mechanisms are responsible, at least in part, for the temporary storage of new information prior to the development of a permanent memory engram.

A generalized kind of learning can be said to have taken place whenever the nervous system functions in a different manner following a period of activity. The phenomenon of posttetanic potentiation can be cited as merely one example of this type of learning. Thus when the presynaptic limb of a monosynaptic reflex arc is stimulated for a prolonged interval at a high frequency, a hyperexcitability of that reflex develops which may persist for several hours. It has been suggested that this phenomenon might provide a useful biologic model in which to study the mechanisms of synaptic plasticity in general and the structural basis of learning in particular. Similarly, habituation has also been suggested as a model for such investigations.

Mechanisms Involved in Long-Term Memory. Although the precise nature of the long-term memory engram remains an enigma, the fact that such memories are quite resistant to physical injury of the brain (e.g., as through concussion) as well as to electric shock would suggest that permanent memory engrams develop as the consequence of actual morphologic and/or biochemical changes within the brain. Furthermore, the time interval required for the development of a permanent memory engram (or consolidation of a temporary memory trace) would tend to substantiate the hypothesis that physicochemical alterations are involved in the process of long-term storage of information as memories.

It has been demonstrated beyond doubt and in many species that the central nervous system can be modified structurally, chemically, and functionally by experience, and that the stimuli producing these modifications are effective regardless of whether they arise within the external or internal environments.

At the gross level, it was observed nearly two centuries ago that animals subjected to a period of intensive training exhibited visibly more complex cerebellar convolutions than did untrained siblings of the same species. Subsequently it has been demonstrated clearly that the total mass of the cortex is related to the learning process. For example, rats which were trained to perform various activities, or which were exposed to visually stimulating or physically complex environments, had somewhat thicker and heavier cerebral cortices than did litter mates maintained under isolated or monotonous conditions.

Careful study of electron micrographs made on sections of brains taken from rats which were subjected to a stimulating environment has revealed that the total number of spines on the dendrites of cortical pyramidal cells is considerably greater than the number of dendritic spines found on similar neurons in the brains of rats maintained in an "impoverished" environment.

The cell bodies of cortical neurons from rats exposed to a stimulating environment were larger than comparable cells of rats maintained in a monotonous environment. Similarly the total number of glial elements present in the cortex increases significantly when sensory experience is enriched.

Furthermore, it has been shown that the cross-sectional area of the synaptic junctions in the occipital cortex of rats exposed to a stimulating environment were about 50 per cent larger than those present in the cortices of rats from a monotonous environment. The rats which had been deprived of a rich sensory experience, however, exhibited a quantitatively smaller number of synapses per unit area of brain tissue. Still other experiments have confirmed that there is an increased area of synaptic contact in rats that have had a wide prior sensory experience, and that an increase in the area of synaptic contact is related inversely to the total number of synapses per unit mass of tissue. These morphologic observations tend to support the contention that learning and memory are due, at least in part, to a distinctive pattern of addition as well as deletion of synaptic contacts between individual neurons concomitantly with reciprocally related variations in the total area of each synaptic junction. Furthermore, it appears that these processes may take place simultaneously, with the net result that the functional contacts between individual neurons in the brain are subject to considerable variation in number depending upon prior experience. It must be reiterated that the total number of neurons present in the nervous system does not change regardless of experience; however, studies such as were cited above clearly indicate that the cerebral neurons are capable of adapting morphologically to changes in their functional state, and that the selective morphologic alterations which take place at the synaptic junctions during the learning and storage of memories may represent an encoding of information at the morphologic level.

The visible morphologic changes noted above clearly reflect the fact that biochemical alterations must accompany the learning and storage of new information. What, then, can be said of the specific biochemical changes that have been found in the brains of animals (rats) following their maintenance in a highly stimulating environment, when these values are compared to the levels of similar components derived from the brains of suitable control animals? The occipital cortex of rats that were exposed to an enriched environment contains quantitatively higher levels of total protein, and in particular the levels of the enzymes, acetylcholinesterase, cholinesterase, and hexokinase are elevated. The quantity of deoxyribonucleic acid (DNA) per milligram of tissue was found to decrease significantly, whereas the level of ribonucleic acid (RNA) decreased to an insignificant extent. Therefore the ratio of RNA to DNA increased significantly in rats subjected to a stimulating environment.

The facts summarized briefly above leave no room for doubt that learning and storage of new information can produce definite morphologic and biochemical changes in the brain, although the mechanisms that underlie these processes remain completely

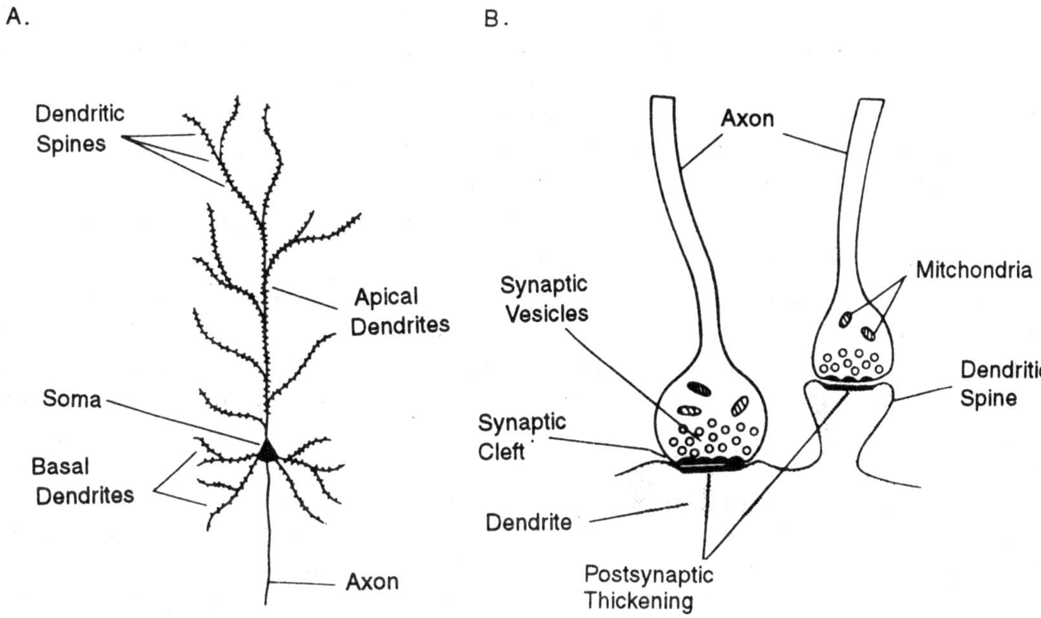

Fig. 8.11. A. Pyramidal neuron of cerebral cortex illustrating pattern of dendritic spines. B. Synaptic junctions directly between an axon and a dendrite (left) and between an axon and a dendritic spine (right).

obscure, as does the mechanism underlying the recall or association of stored information, sometimes in response to specific stimuli or cues.

Insofar as the form in which learned information may be stored in the brain is concerned, a number of investigators have claimed that several specific and different biochemical compounds are synthesized in the brain in response to the stimulus of experience, and these compounds in turn are responsible for all of the enormously complex phenomena related to learning and memory. Thus peptides, proteins, glycoproteins, and RNA all have been implicated as "memory molecules" by various workers. It also has been claimed that learned information can be transferred from trained to naive animals by injection of suitable extracts prepared from the brains of the former. The evidence for these statements at present is interesting and at best circumstantial, but hardly compelling.

There is no doubt that polypeptide, protein, glycoprotein, and ribonucleic acid molecules each has the potential to store an enormous amount of coded information. It is also true that RNA serves as the template for synthesis of specific protein molecules, and that neurons synthesize more protein than any other cell type in the body. Furthermore it can be demonstrated clearly in animals that chemical agents which block protein synthesis also inhibit the consolidation of long-term memory engrams, but do not block memory for short-term learned responses. It is clear that protein synthesis (hence RNA activity) must provide at least a part of the mechanism which results in the formation of long-term memory engrams. However, such studies afford no insight whatsoever as to how such a chemical mechanism operates in detail, since one is studying a general physiologic process rather than a specific memory. Nevertheless the clues yielded by such biochemical studies provide data that ultimately will be of assistance in resolving the problems of memory functions, insofar as chemical effects on synaptic transmission (i.e., neurotransmitter release) and other aspects of this phenomenon are concerned.

From a neurophysiologic standpoint, it is clear that the phenomena of learning and long-term memory do not involve merely the formation of new functional circuits or pathways which are localized in one portion of the brain or another, and which discharge on cue when appropriate stimuli are administered. On the contrary, there is considerable evidence which indicates that memory traces are redundant, and thus may be stored in multiple loci in the brain. It is equally clear that the presence of cortico-cortical circuits is essential to normal learning and memory processes. One fact is evident, however. Learning causes the functional synchronization of large numbers of neurons that may be located in widespread cortical areas and in turn this process involves excitation of some of these neurons together with a concomitant inhibition of others, so that specific patterns of neural activity are evoked in the brain, and these patterns of neural discharge have been postulated to give rise to specific memories.

At present, it is evident that the factual information concerning the mechanisms which underlie learning and memory are fragmentary at best. Ultimately, however, these phenomena will have to be explained in terms of biochemical as well as biophysical mechanisms, because neither of these two processes operates in a mutually exclusive fashion in any single living cell, let alone in the entire nervous system.

Some years ago synaptic transmission was thought to be a chemical process by some investigators, and a wholly bioelectric process by others. Subsequently it was learned that bioelectric and biochemical mechanisms, acting in a coordinated fashion, both were responsible for normal synaptic transmission. It would be most surprising if learning, memory, and the recall of stored information did not involve a similar functional cooperation between biochemical and bioelectric processes in widespread areas of the central nervous system.

9

Sensation

In discussion the general functions of a nervous system we have noted that it is concerned with the collection of impulses due to stimuli which arise in the environment of the individual and from various parts of the body. A certain number of these impulses reach consciousness and give rise to sensations.

All sensations experienced normally depend on the stimulation by an appropriate stimulus of nerve-endings which are adapted to receive certain kinds of stimuli or to appreciate a special quality of the environment. These nerve-endings have, for the special stimulus for which they are adapted, a lower threshold than have the nerve-fibers themselves, and make it possible for a nerve impulse to be set up by a degree of stimulation which would not otherwise be effective. For example, a degree of pressure which would not affect the ulnar nerve (the "funny bone" of the elbow) will cause a sensation of touch if applied to the nerve-endings of that nerve in the little finger.

Nerve-endings have been developed for the appreciation of a large variety of stimuli, e.g., light and colour, sound, smell, pressure. It is convenient to leave the detailed study of these to later chapters, since in some instances, e.g., the ear and the eye, the specialised nerve-endings have become much elaborated.

The *stimuli* most not only have a special quality but must be of adequate strength. Too light a touch, too faint a sound, will produce no effect on consciousness. The strength of stimulus which just suffices to evoke a sensation is called the *liminal* (from limen, a threshold) value of the stimulus, or its *absolute threshold*.

Stimuli must also have a minimal duration as we have seen in regard to excitation. This is well seen in relation to the eye. Cinematograph pictures appear continuous because they are changed so rapidly, and if this does not occur flicks are seen. We are also familiar with the saying that the quickness of the hand deceives the eye.

Similarly, the difference between two stimuli must not fall below a certain minimum in order that the difference may be appreciated. If two musical tones are of too nearly identical pitch, if two colours are of too nearly identical hue, the difference may be imperceptible. There is, therefore, a liminal value for a stimulus difference. This is known as the differential threshold of the stimulus.

Weber's law states that the just appreciable difference between two stimuli depends on the ratio of that difference to their magnitudes, and not on the absolute difference between their magnitudes.

Weber's law is but an expression of everyday experience. A rush-light will brighten a dark cellar, but its presence is unfelt in sunshine. So, too, if a room be lighted by 100 candles, and if one candle more be brought in, the increased illumination produced by the extra candle would be just perceptible to the eye. But if a room were lighted by 1000 candles, no appreciable difference would result from the introduction of an extra candle. Ten candles would have to be introduced, in order to effect a just noticeable difference. In each case a difference of one-hundredth of the original strength of stimulus is needful to cause a just appreciable difference in the sensation; and this is in accordance with Weber's law.

For light, the fraction is about $\frac{1}{100}$; for noise, it is about $\frac{1}{3}$; for cutaneous pressure, it varies between $\frac{1}{30}$ and $\frac{1}{10}$; for weight, between $\frac{1}{70}$ and $\frac{1}{40}$, in various parts of the body.

A sensation requires an appreciable time for its development. Part of this time is spent at the end-organ on which the stimulus acts, part in conveying the nervous impulse along the sensory nerve to the brain, and part within the brain itself. This *latent period* varies in length according to the sensation; e.g., it is longer for sight than for sound, and longer for pain than for touch.

The sensation outlasts its stimulus. Such *after-sensations* are particularly noticeable in the case of sight. If we look at an object intently we can continue to see it for a time after we close our eyes.

The Impulse.— The evidence appears now to be complete that the nerve impulse is identical in nature in all nerves. The impulse set up in the optic nerve by light is the same as that set up in the auditory nerve by sound.

The difference in sensation recognised by the individual must be due to the "analysers" in the central nervous system. The impulses reaching certain analysers, such as those of sight, are interpreted as light however the impulse is set up. This was termed by Muller "*The Law of Specific Nerve Energies.*" The term energy is a bad one, and is not used in a modern physical sense, but the law simply means that every sense-organ, however excited, gives rise to its own specific sensation. However the retina or optic nerve is stimulated light is appreciated. Mechanical, chemical, or electrical stimulation of the chorda tympani causes a sensation of taste. These observations have been made during surgical operations.

A great deal of investigation of the action potentials which are the basis of the various kinds of sensation have been carried out by Adrian, Matthews, Bronk, Rijlant and others, using wireless valve amplifiers and oscillometers or cathode-ray oscillographs. In every case it is found that the stimulation of a receptor brings about a series of discharges which may vary much in their duration and in their frequency, from 5 to 300 per second. The more rapid the rise of intensity of the stimulus the greater the frequency of discharge. Thus the more rapidly the finger is pricked the greater the sensation. The frequency and duration of the responses are different from different regions.

An interesting phenomenon is that of *adaptation*, in which it is found that if a stimulus is continued, impulses are no longer set up in the nerve. This is well shown in Fig. 9.1. Thus is explained why a needle hurts while it is being inserted into the skin but not after it is in. This adaptation appears to depend on the end-organs concerned. In some, such as those of the skin, or Pacinian corpuscles, adaptation occurs rapidly, while in the nerve-endings of muscle it is very slow, a fact which no doubt permits the muscle when subjected to prolonged stretching to send out the sustained impulses so important in posture.

Intermittent stimulation, as might be expected, reduces adaptation. For example, although the response for a single blast of air on the skin is over in 1/5 second, intermittency not exceeding 200 per second will maintain a burst of impulses at that rate. This is important in relation to the importance of air movement in ventilation.

Adaptation is seen in many of our common sensations. The same room feels warm to a man who enters it from the street, and cold to another who has been in a conservatory. The hot bath appears to get more rapidly cooler than it actually does, while if one hand is placed in cold water and the other in hot water at body temperature may appear warm to one hand and cool to the other. Herring calls the point of adaptation to temperature " the physiological zero." Thus the temperature of the mouth and the lips may actually differ by several degrees, yet neither of them will feel hot or cold because each is at the physiological zero temperature. Sensations of warmth or cold arise when the physiological zero is altered: they persist until a new zero is formed; according to Rivers and Head, adaptation to temperature is impossible when epicritic sensibility is absent. So, too, heavy weights feel unduly heavy after light weights, and *vice versa*.

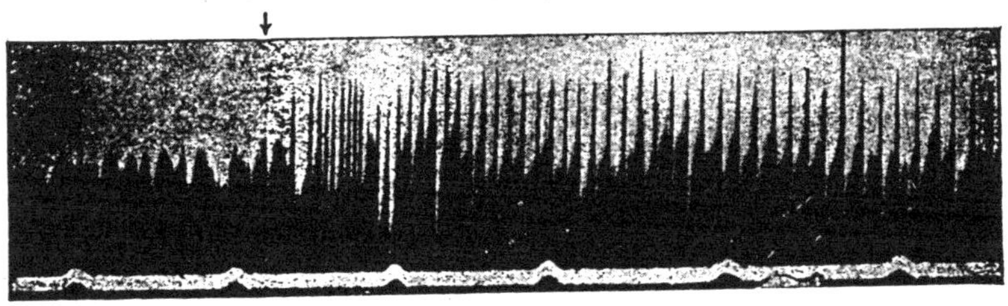

Fig. 9.1. Record of action-potentials from an afferent fiber from a muscle. At the arrow tension was placed on the muscle. Note the burst of impulses with some adaptation—which, however, is never complete—as shown by the continuance of the impulses.

When false teeth or spectacles are first worn, their contact is well-nigh unbearable; yet later, through adaptation, the discomfort vanishes.

The impulse when set up passes into the central nervous system by means of *afferent nerves.* In the case of the cranial nerves, some are wholly sensory. In the case of the trunk and limbs, the impulses pass along fibers which become incorporated in mixed nerves and pass into the spinal cord by way of the posterior roots. Some of the impulses bring about, as we have seen, reflex movements, and may nerve reach consciousness, e.g., the impulse set up by slight pinching of the finger during sleep. The majority of the stimuli, however, during the waking hours and even during sleep, are strong, and the impulses which they generate pass up the spinal cord to the brain (see Sensory Pathways).

Impulses from Muscles.— Investigations (Matthews) tend to show that there are characteristics of discharge corresponding to the four classes of nerve-endings already described, but we do not know with certainty which come from which, nor what functions each subserves, but we know that, in addition to afferent impulses which are appreciated as pain in muscle, there must be those which are concerned with the appreciation of length and tension. An interesting point is the fact that the impulses from an extensor muscle of a decerebrate animal in rigidity cease when the muscle is caused to contract more actively.

A single sense-organ in a muscle has been found to set up impulses with a frequency of 30 per second. This has been discovered by using the sternocutaneous muscle of the frog, and by successively cutting off fibers to leave only one muscle- spindle. There is an increase in the frequency of the impulse with the logarithm of the load and frequencies from 5 to 500 have been recorded. There is, as we have said, little adaptation to stretching.

Impulses from the Skin.— These are characterised by being of very short duration, about 0.2 sec., the nerve-endings of the skin becoming very rapidly adapted, as the adaptation to skin sensation suggests. Pain from section of the skin is therefore short-lived unless the injured part is stimulated further by movement.

Impulses causing Pain.— Pain is experienced from stimulation of any sense to excess, but most commonly when there is actual damage to tissue by severing or burning of the skin or from excessive tension or oxygen-want of internal tissues.

There has been considerable debate as to whether or not there are special nerve-endings. We know many sensations in excess will produce pain, and it has been pointed out by Herring that it would be rather remarkable if there were special endings in internal tubes such as the ureter, from which there is normally no sensation at all. On the other hand, in favour of the view that there are special nerve-endings is the fact that in certain regions of the body, e.g., the cornea, where there are no specialised nerve-endings but only the terminal ramifications of nerves, pains is felt, while it has long been known that there are pain spots in the skin which are sensitive only to pain, also a jet of air does not appear to produce pain although it sets up impulses of 300 per sec., and obvious harmful stimuli often set up impulses of low frequency in the small C

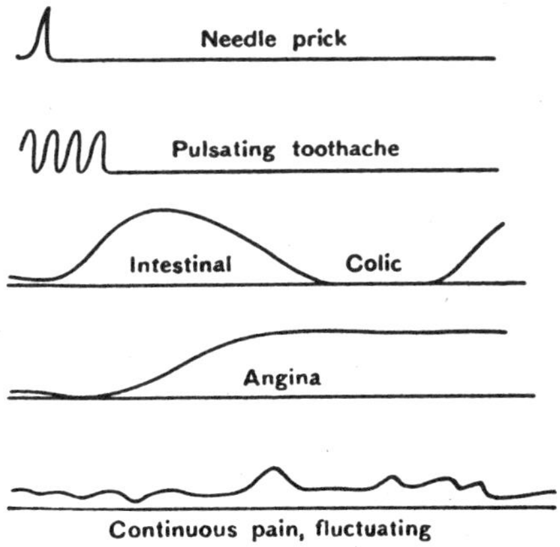

Fig. 9.2.

fibers. As we shall see, too, it is well established that in the cord the fibers carrying pain (like touch and temperature) become collected into distinct bundles or tracts.

The difference between touch and pain is seen when a needle is placed on the paw of an anaesthetised animal and forced into the skin, the action potential being recorded from the nerve to the part. When the paw is touched there is a short burst of impulses, but when the paw is pricked there is a much longer burst of impulses. Both types of stimulus show adaptation, but pain less than touch. The frequency of the discharge for pain may vary from 5-100 per sec. It is not uniformly high as it would be if it were due to stimulation of any kind of receptor.

It seems likely that the *extent* of the sensation is determined by the number of fibers thrown into activity, but the intensity of the sensation depends on the frequency of the discharge set up. As we shall see later, the interpretation of the nature and the value of the stimulus to the animal depends on the cerebral cortex, but as seen in the spinal reflex harmful stimuli are at once acted upon by the spinal cord. The evidence would appear to indicate that while there are special receptors for pain, the excessive stimulation of other sensory impulses may produce a gross disturbance analysed as pain. This would obviously have the advantage of protecting the sensory endings concerned, as in the case of light, for looking at the sun may cause detachment of the retina. Adrian concludes that " it is probable that there are no hard-and-fast divisions into pain endings and touch endings or free endings and encapsulated endings," but thinks there is no doubt that the endings are mainly free and that few of the encapsulated endings give rise to pain.

It would seem, too, that the stimulus for pain must attain a certain massiveness before it produces a sensation, whether it is stimulating a free nerve-ending or a nerve-ending subserving some other sense.

Pain in muscle is of special interest as it occurs in a variety of common conditions of which the most important are those due to inadequate blood-supply. Experimentally it can be conveniently produced and studied by occluding the arterial supply to a limb by means of a sphygmomanometer cuff. The pain is increased by use of the muscles of the limb, but the degree of pain is determined by the amount of use rather than the tension produced. Thus the pain is not increased by short-lived but severe tetanus of the muscles, it is made worse, however, according to the duration of the contractions. On the other hand, it is not relieved by stopping exercise of the part, but the pain at once passes off if the circulation is released.

These facts led Lewis to postulate that a "P" pain substance was released, and in view of the fact that lactic acid accumulates during oxygen-lack it seems likely that it may be the substance or, at least, be concerned.

Pain in muscle occurs typically in occlusion of the coronary arteries, and the pain so produced is said to be the most severe known to man. It occurs, too, in the legs when there is spasm of the arteries, and leads to great pain in walking which is relieved by sympthectomy. The pain of fatigue and cramp is probably of a similar nature. Embolism of the mesenteric vessels produces pain, but occlusion of the vessels of non-muscular organs, such as the lungs or spleen, is not painful, but its results are found by post-mortem.

Much pain, such as that of rheumatism, is located in muscle, but is really due to a low-grade inflammation and possible oedema of the fibrous tissue in its structure or vicinity. Such pain is usually benefited by exercise. Also it is claimed that pain can be produced by the hernia of fat through fascial planes, and certainly nodules can sometimes be felt. Much pain is ascribed to muscle which is really due to bruising of joint surfaces and the setting up of protective spasm of adjacent muscles.

Stiffness after unaccustomed exercise or local cooling produced by draught, which produce vasoconstriction of a temporary and less severe nature, would seem to be due to a local accumulation of metabolism which leads to increased capillary permeability and engorgement of the tissue with exuded plasma. This may be aggravated by actual tearing of tissues in the case of unaccustomed usage. Such pain usually is slow on its onset and lasts fore a few days. Our knowledge of such pain has also been much illuminated by Lewis, who found that the injection of saline solution into muscles, fascia, and joints produced diffuse pain which could be localised only with difficulty. This is common experience.

Varieties of Pain.— Pain is affected by a variety of circumstances which may alter its character. One burst of impulses is appreciated as a single stab of pain, such as that of a pin-prick. If tension is produced by the accumulation of pus in a confined space, such as the socket of a tooth or in a finger, the arterial pulse may be communicated to the nerve-endings and the pain assumes a throbbing character. If the tension is produced by peristaltic waves the pain is intermittent, such as that produced by taking a purgative, or by the passage of a stone down the bile-duct or the ureter. This pain is known as colic and its intermittence is an important point in diagnosis. Much pain, especially that following injury, is aggravated by movement. The pain which results from arterial blockage is sustained, while neuritic pains from inflammation of nerves tend to be irregular.

Other physiological considerations also affect pain. Thus pain in a joint or a muscle may be produced only if the part is moved; a pain in a frontal sinus or a maxillary antrum tends to be worse in the afternoon as the sinus fills with fluid. Pain in the alimentary canal may be definitely related to food. The pain of a gastric ulcer is immediate on the taking of food, while that caused by a duodenal ulcer occurs about two hours after the meal, when the stomach is empty. Spasm of the colon is most liable to occur in the early hours of the morning, when the late meal of the day has reached that area and sympathetic activity is at its lowest. Ulcerated colon produces excessive pain in defaecation. Pain due to inflamed pleura occurs during inspiration. All these considerations assist in determining the cause of any given apin and this is still further helped by palpation or tapping of the appropriate part, for as we shall see in regard to sensation, the patient's localisation may be quite fallacious. Thus tapping of the teeth may determine which tooth may be responsible for a facial neuralgia, and a point of maximum tenderness assist in the diagnosis in many conditions.

The Nerve Fibers Concerned with Cutaneous Sensation

When a cutaneous nerve is cut or crushed all sensation from that part is abolished, but if the two cut ends are sewn together it returns. At first the sensation tends to be crude and confused—that is to say, the patient does not appreciate the full grade of sensation. He may, for example, appreciate pain or crude heat or cold, but is less able to distinguish finer degrees of touch and temeprature. The sense of touch is not, however, lacking if he is carefully tested. At one time it was thought possible to divide sensation into protopathic or crude sensation and epicritic or discriminate sensation. There is no real basis for this, for the apparatus for the discriminative appears to be present at the early stage, only the patient has not learnt to use it. In some cases it is easy to imagine, as pointed out by Sharpey-Schafer, who repeated the experiment of Head and others of severing a cutaneous nerve in himself, that nerve-fibers may grow into the wrong end-organs. At the same time stopford has emphasised that there is no doubt that a crude mechanism for protection is dependent on the thalamus, and later, with the development of the cortex, a better system of perception and discrimination develop.

Various attempts have been made to determine by which nerve-fibers the various sensations travel. As we have seen, fibers vary very much in size, and the large A fibers transmit impulses very much quicker than the smaller. Gasser especially has compared the effect of various prosmaller. Gasser especially has compared the effect of various procedures in the impulses carried in the nerves of anaesthetised animals and compared them with the disappearance of sensations in man. These are as follows:

Asphyxia produced by an armlet	Touch pressure (B), cold, warmth, pain (C).

Cocaine produced by an armlet	Cold, warmth, pain, touch.
Cold produced by an armlet	Cold, touch, pain, warmth.

Generally, however, less information has been obtained by such studies than was hoped for, but it is generally agreed that impulses set up by pain pass at least by A and C fibers (Zottermann).

Drugs.— Cocaine applied locally depresses all forms of cutaneous sensibility, but especially the true tactile sense; carbolic acid acts similarly but less strongly. Chloroform produces a temporary burning sensation, and then blunts sensibility, especially to temperature changes. Menthol produces a feeling of local cold because it first causes hyperaesthesia of the end-organs for cold; this is followed by a depression of the activity of these organs, together with that of those subserving other forms of cutaneous sensation.

Speech

The discovery of a part of the cerebral cortex which was specially associated with speech was one of the first steps towards cerebral localisation. The French physician Broca stated that right-handed patients who died from cerebral embolism, and who had, previous to death, lost the power of speech, had commonly damage in the region of the pars triangular is of the inferior frontal convolution. Modern clinicians, however, tend to look upon Broca's statement as little more than a guess, at first taken too seriously.

Subsequently, Marie and Moutier pointed out that loss of speech may occur with lesions of other parts of the brain and that the loss may be confined to certain parts of speech; thus, the individual may be unable to read aloud, to write to dictation and the like, without any other part of speech being seriously affected. Few will go so far as to suggest, as did Marie, that Broca's area has not a special relation to speech; indeed, there is overwhelming evidence that it has. Head went to the other extreme, and has almost denied that it is possible to differentiate *aphasia*, i.e., loss of speech, into isolated affections of speaking, writing, etc., due to destruction of visual, auditory, or motor areas.

The Formation of Speech.— Probably all these views may be reconciled when we consider how speech is evolved in the individual. Speech in its wide sense may be considered the mode of interchange of ideas between oneself and one's fellow-creatures. It may be looked upon as depending upon three distinct mechanisms.

I. *A Receptor Mechanism* which may involve any sensation, although normally hearing and seeing are utilised. In close relationship to the cortical centre for these sensations are the association areas, in which memories of sensation appear to be stored. Thus, in the second and third temporal convolutions are stored the names of objects and these are lost if this region becomes the seat of disease, e.g., abscess secondary to inflammation of the middle ear.

2. *Association Mechanism.* Our knowledge of this mechanism is, as yet, quite crude, and we cannot relate its facts in any detail to anatomical areas, but from a study of disease a large amount of interesting material has been collected.

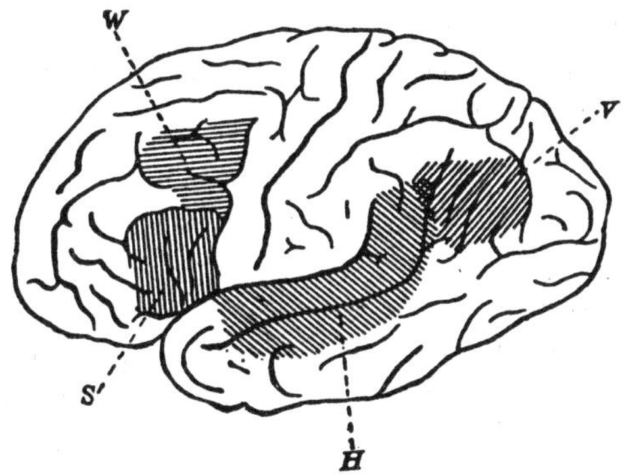

Fig. 9.3. Lateral view of the left cerebral hemisphere of man (after Donaldson). V is the cortical area damage to which produces "word blindness"; it is situated in the angular gyrus, and is called the *visual word centre*. H is the area in the superior temporal convolution, called the *auditory word centre*, damage to which produces "word deafness." S is Broca's convolution, damage to which produces loss of audible speech (motor aphasia); just behind is the motor area for the movements of the tongue, vocal cords, etc., concerned in speaking; Bastian termed it the *glosso-kinasesthetic area*. The area W, called by Bastian the *cheiro-kincesthetic area*, is the corresponding region concerned in hand movements, damage to which abolishes the power of writing (agraphia).

There is general agreement, however, that in right-handed persons the area concerned is on the *left side* of the brain, within a well-defined cortical region extending from the lower and posterior part of the frontal lobe, by the island of Reil, to the temporal and lower parietal and occipital region. Of this region, it is clear that the anterior part is concerned with expression, and the posterior part, or area of Wernicke, with reception.

To each sensation is attached a certain significance according to the circumstance in which it is experienced. If an idea has to communicated, or a reply made, the impulse passes to that part of the association mechanism concerned with expression, where the proper means of expression is determined. Broca's area (as its histological structure suggests) may be considered an association area in close relation to the vocal effector mechanism.

3. *An effector Mechanism.*—The message is then conveyed to the appropriate part of the motor cortex concerned with the vocal organs, but it may be, according to circumstances, the area for hand movements or any other part. A nod of the head, or placing a finger to the mouth, may be even more significant than a

spoken word. It is, then, fairly easy to understand why it is that certain parts of the general speech mechanisms may become impaired, leaving other parts normal. Head does not consider that an aphasic individual is ever quite normal mentally, nor, indeed, can this be expected, unless the disease is limited to a small area of the motor cortex. When we learn to speak, we learn to think and to form ideas by a similar mechanism, and we know how impaired the general mentality of a deaf person may be, simply because he has not the normal facility of communicating with his fellows.

The effect of any given lesion on mentality will then depend on how the individual has acquired his knowledge. If, for example, there is a lesion of the association fibers connecting the visual association area to the motor area for the vocal organs, not only will the individual be word blind, i.e., unable to read aloud, but probably other associations and ideas, which depend on knowledge acquired by reading, will be affected, although he may reply quite well to verbal questions, and knowledge acquired by hearing may be unaffected.

The Voice

The fundamental tones of the voices are produced by the current of expired air causing the vibration of the vocal cords, two bands contained in a cartilaginous box placed at the top of the windpipe or trachea. This box is called the *larynx*. The sounds produced here are modified by other parts such as the tongue, teeth, and lips.

The human musical instrument is often compared to a reed organpipe: certainly the notes produced by such pipes in the *vox humana* stop of organs in very like the human voice. Here there is not only the vibration of a column of air, but also of a reed, which corresponds to the vocal cords in the air-chamber composed of the trachea and the bronchial system beneath it. The pharynx, mouth, and nasal cavities above the glottis are resonating cavities, which by alterations in their shape and size, are able to pick out and emphasise certain component parts of the sounds produced in the larynx. The natural voice is often called the *chest voice*. The *falsetto voice* is differently explained by different observers; on laryngoscopic examination, the glottis is found to be blown open; it is probable fibers of the thyroarytenoid muscle are in contraction.

Musical sounds differ from one another in three ways :

1. *In pitch.*— This depends on the rate of vibration; and in a string, the pitch increases with the tension, and diminishes with the length of the string. The vocal cords of a women are shorter than those of a man hence the higher-pitched voice of women.

2. *In loudness.*— This depends on the amplitude of the vibrations, and is increased by the force of the expiratory blast which sets the cords in motion.

3. *In "timbre."*— This is the difference of character which distinguishes one voice, or one musical instrument, from another. It is due to admixture of the primary vibrations with secondary vibrations or overtones. The range of the

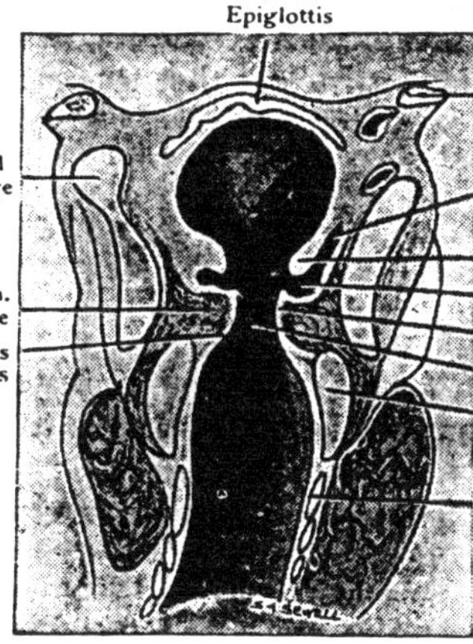

Fig. 9.4. A vertical section through the larynx. It emphasises the fact that the vocal cords are not in reality cords but the apices of sharp folds. Note the valvular appearance of the laryngeal folds. The vocal cords prevent the entry of air into the chest, the ventricular bands hinder the exit or air.

voice is seldom, except in celebrated singers, more than two- and-a-half octaves, and for different voices this is in different parts of the musical scale.

Records may now be taken of the voice with accuracy as in the making of gramophone records, but the magnification required is such that they do not lend themselves readily to reproduction here.

Vocal Speech

Speech is due to the modification produced in the fundamental laryngeal notes by the resonating cavities above the vocal cords. By modifying the size and shape of the pharynx, mouth, and nose, certain overtones or harmonics are picked out and exaggerated: this gives us the vowel sounds; the consonants are produced by interruptions, more or less complete, of the outflowing air in different situations. When the larynx is passive, and the resonating cavities alone come into play, we get whispering.

For detailed description of the larynx, reference should be made to a text-book of Anatomy. It is composed of the thyroid cartilage, the prominence in front of which constitutes Adam's apple, the cricoid cartilage and the two arytenoids, together with several minor cartilages. These are all held together and to the neighbouring structures by fibrous tissue and muscle.

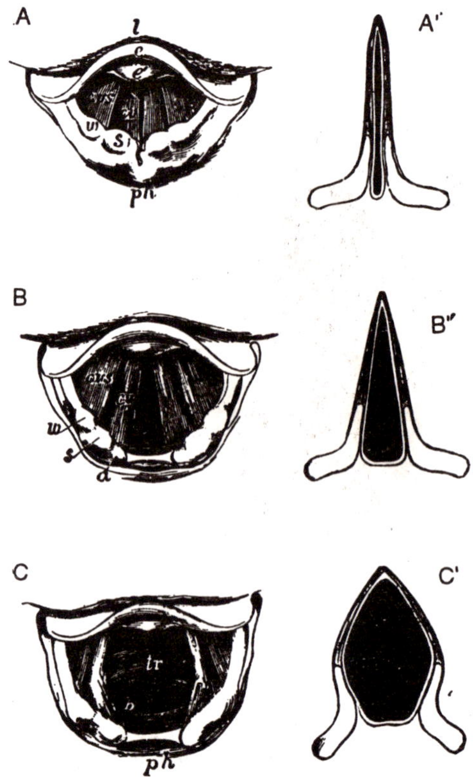

Fig. 9.5. Three larynxgoscopic views of the superior aperture of the larynx and surrounding parts. A, the glottis during the emission of a high note in singing; B, in easy and quiet inhalation of air; C, in the state of widest possible dilatation, as in inhaling a very deep breath. The diagrams A, B′, C′ show in horizontal sections of the glottis the position of the vocal cords and arytenoid cartilages in the three several states represented in the other figures. In all the figures so far as marked, the letters indicate the parts as follows, viz.: *l*, the base of the tongue, *e*, the upper free part of the epiglottis; e′, the tubercle of the epiglottis; *ph*, part of the anterior wall of the pharynx behind the larynx; in the margin of the aryteno-epiglottidean fold, *w*, the swelling of the membrane caused by the cartilages of Wrisberg; s, that of the cartilages of Santorini; *a*, the tip summit of the arytenoid cartilages; *CV*, the true vocal cords or lips of the rima glottidis; *cvs*, the superior or false vocal cords; between them the ventricle of the larynx; in C, *tr* is placed on the anterior wall of the receding trachea, and *b* indicates the commencement of the two bronchi beyond the bifurcation which may be brought into view in this state of extreme dilatation.

Movements of the Vocal Cords

In Respiration.—The position of the vocal cords in ordinary tranquil breathing is so adapted by the muscles that the opening of the glottis is wide and triangular. The glottis may remain unaltered during ordinary quiet breathing, though in some people it becomes a little wider at each inspiration, and a little narrower at each expiration. In the cadaveric position the glottis has about half the width it has during ordinary breathing; during life, therefore, except during vocalisation, the abductors of the vocal cords (posterior crico-arytenoids) are in constant action. On making a rapid and deep inspiration the opening is widely dilated and somewhat lozenge-shaped.

In Vocalisation.— At the moment of the emission of a note the chink is narrowed, the margins of the arytenoid cartilages being brought into contact, and the edges of the vocal cords approximated and made parallel; at the same time their elasticity is regulated by contraction of the thyro-arytenoid muscles.

The approximation of the vocal cords also usually corresponds with the height of the note produced; but the width of the aperture has no influence on the pitch of the note, as long as the vocal cords have the same tension; only with a wide aperture the tone is more difficult to produce and is less perfect, the rushing of the air through the aperture being heard at the same time.

No true vocal sound is produced at the posterior part of the aperture of the glottis, namely, that which is formed by the space between the arytenoid cartilages (pars intercartilaginea).

The exact part played by the mouth and vocal cords is well seen when the larynx is removed for cancer. By attaching a reed-like apparatus to the upper end of the trachea to make the fundamental note and leading it to the mouth by another tube, an almost normal speech can be produced. Such patients can also be taught to speak by eructing swallowed air from the stomach.

The Physiology of Conscious States

In physiological considerations of sensation and voluntary movement it is usual to take consciousness for granted, for we are far from understanding its exact nature. Consciousness belongs academically to the realm of Psychology, but it is becoming abundantly clear that there is no hard-and-fast line between the subjects of Physiology and Psychology. In considering the protective reflexes and also the conditioned reflexes, by which animals learn by experience, we have seen a whole host of activities which the uninitiated might have thought to be dependent on consciousness. We have seen that although consciousness may be necessary for the establishment of such conditioned reflexes, it is certainly not necessary for their operation once they have become "fixed" in the nervous system, and we can certainly learn without conscious effort, as in the case of advertising posters.

Consciousness may be defined as an awareness of the existence of oneself and of the external world, and the evidence is very complete that it is dependent in man on the occurrence of a given amount of oxidation taking place in the cerebrum. Without such chemical changes we know that nerve-cells cease to function and die. We can say, from a study of the changes in electrical potential of the brain, that consciousness is a correlate of the activity of cerebral nerve-cells, and we are aware of certain streams of impulses which pass through the cerebrum provided they are of sufficient magnitude, whether they occur during the awake or sleeping state. If they are present when we are asleep a dream results, but then we are not completely aware of our immediate environment.

It seems most probable that the state of consciousness varies throughout the animal kingdom but in man alone has reached a stage of evolution which makes it possible to form mental concepts of which that of mind, as an abstract or spiritual entity, is the most important. The emotions appear, for the most part at least to depend on instinctive drives very akin to reflex actions, and it is evident that many of the responses to such emotions are conditioned like reflexes. How conditioning, the emotions and the activities of the mind are correlated and affected feelings and conduct are discussed in *Sane Psychology*, a biological introduction to Psychology by the same author and publisher at this book.

In the past the subjects of Physiology and Psychology have been almost poles apart because those whose outlook commenced with the immaterial entity, mind, could see little or no need for the nervous system or any of its workings. It is, however, slowly becoming apparent that not only has mind a profound effect on body but the body greatly influences mental processes, with result that with a saner and more balanced appreciation of the facts the boundaries between Psychology and Physiology are fast disappearing.

Loss of Consciousness

Although we do not know exactly what consciousness is, we know that it depends on a number of entities which are of great importance in practical medicine.

1. *The Physical Integrity of the Brain.*— We know that if the cerebrum is damaged extensively consciousness is lost. This loss may be temporary and may result from a sudden blow, such as the "knock-out" in boxing. This is believed to be due to a sudden raising of the pressure in the cerebrum and the production of vascular spasm causing cerebral anaemia. (Trotter, Souter.) Temporary unconsciousness is known as *concussion*.
2. *The Oxygen Supply to the Brain.*— Any condition which reduces the oxygen supply to the brain produces unconsciousness. The oxygen may fail because the blood supply is deficient or the blood itself may not contain sufficient oxygen.

A state of semi-consciousness may be produced by over-breathing. In this case the blood contains sufficient oxygen, but the loss of carbon dioxide prevents it from dissociating to the cerebral cells, and this is accentuated by any procedure which tends to lower the arterial blood-pressure, such as expiration against resistance (Hemingway).

A large variety of procedures and circumstances may produce a failure of the cerebral circulation. It may be produced by compression of the carotid vessels (a dangerous procedure), a fall of blood-pressure such as results from haemorrhage or from loss of the normal activity of the vasomotor centre, all of which cause a rapid loss of consciousness. If temporary this is known as fainting. It becomes evident that strangulation or section of the carotid arteries in the neck is a much less painful form of death than commonly supposed. There is evidence that in right-handed persons consciousness may depend particularly on the left frontal lobe, occlusion of the blood supply to this region is particularly effective in producing unconsciousness.

Cerebral compression is a state of increased intracranial pressure of great practical importance. It occurs as a result of cerebral tumour and cerebral haemorrhage, but most commonly from a blow on the head resulting in damage to the middle meningeal artery in the parietal bone and bleeding into the skull.

Whenever the intracranial pressure rises above that of the capillaries or veins, the cerebral circulations ceases and unconsciousness is produced. Death occurs when sufficient blood accumulates to force down the medulla into the foramen magnum.

3. *A reduction of the fuel supply* to the brain produces results similar to those of deficient oxygen supply, since both allow the "cerebral fires" to go out. This

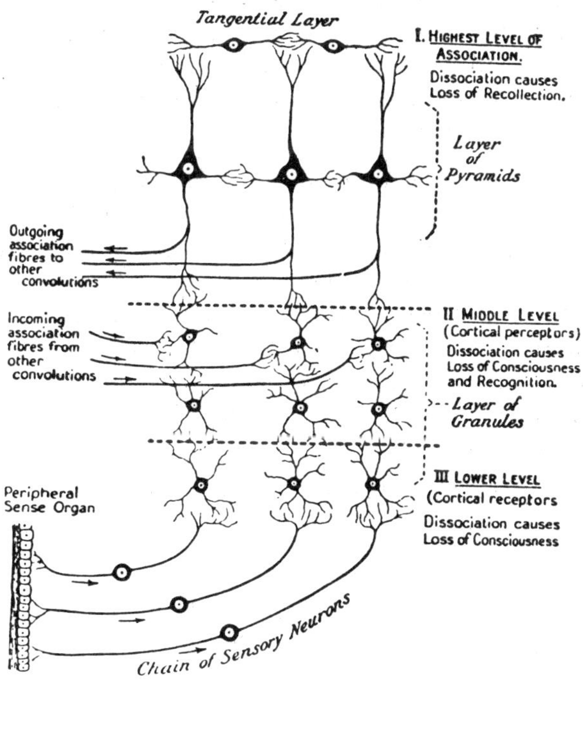

Fig. 9.6. Diagram to illustrate levels of association. This figure if taken absolutely suggests that all three levels are in the same part of the cortex. This is not the case. Moreover, it is possible that the lower levels may be sub-cortical.

occurs if there is insufficient glucose in the blood to be oxidised, as in hypoglycaemia from an excessive dose of insulin, when convulsions or unconsciousness may supervene.

4. Unconsciousness or coma also results from diseases in which *toxic products* are abnormally produced or are retained, as in diabetes mellitus or nephritis. The poisonous substances probably act directly on the cerebral cells.

Consciousness is associated with the activities of the nervous system to differing degrees, and it is possible to indicate this diagrammatically, although it must be understood that there is no hard-and-fast line between the different levels.

Sleep

We are familiar with sleep but its exact nature is not clearly understood.

The first two hours of sleep are always the most profound; later on, relatively weak stimuli will cause awakening. Of the parts of the central nervous system, the spinal cord is always less deeply affected than the brain, but even the brain is never entirely irresponsive, and unless slumber is very profound, dreams are the subjective result of external stimuli. Sensations of sound appear to be the last to disappear as sleep comes on, and the first to be realised on waking.

Changes which Occur During Sleep.— During normal sleep there is general reduction of sympathetic activity as indicated by constriction of the pupil, slowing of the heart, slight fall of blood-pressure, and an increase in the volume of the limbs. If the subject falls asleep on a special balance (Mosso), the head end is found to become appreciably lighter, indicating that blood has been withdrawn from the brain. This is confirmed by the fact that if the brain of a man is observed during sleep, it is seen to retract slightly from the trephine opening in the skull. It may be noted, too, that a similar phenomenon is produced by narcotic drugs which produce sleep. The waves of the encephalogram (see below) are at first increased and then decreased as sleep deepens.

It is known, too, that conditions which reduce sympathetic activity favour sleep, namely warmth, comfort, and the reduction of sensory stimulation by quiet and darkness, while their absence prevents it.

How far the reduction of sympathetic action is the cause of, and how far the result of, sleep is a difficult problem.

A further complication is the recognised fact that fatigue, especially of the muscles, provided it is not excessive, also promotes sleep. This may also tend to cause the accumulation of blood in the fatigued muscles, but it is possible that the chemical products of fatigue may be sleep-promoting. Some investigators claimed to have isolated specific sleep-promoting substances. It used to be considered unlikely that such chemical substances are responsible because of the fact that the awakening from sleep may be a very rapid event. It is, as we shall see, just possible that the localised accumulation of a substance like acetylcholine, which, as we have seen, is very rapidly destroyed, may be responsible.

It has been suggested that cerebral anaemia is the cause, the sleepiness that follows a heavy meal is attributed to the mechanical effect of a dilatation of the abdominal vessels in producing a diminished blood flow through the brain; while the sleep that normally comes on at the end of the day might be considered due to cerebral anaemia following dilatation of the blood vessels of the skin, such dilatation being due to vasomotor fatigue. Studies of experimental sleep suggest that the cerebral changes are the primary cause. There is also a fall of the blood calcium in normal sleep and in that produced by sedatives and hypnotism.

Experimental Sleep.— Sleep may be produced experimentally in a number of ways, notably by depressing the sympathetic, e.g., by the injection of ergotamine into the third ventricle of the brain, or by stimulating the parasympathetic by raising the pressure in the carotid sinus by connecting it, when isolated from the circulation but with its nervous connections intact, to an external pressure system. This latter procedure, it should be noted, reduces the activity of the knee-jerk and causes muscular relaxation.

The injection of dilute calcium chloride into the third ventricle has also been found by Demole to produce sleep. This effect is antagonised by the injection of potassium chloride.

Hess, Professor of Physiology in Zurich, found that stimulation of the mid-brain by a slowly rising and falling current also caused sleep, and has suggested the existence of a sleep centre in the region of the floor of the third ventricle. He found that the injection of calcium chloride into the region of the tuber cinereum also produced a sleep reversible by potassium chloride. The view that the mid-brain is specially concerned in sleep is supported by the fact that detailed post-mortem study, by Economo, of sleepy sickness (encephalitis lethargica) shows evidence of the effects of an inflammation in this region. The disease is characterised by prolonged apparently normal sleep, from which, however, it is always possible to waken the patient.

Considerable attention has been given to the *inhibition theory* of Pavlov, who has been able to produce experimentally in dogs a condition resembling normal sleep. He considers that normal sleep and hypnotic sleep are much more closely related than has been usually thought, and that both are due to the irradiation of inhibition. The subject has already been dealt with under "Conditioned Reflexes." This view makes it possible that the inhibitory process need not occupy the whole of the cortex at a given time, and thus gives interesting explanations regarding sleep-walking, dreams, persistence of the sense of time during sleep, etc. Incidentally, it suggests that the popular idea that certain individuals are at times only half awake has some scientific justification.

It is not, however, agreed by psychologists that hypnotic and normal sleep are so alike as Pavlov claimed.

The view that sleep depends on the activity of a localised part of the brain is supported by Ranson, who produced sleep by section of the lateral hypothalamus in monkeys. This view does not contradict that of Pavlov but rather supports it, for we know that parasympathetic activity is very commonly conditioned. As examples we may take the secretion of saliva, vomiting, constriction of the bronchi in asthma, and erection of the penis. The exact relationship of this "sleep centre" to the sympathetic is unknown. In this connection it should be noted that sleep occurring naturally or produced by narcosis, provided the narcotic does not stimulate, is always associated with diminished sympathetic as distinct from parasympathetic action. The pupil is constricted, the heart slowed, and digestion continues.

The Cause of Sleep.— In conclusion, we say that sleep occurs when certain parts of the cerebrum are inhibited, but that the inhibition is facilitated by states which promote cerebral anaemia or a generalised reduction of sympathetic activity. From a practical point of view it should be remembered that states, e.g., sensory stimulation or cold which cause increased sympathetic activity, are liable to prevent sleep. Thus the hot-water bottle is justified.

The Relation of the Action of Narcotics and Anaesthesia to Sleep

Many attempts have been made to relate the action of drugs which produce unconsciousness to sleep. It is well recognised that the sleep produced by narcotics is restful and beneficial, but it may be that they facilitate or initiate normal sleep. This sometimes occurs during the induction of anaesthesia. It will be realised that a narcotic only differs from an anaesthetic by convention. With the anaesthetic the unconsciousness is deeper and more easily reversible.

There can be no doubt that, as shown by Demoor, little round swellings are produced on the dendrites by the action of anaesthetics and narcotics and the Nissl bodies of nerve-cells are no longer so easily stained. Many have tried to prove that such drugs produce unconsciousness by reducing cerebral oxidations, but the evidence for this is, however, so very slight that it may be ignored (see Henderson, 1930, and Pask, 1941). Some anaesthetics may act by becoming dissolved in the fatty cell envelopes, and certainly the effect of the older anaesthetics was usually proportional to their fat solvency. This constituted the basis of the well-known Meyer-Overton hypothesis. Several of the newer anaesthetics and narcotics are, however, not specially fat soluble and it now seems more probable that they act on enzyme systems in the cells or, as suggested by Moore and Roaf, by making some unstable compound with the cell protein. It might be that the drugs interfere with humoral transmission between the neurones of the cerebrum. However such drugs act, it is evident that neither they nor sleep do the same permanent harm as does prolonged deprivation of oxygen.

The Effect of Loss of Sleep.— It should be recognised by the public that sleep is the period of anabolism, repair, and growth, and a large allowance is therefore necessary in growing children, who, amongst the lower classes, are often seriously harmed by insufficiency of sleep.

A thorough investigation of the effect of sleeplessness in adults was made on himself and his colleagues by Kleitman of Chicago; they voluntarily went without sleep for periods varying from 40 to 115 hours. They could easily remain awake when actively engaged, but became drowsy when sitting and feel asleep immediately on lying down or on complete muscular relaxation. It is remarkable how normal they remained otherwise;

their blood, urine, etc., were examined, as was also the condition of their heart, respiration, blood-pressure, temperature, appetite, digestion, basal metabolism, and reflexes. Any departures from the normal, if present at all, were trivial; subjectively the feeling of sleepiness was alone marked; ability to do mental arithmetic was unimpaired. The most essential factor in causing sleep in muscular relaxation; this causes a loss of proprioceptive reflexes which in activity are always in action.

The effect of loss of sleep not exceeding one night has been shown experimentally to have a beneficial effect during the first half of the following day, but thereafter there is a fall in efficiency which, in spite of sleep, may not be fully recovered for three days.

Experimental studies show also that although during the first three hours sleep is at its deepest, it is not so recuperative relatively as the later five hours of lighter sleep. It would seem then that the duration is more important than the depth of sleep.

The Electrical Reactions of the Cortex

Modern methods of amplification by means of valves have made it possible to study the action potentials of the cortex which occur during activity. These may be recorded direct from the brain of a lightly anaesthetised animal or from the scalp of man. During sleep or deep anaesthesia there is almost complete "silence," but during consciousness or light anaesthesia various rhythmical changes in potential are recorded-notably the Berger rhythm of the human electro-encephalogram. External stimuli sometimes synchronise independent normal rhythms.

These electrical changes appear to be the result of groups of neurones in action—for it can readily be shown that the changes in special regions of the brain become increased or altered when corresponding sensory nerves are stimulated. For example, the occipital cortex becomes active when the eye is stimulated, but the inherent Berger rhythm is abolished. There seems little doubt afferent impulses are also concerned in the production of the electrical changes, for a section of the brain stem reduces the waves to those of deep sleep, which are due to a slow synchronous discharge mainly of the occipital cortex. The alpha waves of Berger are reduced by mental activity or attention to any special stimulus. The waves in a newly born child asleep are large and simple, but when it wakens irregularities appear as if the simple waves are broken up by impulses which result from sensory impressions from the environment. As a subject falls asleep the waves are increased and in bursts, but later are reduced. Narcotics, anaesthetics, and hypnosis produce similar effects. Other waves and rhythms have also been described from other parts of the cortex. Dreams and epilepsy are associated with marked increases in the electrical changes.

It will, of course, be realised that these changes in electrical potential occur spontaneously, but fundamentally we may look upon them as produced similarly to those which may be recorded from the cortex when various sensory nerves are stimulated.

Voluntary Movement

When a decision is made to make a certain movement it is convenient to look upon

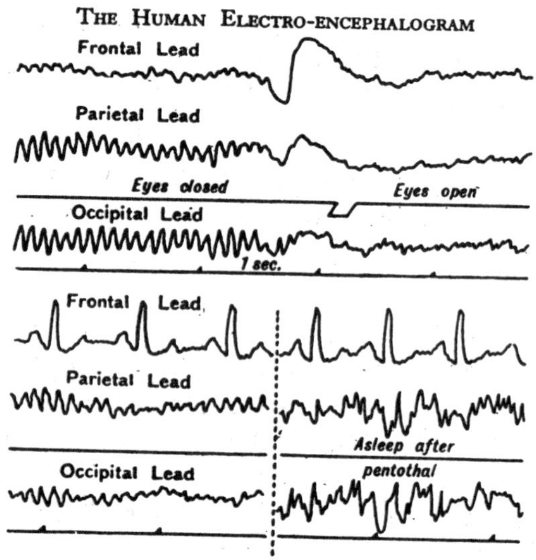

Fig. 9.7. Encephalograms taken in subjects in different states. Note the special activity of the occipital cortex.

the effective impulse as starting in the motor area of the cerebrum and passing down the pyramidal tracts. These arise in the larger pyramidal cells of the precentral gyrus. Thence the fibers converge, like the frame of a fan, through the corona radiata to the internal capsule, where the fibers become bunched together between the lentiform nucleus externally and the thalamus and caudate nucleus on the inside. In horizontal section, the internal capsule appears bent. The pyramidal tracts lie at the bend and in the anterior two-thirds of the posterior limb, and from before backwards the fibers are arranged in order for the head, arm, trunk, legs. The posterior third of this limb is occupied by sensory fibers on their way from the thalamus to the cortex and by the final visual and auditory path. The anterior limb of the capsule is occupied by fibers passing from the frontal lobe to the pons. The importance of this arrangement lies in the fact that a destruction of the fibers very readily occurs as a result of cerebral haemorrhage in this region, and the localised paralysis which results depends on the actual damage done.

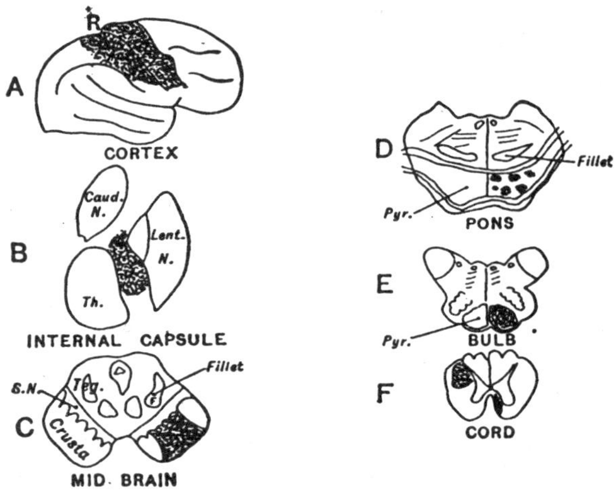

Fig. 9.8. Degeneration after destruction of the Rolandic area of the right hemisphere. The back degenerated area shows the position of the pyramidal tracts throughout its course.

These anatomical details have been ascertained by studying the detailed effects of destruction of the motor area.

In the crus the fibers occupy the middle of the region in front of the substantia nigra (S.N); in the pons the fibers are more scattered, but in the medulla they become again concentrated in the anterior aspect. In the lower part of the medulla most of the fibers cross to the opposite side at the decussation of the pyramids, the *crossed pyramidal tract* occupying the lateral column of the cord until it reaches its destination. In the lower part of the cord where the cerebellar tracts are small the pyramidal tracts extend to the lateral margin of the cord. The fibers of the tract end by arborising round internuncial cells in the region of the posterior horn (not the anterior), whence they are relayed to the anterior horn cells, whose axons pass out from the spinal cord to the muscles, etc. Some of the pyramidal fibers do not cross but remain as the *direct pyramidal tract* in the anterior aspect of the cord throughout, crossing, however, at intervals as far down as the lower thoracic region. Throughout its course in the brain the pyramidal tract gives off fibers via sensory cells (such as those in the substantia nigra) to the cranial nuclei.

The pyramidal tract is not found in all vertebrates below mammals, and its fibers are few in the lower mammals. In rodents they lie in the posterior columns. The direct pyramidal tract is found only in man and in the higher apes.

The rubrospinal tract lies and functions in close association with the pyramidal tracts and, as we have seen, if it is cut, together with the pyramidal tracts, decerebrate rigidity results. It has its origin in the red nucleus, crosses in the mid-brain at the decussation of Forel and ends by synapsing in the lateral grey matter of the cord. It is an afferent pathway of the cerebellum. Other descending tracts are the olivo-spinal tracts which may be concerned with equilibrium, and the *vestibulo-spinal*, responsible for antigravity reflexes.

In clinical work of pyramidal cell and fiber are commonly known as the *upper motor neurone*, while the anterior horn cell with its axon is known as the lower motor neurone.

Destruction or damage to the pyramidal tracts results in paralysis of the particular part of the body supplied. If above the decussation of the pyramids in the medulla, as it commonly is in cerebral haemorrhage, the paralysis is on the opposite side of the body, although it may affect the muscles of the same side of the face. If the motor area is damaged, as it may be at birth, paralysis of a single limb may occur. Even when both limbs of one side are affected (haemiplegia), the trunk, chest, and abdomen which are bilaterally innervated usually escape. The state of the muscles is somewhat reminiscent of decerebrate rigidity, the paralysed muscles have excessive tone (spasticity) and the deep reflexes of the part are increased.

Damage to the tracts in the spinal cord is less common. It may occur in injury and disease, e.g., tumour. In such conditions the interference with voluntary movement is, as a rule, accompanied by impairment of sensation also.

Useful voluntary activity does not, however, depend solely on the motor pathway. It depends also on sensation, and it must be realised that diagrams are merely convenient ways of conveying a mental picture. All the evidence appears to indicate that when we move, say an arm, a shower of impulses is sent down the pyramidal tract to the anterior horn cells moving the essential muscles concerned, but that such contraction sets up at once groups of reflexes which modify the activity of the muscles and the associated muscles.

No doubt the cerebro-cerebellar connections, via the pontine nuclei, also play a part, but how they do so can only be conjecture. Possibly impulses pass down these pathways at the same time as they do the pyramidal tracts.

It is, however, to be understood that to consider the voluntary impulse as beginning in the motor area is merely convenient, as it is the first point which we know of accurately. No doubt, impulses reach this area from the association areas and there is evidence that the frontal area may be specially concerned (Kinnier Wilson). The close relationship of the sensory to the motor area suggests that many of the stimuli come from the sensory area and there is little doubt that many of our so-called voluntary actions are more in response to direct sensory stimulation than at first sight appears. It is of interest also to observe

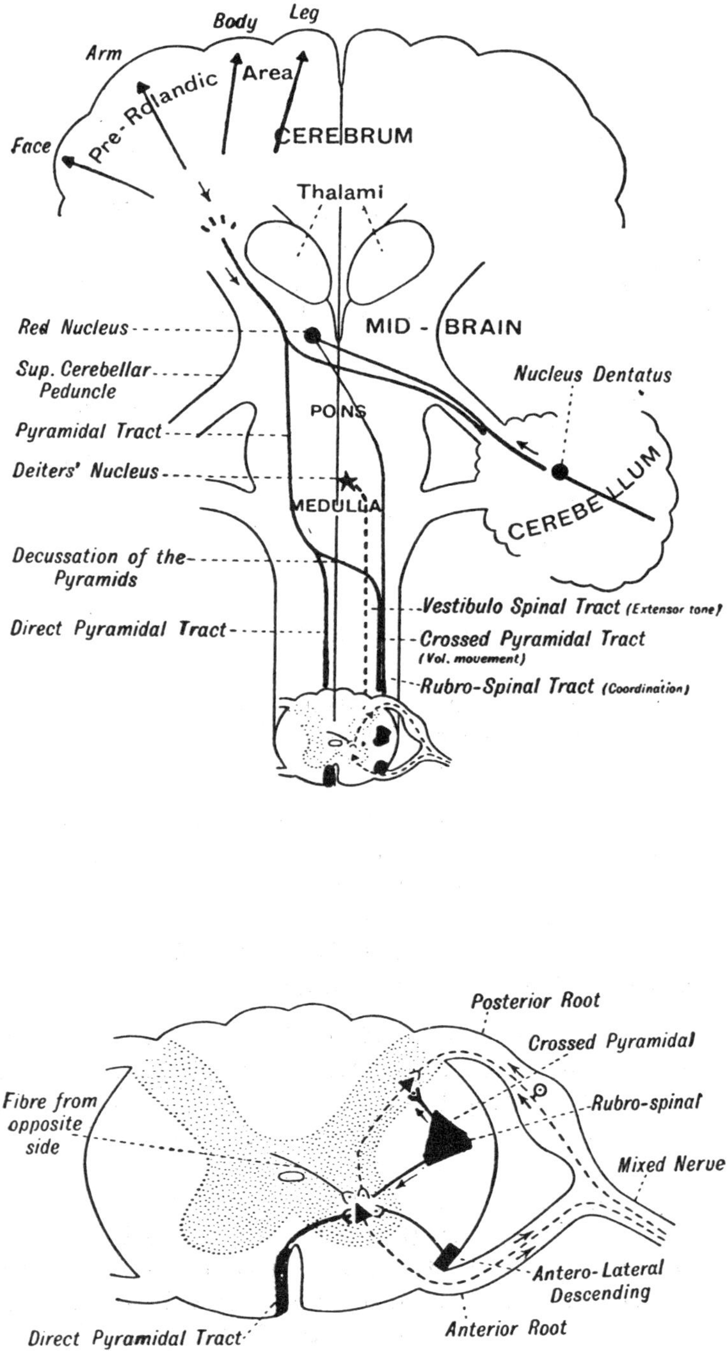

Fig. 9.9. Main efferent paths in central nervous system.

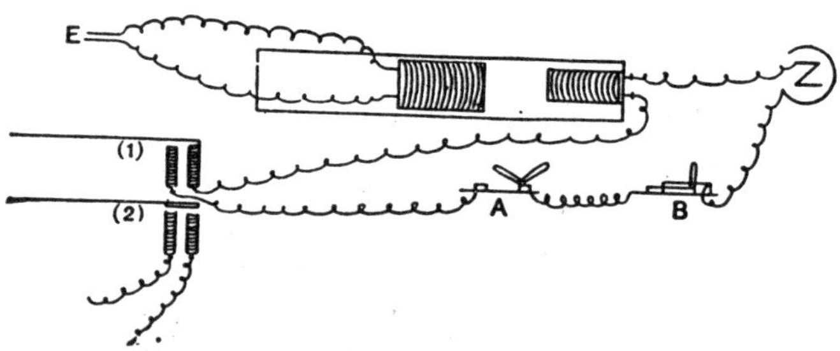

9.10. Diagram of apparatus for recording reaction time.

that repetition of voluntary movement to a given stimulus (seen in taking reaction times) does cause an increased speed of response, while drugs, e.g., bromides, and diseases, e.g., myxaedema, affect voluntary activity and reflexes.

Reactions Time in Man.— The term reaction time is applied to the time occupied in the central nervous system in that complex response to a prearranged stimulus in which the brain as well as the cord comes into play. It is sometimes called the *personal equation*. It may be most readily measured by the electrical method, and the diagram (Fig. 9.10) illustrates one of the numerous arrangements which have been proposed for the purpose.

In the primary circuit two keys (A and B) are included, and an electro-magnetic signal (I), arranged to write on a revolving cylinder (fast rate). A time marker or chronograph (2), marking I-I00ths of a second, is placed below this. The experiment is performed by two persons C and D. The key A, under the control of C, is opened. The key B, under the control of D, is closed. The electrodes E are applied to some part of D's body. C closes A. The primary circuit is made, and the signal (I) moves. As soon as D feels the shock he opens B, the current is thus broken, and the lever of the signal returns to rest. The time between the two movements of the signal (I) is measured by means of the time-tracing written by chronograph (2). From this, the time occupied by transmission along the nerves has to be deducted, and the remainder is the *reaction time*. It usually varies from 0.15 to 0.2 second, but is increased in:

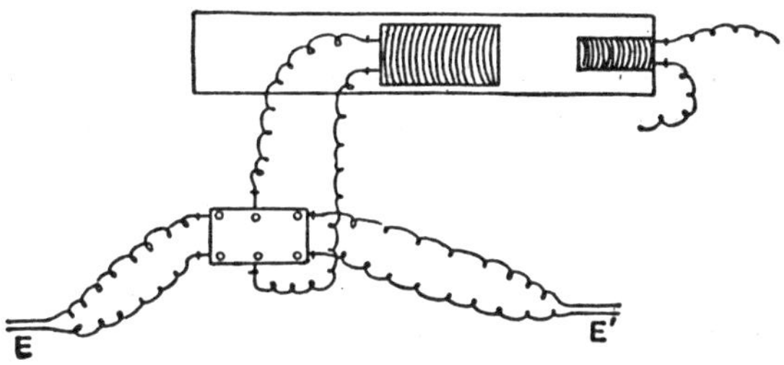

Fig. 9.11. The dilemma.

The Dilemma.— The primary circuit is arranged as before. The wires from the secondary coil lead to the middle screws of a reverser without cross wires. To each pair of end screws, a pair of electrodes E and E′ pass; these are applied to different parts of D's body. It is arranged that D is to open B, when one part is stimulated, but not the other, C adjusting the reverser unknown to D. In these circumstances the reaction time is longer.

The reaction time in response to various kinds of stimuli, sound, light, pain, etc., varies a good deal; the condition of the subject of the experiment is also an important factor.

The Role of Afferent Impulses in Voluntary Movements

Although, as we have said, voluntary movements are conveniently looked upon as commencing in the motor cortex of the cerebrum, afferent impulses play a large part in their initiation and accurate execution.

In the first instance, our decision to make any movement is almost invariably the result of an impulse from the external environment, which causes us to make the movement at a given time. Similarly, afferent impulses may cause us to move the part in a certain direction.

If the movement involves balance, all the impulses from the eyes, from the labyrinth, and from the muscles themselves determine the extent to which movement may be made and the necessary adjustment which is required to maintain equilibrium.

The impulses from the muscles themselves are of special importance in grading and co-ordinating. This is well seen when there is, as in tabes, disease of the posterior horns and posterior nerve roots. The patient is unable to judge exactly when his feet reach the ground in walking, his gait is therefore stamping and gives the name locomotor ataxia to the condition. All such impulses from the muscles are coordinated in the cerebellum, but how exactly they are linked to those of the pyramidal tract is unknown.

Finally, afferent impulses may bring voluntary movement to an end as is well seen in the "Halt" of the drill instructor.

It is of interest to note in conclusion that when the sensory nerves are cut or damaged there is a disinclination to move the part. If the trigeminal nerve is cut (for neuralgia) the patient does not move his face unless specifically asked to do so. Similarly there is in tabes a lack of desire to move, and a similar state has been noticed in animals whose posterior roots are cut.

The Cerebellum

The cerebellum consists of a central lobe known as the vermis which connects two hemispheres, but unfortunately the usual anatomical descriptions bear no relation to function. Its outer cortex of grey matter is even more infolded than that of the cerebrum, and in the white matter of each hemisphere are situated masses of grey matter of which the most important are the dentate nuclei. The grey matter is peculiar in possessing the cells of Purkinje, each of which has a bush-like dendron.

The connections of the cerebellum to the rest of the brain are by means of its *three peduncles* in which are the nerve-fibers which subserve its various functions, but the exact function of all these connections is by no means clear.

The *inferior peduncle* (I.P.), or restiform body, is composed of ascending fibers which pass into it—(I) from the cerebellar tracts of the same side, and (2) from the olivary nucleus of the opposite side; (3) from the nucleus gracilis and nucleus cuneatus of both sides (external and posterior arcuate fibers); (4) from the vestibular nerve, or from the nuclei in which it terminates in the pons.

The *middle peduncle* (M.P.) is formed of fibres which originate from the cells of the nucleus pontis: they pass from one side of the pons to the opposite cerebellar hemisphere.

In the higher mammals, which use their forelimbs freely, these connections are of special importance as the impulses from the motor area of the cerebrum pass through thiw way *via* the nuclei pontis.

The *superior peduncle* (S.P.) consists of (I) the axons of the cells of the nucleus dentatus and (2) fibers of the indirect spino-cerebellar tract. The axons arising from the nucleus dentatus decussate in the mid-brain with those of the opposite side, give off descending branches which terminate in the nucleus of Deiters, and furnish collaterals to the red nucleus and third nerve nucleus; they are then continued upwards to the optic thalamus. From the red nucleus the rubro-spinal tract arises decussates with its fellow in the mid-brain, and descends to the spinal cord. From the optic thalamus a relay of fibers passes to the cerebral cortex.

Thus it will be seen that each half of the cerebellum receives impulses from the joints and muscles, mainly from the same side, *via* the spinocerebellar tracts; from the labyrinth by means of the vestibular nerve of the same side; and from the cerebral cortex of the opposite side through the fronto-pontine tract and the nucleus pontis. Since the

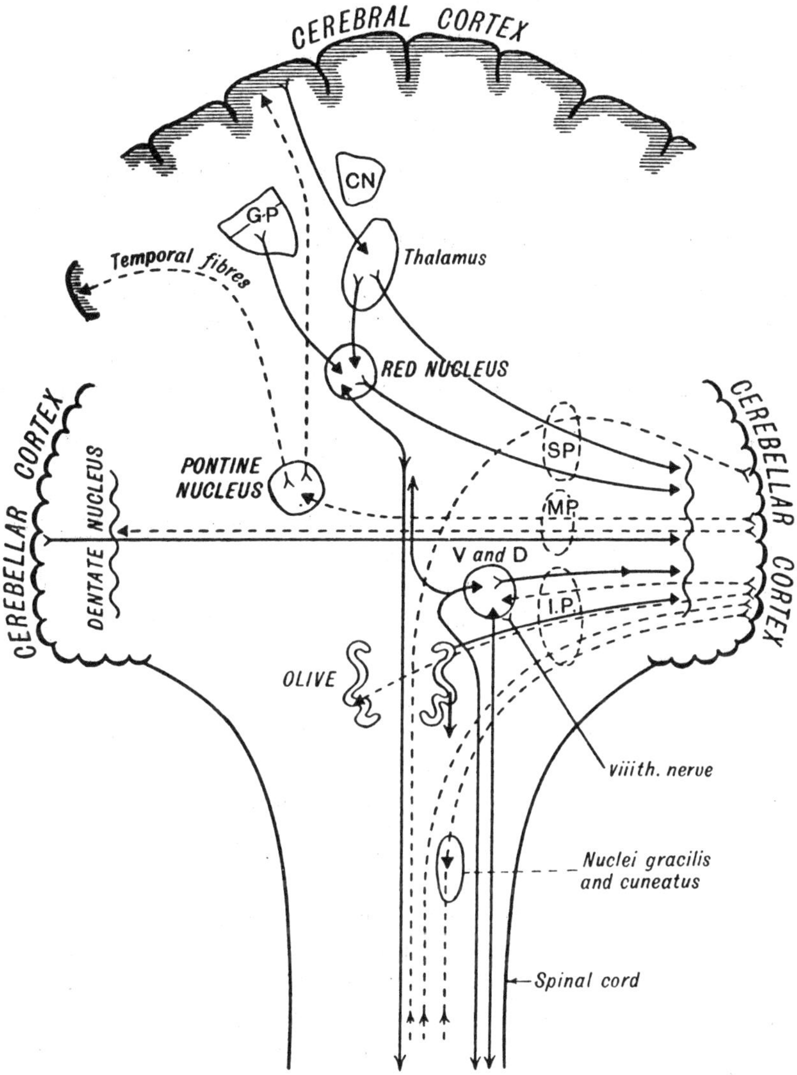

Fig. 9.12. The main connections of the cerebellum on one side. Dark lines = efferent and broken lines = afferent paths.

axons of the Purkinje cells of the cerebellar cortex end in the nucleus dentatus, the axons of which form a large part of the superior peduncle, one hemisphere of the cerebellum furnishes efferent impulses to the opposite cerebral hemisphere *via* the optic thalamus and to the same side of the spinal cord through the rubro-spinal tract; the impulses to the spinal cord must therefore cross the middle line twice. The cerebellum, through its superior peduncle, also gives impulses to the third nerve nucleus; the important part played by the cerebellum in the co-ordination of eye-movements is thus readily understood.

The *function of the cerebellum* was first pointed out by Flourens, who showed that the cerebellum is, as has been indicated already, the great centre for the co-ordination of muscular movement—that is, the harmonious adjustment of the working of the muscles; in doing so the cerebellum co-operates intimately with the postural mechanisms already described and with those responsible for voluntary movement.

Fulton describes it as a vast organ of the motor system lying downstream in the reflex arc from the cerebral cortex. There seems to be little doubt that it is particularly concerned with co-ordinated movements which have been acquired.

Methods of Study.— The functions of the cerebellum may be inferred from (I) its development, (2) its nervous connections, (3) the effects of extirpation in animals or removal for tumour in man, (4) by studying the effects of disease, and (5) by studying the electrical potential changes which are produced by various peripheral stimulation.

These functions fall into three main groups: (I) equilibration, (2) standing, (3) the co-ordination of muscular movement.

1. A study of its development in animals indicates that the organ is developed as an extension from the vestibular nucleus. It earliest developed part or paleocerebellum (the flocculus and nodule) has therefore special connection with the vestibular part of the 8th nerve and is concerned with equilibrium. In fishes and birds this is well seen.

2. With the development of legs and the antigravity mechanisms the cerebellum becomes concerned with the impulses from muscles, especially from the limbs, and the spino-cerebellar tracts make their appearance and are associated with the development of new parts in the middle of the organ known as the paraflocculus and the pyramid. Students should refer to textbooks of Anatomy at this point.

3. In the higher mammals in which free movement of the limbs, apart from standing and walking, becomes an established feature, the cerebellum takes on a still larger function in regard to co-ordination of muscular movement, and new afferent connections *via* the thalamus and efferent connections *via* the pontine nuclei between the cerebellum and the cerebrum become established. A new portion or neocerebellum (The Body) grows again into the middle of the existing cerebellum and becomes its largest part, but a study of the electrical potentials of this region suggests that its function is largely associational. (See Localisation of Function below.)

As its development suggests the *effect of removal* in animals depends very much on the animal used and the use it makes of its muscles.

From the above we should expect that a lesion of the flocculonodular lobe should give rise to disturbances of equilibrium without necessarily any of limb reflexes or motor activity, whereas tumours of the body or the pathways to it will be expected to affect primarily coordination of muscular movement and produce tremor.

Lesions of the primitive flocculo-nodular lobe or tumours of the nodule give rise to a loss of equilibrium of the trunk, but there are no tremors and no disturbances of reflexes.

Flourens and many others used birds for their investigations because the organ in these animals is relatively large and accessible, and in these animals as in all others the disturbed condition of gait and the co-ordination necessary for flying contrasts forcibly with normal movements but sleepy state produced by removal of the cerebrum.

Removal of the most recently developed neocerebellum or body of the organ results in co-ordination of the voluntary activities of mammals and section of the superior peduncle which connects the organ to the cerebrum has a similar effect. It has also long been known that faulty development of the cerebrum is associated with a similar failure of development of the cerebellum (especially the body) of the opposite side. Removal of the anterior lobe connected with the spinal cord causes an increase of reflexes and of decerebrate rigidity (Sherrington), while stimulation has the opposite effect.

In *man* disease, such as tumour or abscess of the cerebellum, leads to the condition of cerebellar ataxia. This *ataxia* or disorderliness of walking is part of a general disturbance of co-ordination and is specially seen in lesions of the flocculo-nodular lobe, but there is no tremor. There is general weakness (*asthenia*) and loss of tone (*atonia*) of the muscles concerned. The muscles, therefore, feel flabby and the limbs unduly loose and flail-like if moved. The individual is slow and clumsy and cannot bring his movements smoothly to an end. This may be seen if the patient attempts to touch the nose; he not only has difficulty in reaching the nose, but he may strike the nose forcibly, while in attempting to make such an accurate movement the muscles act in co-ordiantely instead of acting smoothly together (*asynergia*). There is also a coarse tremor of the hand and there may be nystagmus of the eyes.

The weakness, if unilateral, tends to render him liable to fall to the *affected side*, since, as we have seen, the cerebellar tracts are uncrossed. The head is commonly rotated to the opposite side.

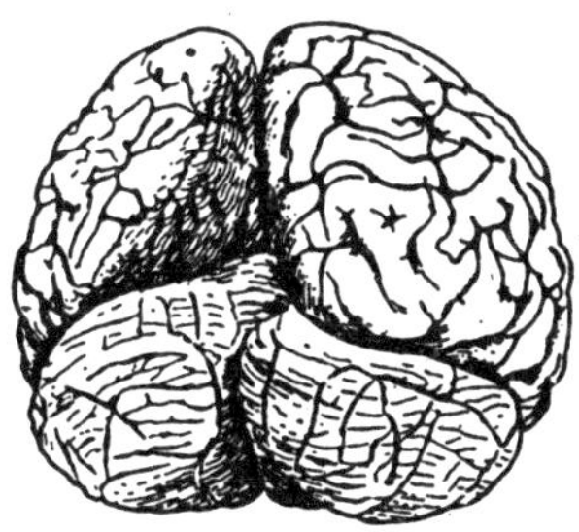

Fig. 9.13. A photograph of a lunatic's brain (Fricke). One cerebral and the opposite cerebellar hemisphere are atrophied.

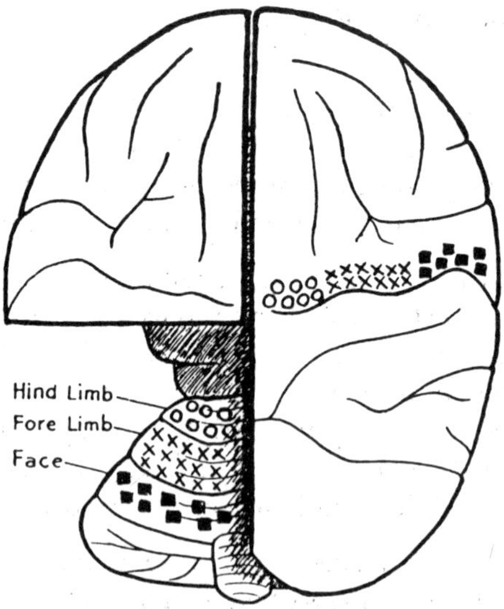

Fig. 9.14. Diagram showing the points of receipt of afferent impulses on the surface of the cerebellum in the monkey and their relation to the cortex.

These facts are no doubt related to the observation that decerebrate rigidity is reduced by stimulation of the superior peduncle, of the anterior lobe or the roof nuclei, while lesions of these regions increase the rigidity, but no localised lesions of this kind have been described in man.

Speech may be similarly affected, being typically staccato in character or laboriously slow. There is also interference with the compensating movement of the eyes, the production of nystagmus and deviation of the eyes. These disturbances result not only from disease of the cerebellum, but also when the paths to and from the organ have been impaired, and may be considered to be due to an asynergy of the muscles concerned. The normal mechanism of the knee-jerk is disturbed. It is less sustained than normally, so that the leg appears to fall limply. The after swing so produced has caused the term pendulum knee-jerk to be given to the response.

Localisation of Function.— Here the method of studying electrical potentials has been of particular value. It has now been shown, especially by Adrian and by Dow, that in the monkey afferent impulses are received on definite areas of the cerebellum, as we have seen occurs in the parietal region of the cerebrum. Pressure on the pad of the foot and its dorsiflexions are particularly efficacious in setting up nerve impulses which can be traced electrically to the cerebellar cortex, bu tactile stimuli and those set up by blowing on the hairs can be similarly traced. The area for the hind limbs is represented anteriorly in the lobus centralis, then the forelimb and the face, especially the vibrissae of the nose region, farther back, the lobus simplex. In each case the pontine fibers are represented more laterally than the fibers from the spinal cord. It would seem that the vermis is concerned with the trunk movements. The bulk of the neocerebellum appears to be of the nature of an association or silent area. As in the case of the motor area of the cerebrum, the afferent area for the forelimb is relatively large.

It has also been possible to relate facts of the cerebrum to the cerebellum. Hampson has picked up potentials in various parts of the cerebellum when sensory areas of the cerebrum are stimulated. For example, impulses pass to the posterior vermis when the auditory area is stimulated.

Recovery from Lesions.— The effects of removal of the cerebellum in animals is, however, not permanent; indeed, dogs in which the cerebellum has been removed recover their normal gait and do not appear otherwise abnormal.

This recovery appears to be the result of other parts of the central nervous system, especially the cerebrum, taking over the functions of the cerebellum, since, if in recovered animals the cerebrum is now removed, the disturbance of gait returns.

These facts emphasise the intimate relationship between the cerebrum and the cerebellum. It seems not unlikely, however, that by greatly facilitating co-ordination movements may become very much easier, and that thereby the cerebrum is relieved of some of its duties. Complicated movements become as a result much more automatic than would otherwise be possible.

Compensating Movement of the Eyes.— Of considerable interest and importance is the movement of the eyes, which takes place automatically when the head is moved, so that they may remain fixed on an object. It may be observed in an animal whose cerebrum has been removed. If the head is moved up, the eyes move down, and *vice versa*. These eye movements depend on impulses from the labyrinth and from the muscles.

Similar movements may be observed in man: for instance, in an individual who attempts to look at passing objects from a rapidly moving train, the eyes appear to jump from one object to another. It would seem that this is a mechanism whereby during movement objects are retained in the retina sufficiently long to be appreciated. By its use if we pass through a station in an express train we see only certain objects distinctly but the rest are a blur. The jump is due to the cerebrum, but the lag behind which permits a series of objects to be focused depends on cerebellar and brain-stem reflexes. The alternation of slow and fast movements of the eyes is known as *nystagmus*. A similar nystagmus, or difficulty in keeping the eyes fixed on an object held at the side of the head, is produced normally by heating or cooling the labyrinth, and is now a test for the efficiency of the latter in suspected disease. We have already remarked the interference with the normal position and movements of the eyes in cerebellar disease.

The Afferent Pathways of the Cerebellum

The cerebellum receives impulses from the spinal cord by way of the direct spino-cerebellar tract (Flechsig) which arises from the cells of Clarke's column within the grey matter of the medial part of the base of the posterior horn. It does not degenerate if the posterior roots are cut. It lies in the dorso-lateral margin of the cord (see fig. 9.12) and passes to the cerebellum by the inferior peduncle.

Arising from Clarke's column also is the *indirect* or *ventral spinocerebellar tract of Gowers*, which reaches the cerebellum by way of the superior peduncle, but some fibers go by the inferior peduncle. It will be observed that the cerebellar tracts do not cross.

The Effect of Injury to the Spinal Cord

The study of paths makes it evident that an injury of, or a tumour pressing on, the spinal cord will affect its motor, sensory and reflex functions. On an accurate study of the changes brought about will depend the power of the surgeon to diagnose the exact position of the lesion and possibly to treat it.

Complete transverse section of the pinal cord may produce immediate death if the operation is performed sufficiently high in the cervical region, for the paralysed muscles will then include those of respiration. The spinal cells from which the phrenic and other respiratory nerves originate are then cut off from the respiratory centre in the bulb above them, and the animal will die of asphyxia. One sees the same thing after severe injury to the upper cervical cord in man, as when he "breaks his neck." It occurs commonly in horses when they fall head first when jumping.

If the injury is sufficiently low down and is not so abrupt that the patient or the animal does not die of shock, a series of typical changes are seen:

1. Loss of motion of the parts supplied by the nerves below the section on both sides of the body.
2. Loss of sensation in the same regions.
3. Hyperaesthesia at the junction of the areas of normal and diminished or lost sensation.
4. There is an initial period of *spinal shock* during which all reflexes are absent, and specially important is loss of control of the urinary bladder which necessitates it being emptied by means of a catheter, a proceeding which is very liable to lead to fatal sepsis of the urinary tract.

In man in about three weeks there may be a considerable recovery of the reflexes, the typical flexor tone and exaggerated spinal reflexes, i.e., flexor withdrawal, appear. Reflex control of the bladder may return although voluntary control is permanently lost. Defaecation also takes place regularly.

5. There is loss of sympathetic control of the blood-vessels and viscera, resulting in generalised vasodilatation and a fall of blood-pressure, but these become re-established later. In animals an exaggerated peristalsis may be seen.
6. Degeneration, ascending and descending, on both sides of the cord.

Hemisection.— If the operation performed is not a complete cutting of the spinal cord transversely, but a cutting across of half the cord, it is termed hemisection. This leads to:

1. Loss of voluntary control of the muscles of the same side below the level of the section.

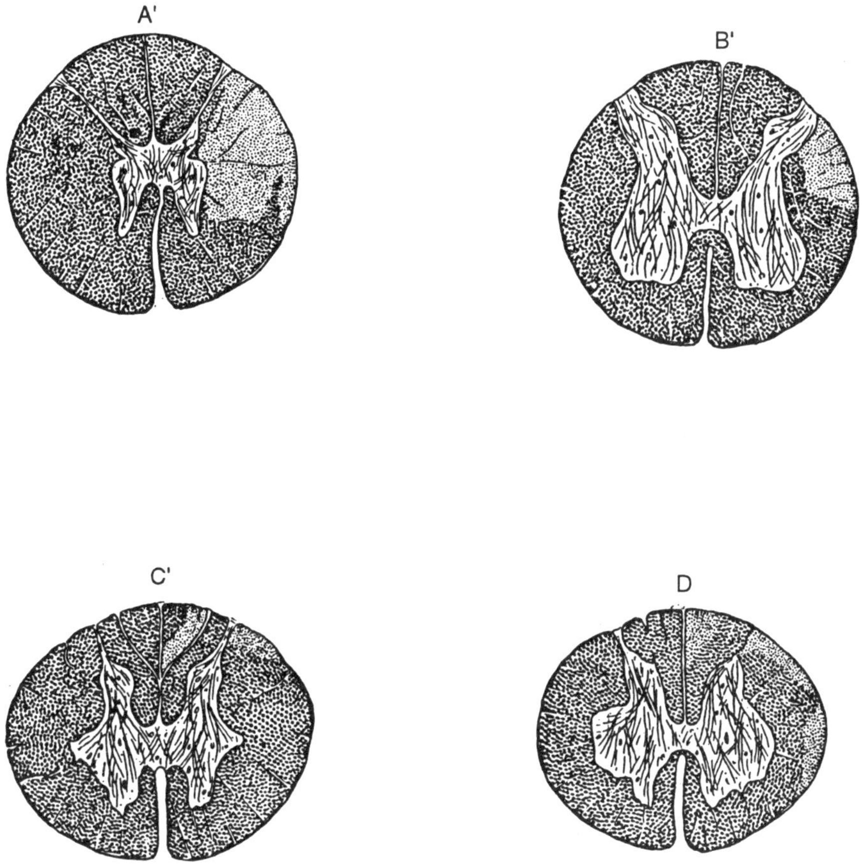

Fig. 9.15. The above diagrams are reproductions of photo-micrographs from the spinal cord of a monkey, in which the operation of left hemisection had been performed some weeks previously (Mott). The sections were stained by Weigert's method, by which the grey matter is bleached, while the healthy white matter remains dark blue. The degenerated tracts are also bleached. A is a section of the cord in the thoracic region below the lesion; the crossed pyramidal tract is degenerated. B is a section lower down (in the lumbar enlargement); the degenerated pyramidal tract is now smaller. C is a section in the thoracic region some little distance above the lesion. The degenerated tracts seen are in the outer part of Goll's column, and the direct cerebellar tract. D is a section higher up in the cervical region; the degeneration in Goll's column now occupies a median position; the degenerations in the cerebellar tracts are also well shown. Notice that in all cases the main degenerated tracts are on the same side as the injury.

2. Loss of sensation below the divided segment, approximately as follows: (a) Loss of joint and muscle sense, of sense of vibration, and of tactile discrimination, on the *same* side as the section; (b) Loss of the sense of pain, heat, and cold on the side *opposite* to the section. The reason for this peculiar distribution of sensory loss is the presence of an inferior and a superior sensory

decussation; the former occurs within the cord as the decussation of the spino-thalamic fibers, the latter in the medulla as the decussation of the fillet.

In man these changes constitute the crossed paralyses of Brown-Séquard, who first described them.

3. Unilateral vasodilatation below the lesion and hyperaesthesia of the nearest healthy skin area above is also seen.
4. The tendon reflexes are at first absent, but subsequently become exaggerated on the same side as the lesion as a result of the loss of the higher inhibition carried by the rubrospinal and pyramidal tracts.
5. Degeneration, ascending and descending, largely confined to the same side of the cord as the injury. The most important of these are shown in the preceding diagrams, the small text beneath which should be carefully studied.

The Functions of the Hypothalamic Region

This region of the brain which lies just below the thalamus and above the mid brain, and adjacent to the floor of the third ventricle plays an important part in the elemental reactions of the body.

1. *Sex.*— It is suggested that the hypothalamus controls the action of the pituitary in regard to sex, but the evidence on the point is not convincing.
2. *Emotion.*— Particularly it is concerned with the reactions to emotion, which are only different from reflexes in that they are more complicated.

It has also been observed by Bard that removal of the frontal cortex by section of the fronto-hypothalamic tracts results in a remarkable condition of rage being produced, e.g., snarling, clawing, lashing of the tail, erection of the hairs, a rise of blood-pressure and heart-rate, and dilatation of the pupil such as might be produced by the injection of adrenaline. When the hypothalamus is removed these symptoms disappear. It is possible to place electrodes in the hypothalamus of an otherwise intact animal, and when the animal has recovered from the anaesthetic to stimulate the region. This also produces the state of rage.

The connections between the hypothalamus and the frontal lobe appear to be somehow concerned in the production of pathological mental depression in man, and patients suffering from this state cheer up when they are cut. Very rarely a liability to anger is observed after the operation.

Normally, like the postural reflexes, the emotions are more or less inhibited by the mediation of higher centres, and it is easy to see how anaesthetics like alcohol may, by paralysing the higher control centres, lead to loss of control of these lower activities. The liability of a partly drunk man to lose such control is well recognised.

3. *Body Temperature.*— There is no doubt also that the hypothalamus is concerned with the control of body temperature, which control is lost if this region is

removed. The region specially concerned appears to be that of the tuber cinereum; damage to it may result in high body temperature. As might be expected, there are secondary changes in metabolic rate, sweating, and in water loss from the body.

4. *Sleep.*— This has already been discussed.

5. *Diuresis.*— Damage to the hypothalamic region is associated clinically with diabetes insipidus, with emaciation, and with Fröhlich's syndrome (see Pituitary).

6. Electrical stimulation of the posterior and lateral nuclei produces sympathetic effects like cardiac acceleration and inhibition of the gut, while stimulation of the mid-line nuclei causes opposite effects. Some have supposed that this indicates that the hypothalamus has some special relation to the autonomic nervous system, but many of these effects can equally well be produced by stimulation of the cerebral cortex (Fulton).

The Function of the Basal Ganglia

The difficulty of removing the basal ganglia such as the caudate or lenticular nuclei, which are large masses of grey matter, has made it difficult to obtain information regarding their function. Evidence has, however, accumulated to indicate that disease of the lenticular nucleus produces motor disturbance of the face resembling laughter, increased reflexes and muscle tone, and in the condition of paralysis agitans or shaking palsy, which is characterised by great tremor of the hands or head, degeneration of the corpus striatum has been found postmortem. It would seem, then, that the region of the basal ganglia probably controls some of the primitive movements.

The evidence is very complete that the basal ganglia receive fibers and presumably impulses from the area in front of the motor area, especially an area in front of the arm area.

It has now become apparent that the basal ganglia are not "silent" as previously imagined, but have an important function in the cerebral cortex. They are also connected to the red nucleus and substantia nigra.

10

Disorders

Clinical Correlates

Derangement of neural functions can range from abnormal neuromuscular transmission to defects in "higher" cortical functions including learning, memory, and affective behavior. Sensory and/or motor defects encompass an entire gamut that extends from mild and transient, through incapacitating and chronic, to rapidly lethal.

From a clinical standpoint, the definition (or diagnosis) of the specific problem at hand is fundamental to the rational therapy or management of any disease entity, and this fact is exemplified with great clarity by many of the nervous disorders which produce specific *symptom complexes*, or *syndromes*. In turn, fundamental neuroanatomic and neurophysiologic considerations are critical to such an evaluation. The classification of neural (and other) disorders according to their etiology not only affords one basis for the diagnosis and subsequent treatment of the individual patient, but also can yield an occasional insight toward the better understanding of the normal functions of particular structures or regions of the nervous system. Thus pathophysiologic events may have their primary origin in congenital, vascular, traumatic, infectious, neoplastic, metabolic, toxic, degenerative, and idiopathic as well as iatrogenic factors. The principal causative agent (or agents) just listed may, in turn, induce one or more secondary adaptive or maladaptive physiologic responses.

The specific topics that were selected for discussion in the remainder of this chapter will serve to illustrate the several points which were brought out in this introduction, as well as to review certain aspects of neuroanatomy and neurophysiology which were presented earlier. The first four principal subdivisions of this section deal with some general as well as specific dysfunctions that involve peripheral nerves, spinal cord, brain stem, and cerebellum. The remainder of this section will be concerned with discussions of a number of particular clinical situations, primarily from the standpoint of the pathophysiology involved.

Lesions and Regeneration of Peripheral Nerves

When a mixed peripheral nerve is severely injured or severed, a complete loss of all modalities of sensation, including proprioception, as well as paralysis of the skeletal muscles that are innervated by that nerve, take place distal to the lesion. The affected muscles are completely flaccid, absolutely no reflex activity can be evoked from the denervated region, and eventually total atrophy of the muscles develops. A comprehensive knowledge of the gross anatomy underlying the ramifications and distribution of peripheral nerves is essential to the accurate diagnosis of lesions in specific nerves.

It is important to realize, however, that not all paralytic conditions are total so that some innervation may remain and the muscle may be weakened but not completely paralyzed, the reflexes can be decreased but not eliminated entirely, and only subtotal atrophy develops. For example, *multiple neuritis* involves an inflammation or partial destruction of peripheral nerves, the lesions may be widespread, and occur on both sides of the body, being most evident in the distal regions of the extremities. Clinically, multiple neuritis is characterized with diffuse, poorly circumscribed cutaneous regions which exhibit marked sensory changes. On the other hand, the neuritis may be localized (mononeuritis) so that it affects only one nerve trunk or a small group of nerves.

Etiologic factors that underlie these neuropathies include chronic intoxication (alcohol, benzene, sulfonamides, carbon disulfide); specific infections (syphilis, meningitis, diphtheria, pneumonia, mumps, tuberculosis); metabolic causes (gout, diabetes mellitus, pregnancy, rheumatism); and nutritional factors (vitamin deficiencies, beriberi, cachectic states).

Following section of a motor nerve to a skeletal muscle, as the nerve degenerates the muscle becomes exceedingly sensitive to the pharmacologic effects of acetylcholine, a phenomenon called *denervation hypersensitivity*. In contrast to skeletal muscle, smooth muscle does not undergo atrophy following denervation but it too develops an acute sensitivity to the chemical transmitter that normally stimulated it while innervated.

When any nerve fiber is cut in two or otherwise damaged irreversibly, the portion of the fiber that has been detached from the soma degenerates, and as this process takes place the fiber loses its myelin sheath. In addition to causing irreversible damage to the part of the fiber distal to the cut, severing the axon from the nerve cell body exerts a deleterious effect upon the nerve cell body per se. Thus the Nissl bodies undergo *chromatolysis* during the several weeks following the injury. During this process, the cytoplasmic ribonucleic acid granules lose their normal staining properties so that they appear to "dissolve" in the cytoplasm. Some of the neurons die and degenerate following chromatolysis, however others recover as RNA synthesis is restored. This *retrograde degeneration* that may accompany chromatolysis provides an important experimental technique for determining the cells from which specific fibers originate in the central nervous system. Thus serial sections made several weeks after placing a discrete lesion can be stained for Nissl substance, and the specific regions which show chromatolysis are indicative of the loci which contain the nerve cell bodies of the damaged fibers.

Following the complete section of a peripheral nerve, the fibers central to the cut send branches outward. These branches are outgrowths from the axon near its cut tip, and as many as 50 may develop from a single axon. Concomitantly the neurilemmal cells of Schwann at the proximal end of the severed nerve proliferate rapidly and migrates so as to bridge the gap between the cut ends of the nerve. The neurofibrils within the proximal end of the nerve divide longitudinally and commence to sprout from the end of the nerve. Some of these regenerating axon tips successfully cross the gap between the severed ends of the nerve and each may enter one ultramicroscopic neurilemmal tubule leading to the peripheral terminals of the nerve, the growth rate ranging between one and four millimeters per day. The entrance of a single regenerating axon into a neurilemmal microtubule that is connected to a sensory or motor terminal apparently is governed strictly by chance, the tubules being empty because of degeneration of the axon. Thus if the severed endings of a peripheral nerve are carefully apposed and sutured, function sometimes can be restored. If, however, the gap between the severed nerve endings is about 3 millimeters wide, the fibers growing outward from the central stump tend to form a dense meshwork which results in a bulbous swelling at the tip of the proximal end of the cut nerve called a *neuroma*. Once this has taken place, functional regeneration is unlikely to occur. Furthermore, if sensory fibers are present in the neuroma, it can be exquisitely sensitive to pressure. Hence, neuroma formation can be a serious complication following limb amputation.

Fibers of the spinal cord and brain do not regenerate to any significant extent following their destruction.

Lesions of the Spinal Cord

Dorsal Columns and Posterior Roots. Tabes dorsalis, a type of neurosyphilis, will serve as an example of a disease which causes bilateral lesions in the dorsal roots of the cord as well as in the posterior funiculi. As might be anticipated from the area of the cord that is affected preferentially, *paresthesias* (abnormal or perverted sensations), including shooting and burning pains, pricking sensations, and formication may be present. The loss of the proprioceptive pathways in the dorsal roots and posterior columns of the cord results in a pronounced failure of muscular coordination or *ataxia*. Consequently, the patient walks with his legs apart, the head is inclined toward the ground, and the eyes are fixed in the same direction. The legs are thrown abnormally high and the feet are slapped down. Vision is essential to maintenance of posture, and the pattern of *locomotor ataxia* that develops in tabes victims is reminiscent of that seen in chronic alcoholics.

The paresthesias and bouts of severe pain that accompany the early stages of tabes dorsalis are caused by irritation of the dorsal roots and posterior columns. As degeneration of the cord continues, a diminished pain sensitivity develops, especially in the testicles and Achilles' tendons (the latter symptom, known as *Abadie's sign*, is presumptive evidence for tabes). The ankle jerk and patellar reflex disappear, whereas the vibratory sense diminishes as the disease progresses. The Romberg sign is positive; that is, the body sways uncontrollably or the patient falls down when standing with the feet close together and the eyes closed.

Anterior Columns. Acute poliomyelitis (Heine-Medin disease or infantile paralysis) is produced by a virus which preferentially destroys the nerve cell bodies of the anterior columns of the spinal cord, particularly in the cervical and lumbar enlargements of this structure. The specific muscles that are paralyzed depend upon the precise distribution of the motoneurons which are damaged irreversibly, and the affected muscles are flaccid whereas their reflexes generally are absent. Several weeks after the infected motoneurons have been destroyed, muscular atrophy develops. This effect may be extensive so that eventually the muscular tissue may be replaced entirely by connective and adipose tissue, and severe physical deformities develop.

Central Gray Matter. Syringomyelia is a condition of unknown origin (i.e., it is idiopathic) in which softening and cavitation take place around the central canal of the spinal cord and brain stem. The affected area of the cord is surrounded by an area of gliosis (i.e., the glial cells exhibit an enormous proliferation, particularly the astrocytes).

Clinically syringomyelia is characterized by muscular atrophy, weakness, assorted sensory defects, evidence of injury to the long tracts, and trophic abnormalities.

Commonly the lesion is found in the cervical enlargement of the spinal cord such that the fibers of the lateral spinothalamic tracts are interrupted as they decussate just ventral to the central canal. Consequently, and as the lateral spinothalamic tracts transmit signals related to pain and thermal sensations from dermatomes that are located bilaterally, the results of syringomyelia can include a loss of pain and thermal sensibility having a segmental distribution in the upper extremities on both sides of the body. However, the spinothalamic tracts from the lower regions of the body are unaffected, therefore no such impairment is present in the lower extremities. Muscular weakness as well as alterations due to involvement of the sympathetic fibers that are located centrally in the cord characteristically accompany syringomyelia.

When the lesion is unilateral, thermal sensations are lost and analgesia develops in the skin that is innervated by, and on the ipsilateral side of, the diseased segments of the cord themselves. The sensations of touch and proprioception are unaffected until later in the progress of the disease. Such a condition, in which one modality of cutaneous sensation is lost whereas others are preserved, at least temporarily, is called sensory dissociation.

If the disease process extends into the medulla oblongata (*syringobulbia*) then signs that the nuclei of the cranial nerves are affected may appear, and when the spinal nucleus of the trigeminal nerve is involved, a characteristic loss of sensation develops over the facial region. The skeletal muscles which are supplied by the ventral column cells of diseased segments become atrophic and functionally weak, such effects frequently being manifest first in the small muscles of the hand.

If the white matter is not involved in the disease process, then the sensory and motor defects produced by syringomyelia are localized and distributed segmentally. On the other hand, if the descending motor pathways are involved in the disease process, a spastic paralysis will develop caudally to the lesion, whereas pressure exerted upon the dorsal columns and spinothalamic tracts will result in a loss of sensation caudal to the lesion. Consequently the actual extent of the sensory loss, its type, distribution, and bilateral representation will vary from patient to patient depending upon the extent to which particular tracts are involved in the disease process.

Since thermal and pain sensations are absent in some areas, the patient with syringomyelia readily can suffer local minor injuries (such as a cut or burn) which go unperceived and thus may develop into serious disorders.

Since the sympathetic nervous centers in the lateral columns of the cord may be involved in the lesion produced by syringomyelia, vasomotor mal-functions and heavy sweating (or no sweating at all) may result. The abnormalities of vasomotor function in turn can lead to trophic disturbances in the periphery due to circulatory inadequacy, including gangrene and ulcers.

Anterior Horns and Pyramidal Tracts. Amyotrophic lateral sclerosis is a fatal condition of unknown etiology which typically involves degeneration of the motoneurons in the anterior gray columns of the spinal cord in addition to bilateral destruction of the pyramidal tracts. Sensory alterations generally do not accompany this disease. Some muscles exhibit weakness and atrophy, whereas others are spastic and hyperreflexic, the specific pattern of neuromuscular defects noted in any particular patient being a reflection of the specific pattern of neural damage in the spinal cord. In its classic form, amyotrophic lateral sclerosis first is manifest by skeletal muscle weakness, atrophy, and fasciculation of the muscles of the hands and arms. Subsequently, spastic paralysis of the legs develop, and the motor nuclei of the cranial nerves may deteriorate as well.

Posterior and Lateral Funiculi. Subacute combined degeneration of the spinal cord involves the white matter of this structure, and practically always is associated with pernicious anemia although it may be related occasionally to other types of anemia or nutritional disturbances. The disease process involves a degeneration of the myelin sheaths of the posterior funiculi and the pyramidal tracts of the cord, although the gray matter usually is not affected. Subsequent to demyelination, the axons are destroyed and the neural elements are replaced ultimately by glial tissue. These pathologic changes are seen most commonly in the pyramidal (corticospinal) and cerebellar tracts as well as in the dorsal columns.

From a clinical standpoint, the major features of subacute combined degeneration of the cord are muscular weakness and spasticity; a deranged sense of position as well as of passive movement of the limbs, defects which in turn underlie ataxia and a positive Romberg's sign; the ability to perceive vibration, as well as the ability to carry out spatial discriminations are lost or impaired to varying degrees.

The paresthesias seen in this condition may include tingling, pricking, and burning sensations which often appear prior to the loss of particular sensory capacities and frequently are related to a peripheral neuropathy that is associated with the primary disease process. Frequently the tendon reflexes are abnormally active since descending motor pathways are involved, but such responses may be lost completely as the disease progresses, provided that the peripheral neuropathy becomes exacerbated sufficiently. A positive Babinski sign (or reflex) is seen bilaterally, when the outer margin of the sole of the foot is stroked from the heel toward the little toe. Normally, such a maneuver elicits flexion of all toes in an adult. However, if the corticospinal fibers are interrupted at any point along their course between the upper region of the precentral gyrus and the muscles of the big toe, the latter structure will dorsiflex, whereas the other toes may (or may not) fan out laterally.

There is no consistent parallel between the extent of the nervous defects exhibited by the patient with subacute combined degeneration of the cord and the degree of anemia that is present. Furthermore, the degeneration is not caused by the anemia per se, despite the fact that the two diseases are associated. This is demonstrated clearly by the clinical observation that the neurologic deterioration proceeds unabated despite correction of the anemia by administration of folic acid. Conversely, progress of the neurologic degeneration can be arrested by the administration of cyanocobalamin (vitamin B_{12}).

Transection of the Spinal Cord. A sudden and total disruption of the integrity of the spinal cord at one level can result either from a traumatic cause (e.g., a stab or gunshot wound or a fracture and spinal dislocation) or from the operation of an acute inflammatory process (e.g., transverse myelitis). In either event, the cord is transected functionally so that an immediately and total loss of all voluntary control over the skeletal muscles caudal to the lesion ensues together with a complete loss of all sensation in the same region of the body.

The term *paraplegia* is applied to the total paralysis of both lower extremities resulting from any lesion of the spinal cord, whereas if the cord is severed completely in the lower cervical region all four extremities are paralyzed, a condition known as quadriplegia. If, on the other hand, the cord is transected in the upper cervical region, death rapidlly ensues as the diaphragm and other respiratory muscles no longer are controlled by impulses from the respiratory center.

The condition of spinal shock which develops immediately following complete interruption of the spinal cord, as well as the progressive return of certain reflexes after cord transection.

Hemisection of the Spinal Cord. When the spinal cord is hemisected laterally, as by a "clean" knife or bullet wound, a condition known as the *Brown-Sequard syndrome* develops. The functional defects seen in this syndrome as well as the damaged structures responsible for causing them can be summarized as follows:

Injury to the fiber tracts that are located in the *same side of the cord* as the lesion produces an ipsilateral motor paralysis (*hemiplegia*) below the lesion, because of pyramidal tract injury. Hence damage to this tract results in the clinical signs of spasticity, some hyperreflexia, loss of superficial reflexes, and the development of a positive Babinski sign.

Concomitantly, damage to the posterior funiculus on the same side of the cord as the injury result in a loss of proprioceptive ability and a loss of the ability to perceive vibrations, as well as a loss of the capacity to perform tactile (touch) discriminations; all of these defects are apparent caudal to the injury on the same side of the body as the lesion. Ataxia cannot be demonstrated clearly because of the muscular paralysis.

Injury to the fiber tracts which are located on the *opposite side of the cord* from the lesion results in a loss of thermal and pain sensations on the contralateral side of the body because of damage to the dorsal (anterolateral) spinothalamic tract. This defect is seen to commence one or two segments below the lesion, because of the fact that the fibers of this tract ascend in the same side of the cord for a segment or two before undergoing decussation to the opposite side.

Damage to the ventral (anterior) spinothalamic tract causes only a slight alteration (or no change whatsoever) in the sense of simple touch.

Only rarely is a lesion located so precisely within the cord as to produce all of the classic signs of the Brown-Sequard syndrome described above. More frequently, the lesions encountered in clinical practice are limited to one portion of the cord, and thus produce an incomplete Brown-Sequard syndrome whose specific signs and symptoms reflect the exact location and extent of the lesion in the patient under examination.

Local Injury to Specific Cord Segments and Nerve Roots. In addition to the clinical states which are caused by destroying signal transmission in the long ascending and descending tracts of the cord, other clinical symptoms can result from injury to specific dorsal and ventral roots at the same level as the lesion. Such symptoms, when present, are of assistance to the physician in localizing the particular segments of the spinal cord that are involved in the case under evaluation.

Thus excitation of fibers in the dorsal root area on the same side of the lesion can induce paresthesias or radicular pain which is localized over the particular segments (or dermatomes) that are innervated by the specific nerve whose root is affected. Similarly, total destruction of dorsal root causes anesthesia over the specific dermatome that is supplied by the affected dorsal root. Conversely, destruction of a specific ventral root causes flaccid paralysis of only the specific skeletal muscles whose innervation is affected, and the sensory innervation of that area is unaffected.

Thrombosis. The anterior spinal artery courses in the ventral median sulcus, and terminal branches of this vessel supply the ventral columns, the dorsal spinothalamic tracts, and the corticospinal (pyramidal) tracts. The posterior columns and dorsal funiculi of the cord receive their blood supply from a pair of dorsal spinal arteries which are independent of the anterior spinal artery. The effects of a clot or thrombosis therefore depend upon which vessel, hence which region of the cord, is affected primarily. For example, a clot, or thrombus, which forms in the anterior spinal artery in the cervical region causes flaccid paralysis, fibrillation, and eventually atrophy of the muscles that are innervated by the motoneurons whose cell bodies are located at the level of the cord where the lesion is located, and which are killed and degenerate following the thrombosis. Pyramidal tract involvement results in violent, involuntary, and sudden bilateral muscular contractions below the level of the thrombus, and this *spastic paraplegia* can be exceedingly painful. Concomitant damage to the dorsal spinothalamic tracts sometimes may result in a loss of thermal as well as painful sensations below the lesion. The onset of the symptoms caused by thrombosis of the anterior spinal artery not only is sudden, but also may be accompanied by severe pain.

Tumors Located Within the Spinal Cord. Neoplasms are classified depending upon their location within the spinal canal. Thus extradural tumors are located outside of the dura mater whereas intradural tumors are located within the dura mater. In turn, intradural neoplasms are located either outside of the spinal cord (extramedullary tumors) or within the spinal cord (intramedullary tumors). There is a definite correlation between the location of a tumor within the spinal canal and its pathologic nature. For example, an extramedullary tumor usually is benign, but can progressively exert pressure on the cord as it enlarges. Generally the nerve roots are compressed first at the tumor grows, and this mechanical factor is responsible for the pain that is manifest over the dermatomes which are innervated by affected roots. Subsequently, and as the tracts within the cord become involved, a complete or partial Brown-Sequard syndrome is exhibited.

The temporal sequence in which particular symptoms appear often can provide an indication as to where the tumor is located. Thus a loss of thermal and pain sensations on the right side of the body followed by spastic paralysis on the left side suggests that the neoplasm has originated around the ventrolateral portion of the cord on the left side. Similarly, a loss of the normal proprioceptive sense on the right side with a subsequent development of spastic paralysis on the left side implies that the tumor is exerting pressure on the dorsomedial portion of the spinal cord on the left side.

Specific neurologic symptoms that may develop subsequent to compression of the spinal cord include sensory loss, disturbances in the operation of the bladder and rectal sphincters, and paresthesias that become exacerbated during physical exercise, coughing, or straining. Localized skeletal motor weakness, paralysis, and muscular atrophy can occur if the ventral (motor) roots or columns of the cord are affected by the tumor.

Nerve fibers can be damaged to various degrees, so that in some instances pressure that is exerted on a nerve or tract may inhibit transmission of impulses, but not cause irreversible destruction of the fibers. Thus the pressure exerted by tumors, blood clots, the edema and swelling caused by traumatic injuries, and/or by displaced intervertebral discs all may produce symptoms that are indicative of spinal cord dysfunction, and yet may prove to be completely reversible following appropriate therapy. The ultimate prognosis, of course, depends upon the extent or severity of the compression as well as the length of time the abnormal pressure has been exerted upon the neural elements themselves, and the same factors obtain regardless of whether one is dealing with the spinal cord or the brain per se.

Lesions of the Brain Stem

The complex structures of the brain stem are located in such a relatively small volume of neural tissue that a restricted lesion generally affects a number of these structures; consequently a bewildering array of clinical signs can result. Hence the correct interpretation of these signs rests on a clear understanding of the neuroanatomy and neurophysiology of the nuclei and fiber tracts. Only three of the many possible syndromes which can result from lesions in specific areas of the brain stem will be described. However, these symptom complexes will serve to illustrate the potential effects of thrombosis, hemorrhage, tumor development, or degeneration in particular areas of this part of the central nervous system.

Basal Portion of Medulla. A number of cranial nerves run near the lateral aspect of the pyramidal tract before they exit from the brain stem. A lesion which includes the nerve as well as the pyramidal tract at one point causes paralysis of the nerve on the same side as the lesion and hemiplegia on the opposite side. For example, a lesion that involves the left pyramid as well as the left hypoglossal nerve produces a right hemiplegia together with a motor paralysis of the muscles in the left half of the tongue. Paralysis of the arm and leg is on the contralateral side to the lesion because the pyramidal tract undergoes decussation to the right side caudal to the site of the lesion. Symptoms of spasticity, including increased tonus of the skeletal muscles, hyper-reflexia, pathologic reflexes, and loss of superficial reflexes, are present. The tongue deviates to the left when it is protruded from the mouth, because of the paralysis of the muscles on the left side of this structure, and eventually these paralyzed muscles will undergo total atrophy.

Another important sign of hyperreflexia that frequently is associated with spastic states in general is clonus, and this neurologic sign may be present when a lesion develops in the basal medullary region (as well as in other parts of the central nervous system). Clonus is manifest when the normal (or physiologic) asynchrony of discharge from the motoneurons involved in a stretch reflex is lost, and thereby a series of jerky, irregular contractions take place in a repetitive manner, and these contractions may be superimposed upon a single tonic contraction. Thus in a hyperreflexive patient, clonus may be initiated by applying a sustained stretch to a muscle, and then tapping on the tendon of that muscle. The tendon reflex which results from this stimulus is followed by a series of irregular twitches which continue for a prolonged interval, provided that the muscle is maintained in the stretched condition.

Clonus is explained by the fact that the stretch receptors are arranged in parallel within the muscle spindle so that a sharp rap on the tendon initiates a synchronous volley of afferent impulses which in turn suddenly discharge the alpha motoneurons to the muscle, also in a synchronous manner. The sudden jerk like contraction which develops then release the spindles from the tension caused by the maintained stretch, therefore they stop firing and the afferent stimulus to the motoneurons is terminated. As a consequence, the muscle now undergoes relaxation so that the spindles once again are placed under tension which leads to the initiation of another synchronous afferent signal discharge which again fires the alpha motoneurons, and the cycle is repeated.

Clonus that persists for any length of time always is symptomatic of hyperreflexia, which in turn indicates damage to the central nervous system, although normal individuals sometimes may exhibit small clonic oscillations of relatively short duration. In normal individuals, of course, gamma efferent discharge to the spindles is modulated by inhibitory (as well as facilitory) impulses from higher neural centers which automatically and continually regulate the net spindle sensitivity. But when lesions are present in higher motor pathways, then the normal balance between excitatory and inhibitory impulses that impinge upon the neurons of the gamma efferent pathway to the spindles is altered in favor of excitation, so that the spindles (and the myotatic

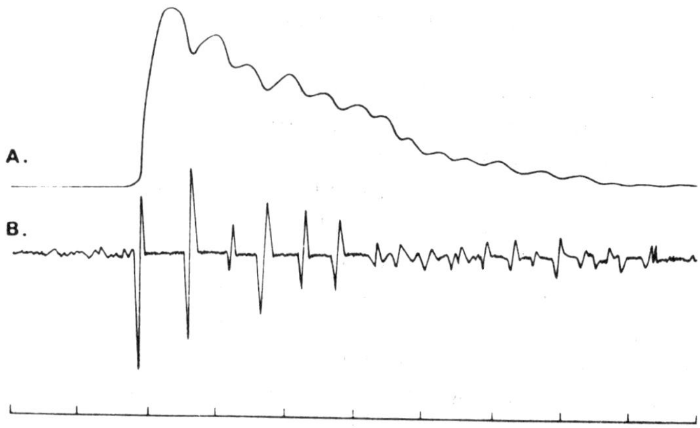

Fig. 10.1. Clonus. A. Mechanical record of contractions. B. Electric record from same muscle (quadriceps). A slight prior stretch of the muscle evoked a tonic reflex discharge of impulses to the muscle as shown by the asynchronous waves to the left in B. Subsequently a tap applied to the tendon of the muscle elicited a sudden sharp contraction (sudden rise in curve A), followed by a characteristic clonic response as indicated in both the mechanical and electric records.

reflexes these structures subserve) become hyperexcitable and the stage is set for clonus to be manifest when an appropriate stimulus is applied.

Ankle clonus affords a specific example of this type of response. This clonic reflex can be evoked in a suitable patient by a sudden, sharp dorsiflexion of the foot, stretch of the gastrocnemius muscle being maintained by placing the hand upon the sole, the opposite hand being held in the popliteal space to support the leg. A rapid, sustained, and repetitive plantar flexion and extension at the ankle indicates a positive response.

In conclusion, it must be stressed that a clonic response is a *neurologic sign* of a lesion that is located somewhere in the motor pathway of the central nervous system, and that it is not a sign of any specific disease.

Upper Portion of Medulla. The presence of a small discrete lesion in the lateral reticular formation of the upper medulla may affect simultaneously the dorsal spinothalamic tract as well as the nucleus ambiguus. If the lesion is present, for example, on the left side, there is a loss of thermal and pain sensations on the right side of the body with the exception of the facial region. These sensory defects occur on the contralateral side of the body because the fibers of the dorsal spinothalamic tract undergo decussation near the point of origin. When the left nucleus ambiguus is destroyed, the voluntary muscles that are innervated by the left glossopharyngeal and vagus nerves are paralyzed. The left side of the soft palate is unable to contract so that difficulty in swallowing becomes apparent. Furthermore, when the patient attempts to speak, the uvula and palate are pulled toward the normally innervated right side of the pharynx, and loss of function of the left vocal cord causes the voice to become hoarse during phonation.

When a lesion of somewhat greater size is present in the same region of the left upper medulla, the tractus solitarius as well as the medial lemniscus may be affected. Thus in addition to the defects noted above, destruction of the solitary tract causes anesthesia of the pharyngeal mucosa on the left side of the oral cavity as well as a concomitant loss of the sensation of taste on the left side of the tongue. Functional interruption of the fibers of the medial lemniscus produces a loss of the proprioceptive and tactile discriminative senses on the right side of the body, in addition to anesthesia for temperature and pain senses on the same side of the body which were incurred following development of a smaller lesion.

Pontocerebellar Angle. When a neoplasm develops from the Schwann cells that form the sheath of the vestibulocochlear nerve as this structure exits from the brain stem, the lateral portion of the caudal region of the pons gradually becomes compressed adjacent to the pontocerebellar angle. The symptoms, which include deafness, a deficiency of normal labyrinthine responses, and occasionally horizontal nystagmus, are progressive and resemble those which follow damage to the vestibulocochlear nerve per se (see also Meniere's syndrome). Subsequently the cerebellar peduncles undergo compression as the tumor enlarges so that cerebellar asynergia (or dyssynergia) becomes evident on the ipsilateral side of the body to the lesion (see next section). Injury to the spinal tracts as well as to the trigeminal nucleus eliminates the corneal reflex and produces a reduced thermal and pain sensibility of the facial region on the same side as the lesion. When fibers of the facial nerve (VII) also are involved a peripheral facial paralysis is also present on the homolateral side of the body as the lesion.

Lesions of the Cerebellum

Characteristically, lesions of the cerebellum or of its pathways are distinguished by *asynergies* (*asynergias, dyssnergias*), that is, a failure in the normal, smoothly coordinated and integrated action among groups of muscles. The general neuroanatomic centers which underlie the regulation of synergistic contractions at the cerebellar level may be summarized briefly. The cerebellar vermis controls the contractions of the bilaterally innervated muscle of the head, neck, and trunk. The left and right cerebellar hemispheres regulate antagonistic (i.e., flexor and extensor) contractions on the same (or homolateral) side of the body. This fact is in marked contrast to the cerebral hemispheres, which are concerned with functions located on the contralateral side of the body. At the spinal cord level the neural centers are essential to the normal bilateral control of muscular activities in the extremities, e.g., walking. The physiologic mechanism which ultimately is responsible for all forms of synergy regardless of the neural center involved is, of course, reciprocal innervation of antagonistic muscles.

The cerebellum is no different from any other organ or structure in that it is susceptible to hereditary (or congenital) defects, as well as to neoplastic, traumatic, inflammatory, vascular, toxic, degenerative, functional, and metabolic derangement. The signs and symptoms of cerebellar dysfunction, as well as of the afferent and efferent pathways to and from this structure, are similar regardless of the etiologic factor (or factors) involved. Furthermore, all of the signs related to cerebellar disorders involve motor functions.

Several types of *ataxia*, or failure of normal muscular coordination, characteristically are associated with cerebellar disease.

First, ataxic disturbances of *gait* and *posture* may be marked. Thus damage to the midline portion of the cerebellum causes difficulty in maintaining a standing, or upright, posture. The loss of equilibrium that is present is caused by a defect in the synergistic action of the muscles and not by a functional defect in the pathway that mediates conscious proprioception. Closing the eyes does not exacerbate this form of ataxia, and the gait is staggering and may resemble that seen in acute alcoholic intoxication. If the lesion is localized in one cerebellar hemisphere, there is a tendency of the body to fall toward the same side as that in which the lesion is located, and if the victim attempts to walk a straight line with the eyes closed, he may swerve or reel erratically toward the side of the damaged hemisphere. Vertigo (dizziness), unsteadiness, and irregularity of movements thus are typical signs of cerebellar ataxia. While walking, the legs are held wide apart, appear loose, and the limb taking the forward step starts to move gradually; but suddenly it is thrown forward erratically and the step ends with the foot thrust to the floor in a stamping movement.

Second, ataxia due to cerebellar damage can be manifest as *decomposition of movement*, sometimes called the "by-the-numbers" phenomenon. That is, a physical action which requires the smoothly coordinated movement of several joints becomes uncoordinated so that the movement takes place in several discrete phases rather than as a smooth continuum. For example, in bringing a hand with food to the mouth, the joints of the wrist, elbow, and shoulder may be moved individually in a jerky fashion rather than as a single, smooth, and synchronized movement. A coarse *intention tremor* may be induced by the movement, and this tremor will disappear once the movement is completed (see also below).

Third, cerebellar damage can result in *dysmetria*. The patient is unable to estimate the range of voluntary movement, so that when reaching a hand toward an object the hand either stops before the object is reached or else it overshoots the goal. For example, when the patient is requested to point a finger directly at one of the examining physician's finger he may point consistently to one side, a phenomenon that is called past-pointing. Similarly the subject may touch his cheek with a finger when asked to touch his nose.

Fourth, *adiadochokinesia* (*or dysdiadochokinesia*) is an inability to stop one movement and immediately start another movement in the opposite directions; i.e., to perform rapidly alternating movements. For example rapid pronation and supination of the hands, tapping of the fingers, or flexion and extension of a hand cannot be carried out by a patient who exhibits this manifestation of cerebellar ataxia.

Fifth, *scanning speech* is caused by asynergy of the muscles used in phonation. The spacing of the sounds is irregular, and pauses, as for punctuation, syllables, emphasis, and so forth are made in the wrong place. Another type of speech defect which may be caused by cerebellar lesions is *dysarthria*; in this instance the speech is slurred and explosive.

In addition to the five general manifestations of ataxia listed above that may be related to cerebellar dysfunction, several other defects can be related to lesions in this region of the central nervous system. Cerebellar damage can result in *hypotonia*, an effect which is manifest by the decreased muscle tone that is evident upon palpation. A *pendular knee jerk* reflex sometimes is observed in conjunction with, and as a consequence of the hypotonia. When this sign is present, the legs swings freely back and forth several times following stimulation of the patellar tendon.

The skeletal muscles which are affected by cerebellar lesions are weaker and undergo fatigue far more readily than do normal muscles, this condition being known as asthenia.

When involuntary movements (or tremors) are associated with cerebellar disease, the tremors usually become evident during purposeful (voluntary) movements, but are absent or decreased when the muscles are at rest. Such movements, called *intention tremors*, are generally caused by lesions which affect the efferent pathways that are located within the superior cerebellar peduncle. The gross movements associated with intention tremors are coarse and irregular (i.e., arrhythmic).

Lastly, cerebellar lesions frequently are accompanied by nystagmus, and such eye movements are induced by the stimulation of vestibular fibers located within the cerebellum by the lesion. Alternatively the nystagmus may be caused by mechanical compression of the vestibular nuclei of the brain stem which are located ventral to the cerebellum.

In conclusion, it is important to reiterate that the left cerebellar hemisphere controls the left side of the body, and the right cerebellar hemisphere controls the right side. Consequently any signs of cerebellar dysfunction on one side of the body reflect a cerebellar defect that is located on the ipsilateral (or homolateral) side of the cerebellum. This fact is in sharp contradistinction to the situation which is present with lesions of the cerebral hemispheres, and which always cause defects upon the contralateral side of the body.

Disorders of the Basal Ganglia

Two general type of defective movements are seen in humans suffering from diseases of the basal ganglia. *Hyperkinetic movements* are seen in athetosis, ballism, and chorea; in these conditions excessive as well as abnormal patterns of movement are present. *Hypokinetic* as well as hyperkinetic movements are seen in Parkinson's syndrome (or disease).

Athetosis, Ballismus, Chorea. There are many similar features among the three dyskinesias (abnormal movements) known clinically as athetosis, ballismus, and chorea. All of these conditions in common exhibit movements that appear to be voluntary, but which are not, and thus are completely beyond the control of the patient. The movements themselves are pronounced and can even become quite violent; however no characteristic tonus changes accompany the movements, as is the case in parkinsonism.

In *athetosis*, the limbs writhe continuously, slowly, and in a sinuous manner. These involuntary movements are particularly evident in the hands and may appear as though these extremities are grasping or performing avoidance reactions. Antagonistic muscles may undergo simultaneous contraction. Damage to the lenticular nucleus and the corpus striatum both have been implicated as sources of the defects which cause the abnormal movements of athetosis.

In *ballismus*, the involuntary movements are quite violent, the limbs being flung wildly about by contraction of the proximal muscles of the extremities. That is, the movements are rapid, hence ballistic. When the movements are restricted to only one side of the body, as frequently happens, the condition is called hemiballismus. Ballismus appears when the subthalamic nuclei are damaged as by a thrombus or hemorrhage. Thus hemiballismus may appear with exceeding rapidity following a hemorrhage in the contralateral subthalamic nucleus.

In *chorea* a considerable variety of rapid and jerky but well-coordinated movements occur continuously. As is the case with the other dyskinesias, the movements are involuntary and are useless insofar as being of some purpose to the patient is concerned.

Parkinson's Syndrome (Paralysis Agitans). This syndrome, originally described by James Parkinson about one and one half centuries ago, has a gradual and insidious onset, progresses slowly, and generally develops in persons in the fifth or sixth decade of life. A number of etiologic factors are known to produce Parkinson's disease, including cerebral arteriosclerosis, trauma to the head, neurosyphilis, cerebrovascular accidents, carbon monoxide or manganese poisoning, or following an attack of endemic encephalitis or influenza. Parkinsonism also can develop as a serious complication of therapy with phenothiazine tranquilizers (iatrogenic etiology), or in many instances the cause simply is unknown (idiopathic etiology).

The principal clinical findings of well-developed parkinsonism are the hypokinetic sign, akinesia (or poverty of movement), as well as the hyperkinetic features of *tremor* and *rigidity*. The absence of voluntary motor activity can be quite pronounced, as the patient experiences considerable difficulty in initiating such movements. There also is a marked decrease in normal *associated movements* that take place unconsciously, e.g., swinging the arms while walking, and the spectrum of facial expression related to the emotional aspects of thought, speech, and language, as well as the normal gestures and motor manifestations of mild mannerisms that are common to everyone.

The rigidity or hyperkinesia of parkinsonism is not spastic, and the myotatic reflexes are normal, although Jendrassick's maneuver (i.e., clenching the hands firmly together) to enhance a weak tendon jerk reflex does not alter such responses in Parkinson's disease.

Passive flexion of an extremity has been likened to bending a lead pipe as the rigid muscles are stiff although somewhat plastic. Occasionally a limb will "give" and then "catch" again in a series of jerks as it is being moved. Hence the terms *lead-pipe rigidity* and *cogwheel rigidity* sometimes are applied to the muscles of a patient having Parkinson's disease.

A clasp-knife effect can be seen when a spastic muscle suddenly loses resistance as it is stretched passively. In Parkinson's disease, however, no such response occurs during passive flexion of the rigid limbs.

The intermittent tremor of Parkinson's disease occurs through regular alternating contractions of antagonistic muscles at a frequency that ranges between two and six contractions per second. In sharp contrast to the intention tremor that is associated with cerebellar lesions, the tremor of Parkinson's disease is most pronounced while the patient is at rest and tends to disappear or be reduced as a movement takes place. Tremors often are of a type called "pill-rolling" and thus involve the thumb, index finger, or wrist. Occasionally a to-and-fro tremor of the head is present. Fatigue and emotional states tend to exacerbate the tremor. The facial expression on the other hand is characteristically fixed and masklike.

The rigidity of the skeletal muscles may be such that the patient has difficulty in arising from a chair, turning around while standing, or turning over in bed. Even normally simple actions such as washing and dressing become exceedingly difficult without assistance, and voluntary movements are carried out sluggishly and with great effort. Characteristically, the posture is stooped, and while walking a *festination gait* is seen. That is, the victim of paralysis agitans leans forward and takes shuffling steps that are quite short, commence slowly, and become rapid as they progress. Frequent rapid accelerations are seen so that the patient "appears to be chasing his center of gravity."

Parkinson's disease cannot be reproduced readily in experimental animals. In humans, however, this condition clearly is produced by diffuse brain damage. In particular, the basal ganglia are involved, although the specific neurophysiologic and neuroanatomic mechanisms that underlie the tremor, rigidity, and poverty of movement that are the principal features of this disease remain obscure. In humans, the parkinsonian syndrome sometimes can be alleviated surgically by additional destruction of the very nuclei whose mal-function underlies the abnormal condition in the first place, an interesting paradox! Thus extirpation of the motor cortex, section of the crura cerebri (cerebral peduncles), posterolateral spinal cordotomy, destruction of the medial globus pallidus, section of the ansa lenticularis, and lesions induced in the ventrolateral thalamic nuclei all have been claimed to diminish the rigidity and tremor of parkinsonism. If nothing else, these facts indicate that an exceedingly diverse and complex pattern of neural elements is involved in the etiology of Parkinson's disease.

During recent years, considerable interest has focused upon a biochemical mechanism for the etiology of Parkinson's disease as well as for the therapy of this disorder. In particular, parkinsonism has been related to an abnormal metabolism of certain amines in the basal ganglia, and perhaps the hypothalamus as well.

Under normal circumstances, the concentration of dopamine in certain parts of the brain is high whereas that of norepinephrine is low. Dopamine (dihydroxyphenylethylamine), is, of course, the normal precursor of norepinephrine, and this compound has been implicated as a neurotransmitter that is involved in motor functions. Under normal conditions the basal ganglia of humans, especially the caudate nucleus and putamen, contain high dopamine concentrations whereas the norepinephrine concentration in these structures is quite low. In Parkinson's disease the dopamine level of the caudate nucleus and putamen falls to about 50 per cent of the normal level. Concomitantly the hypothalamic norepinephrine level also falls somewhat, but not to such a great extent. In addition, several pharmacologic agents that induce undesirable side effects in patients that resemble certain features of Parkinson's syndrome are known to alter the normal metabolism of dopamine in the brain. All of these facts provide some evidence, albeit circumstantial, that the normal metabolism of certain amines in the basal ganglia is deranged in Parkinson's disease, and that the two states may be related causally.

In support of this contention, it has been found clinically that L-dopa (levo-dihydroxy-phenylethylamine), which is the immediate biochemical precursor of dopamine in vivo, is extremely useful in the treatment of Parkinson's disease when administered in a sufficiently large dose. L-dopa, unlike dopamine per se, is able to cross the blood-brain barrier in quantities sufficient to produce a demonstrable increase in brain dopamine concentration.

Epilepsy

Epilepsy is a transient state, a syndrome, and not a particular disease entity. The epileptic state is characterized by abrupt and transitory changes in the normal functions of the brain so that somatic sensory, somatic motor, autonomic, and/or psychic symptoms which may (or may not) be accompanied by alterations in consciousness are manifest. Concomitant changes in the brain waves accompany epileptic attacks, hence profound alterations in the EEG can be recorded during such periods.

From an etiologic standpoint, epilepsy frequently is caused by abnormally functioning brain tissue that results from trauma, infections, or unknown agents (i.e., idiopathic epilepsy). The latter tends to occur in families, hence congenital or genetic factors may be suspected in such instances. The most common factors related to the development of epilepsy in children are birth trauma which may be related to anoxia, head injuries, cerebrovascular accidents, infections of the brain with attendant inflammatory processes, and congenital malformations of the brain.

It should be mentioned that seizures which are identical with those seen during episodes of idiopathic epilepsy may take place in patients suffering from organic brain disease (e.g., intracranial infection, cerebral vascular accidents, tumors). Similar epileptiform attacks also may be precipitated by metabolic defects, such as during hypoglycemia, uremia, and hypocalcemia.

Epileptic seizures may be precipitated in some persons who are susceptible to such attacks by physical events such as auditory, tactile, and visual stimuli, whereas in other patients the seizures occur typically during sleep. Additional factors may participate indirectly in the genesis of epileptic seizures, including a lack of food and sleep, emotional tension, or the ingestion of alcoholic beverages.

The pattern of epileptic seizures in any given patient tends to be stereotyped, although there is a wide disparity in the patterns of attack that are seem among different patients. For example, epileptic seizures may take place in groups over a period of hours or of days. If the seizure arises in the motor cortex, the patient tends to exhibit a temporary paresis known as *Todd's paralysis* following the attack.

Pathophysiology. Considerable research has been conducted on possible biochemical and physiologic mechanisms that could be invoked to explain the pathophysiology of epilepsy, but the fundamental causes that underlie seizures remain obscure. It is clear, however, that seizures are more likely to appear when organic brain damage is present than in persons with a normal central nervous system. Furthermore, histologic examination of the brains from patients who had idiopathic epilepsy usually fails to reveal any specific alterations in the tissue that can be correlated with the functional defect.

Possibly a seizure could be initiated by hyperexcitability of the neurons in one (or more) reverberatory (or oscillatory) circuits, such as might be found in the reticular activating system, any specific lesion being a sufficient stimulus to induce such hyperexcitability. Alternatively, specific neural pathways could become facilitated, hence hyperexcitable, so that synchronous discharges from reverberatory circuits could produce firing in these specific pathways that would lead to the particular signs and symptoms observed.

Presumably, an epileptic seizure could be terminated physiologically by active fatigue of the synapses involved in the circuits responsible for the seizure in the first place, although the sustained attacks seen in status epilepticus might seem to cast some doubt upon this idea. Alternatively, active inhibition through negative feedback circuits might play some role in breaking the cycle of events initially leading to the seizure.

Our current state of ignorance in this area is clearly defined by the vague and speculative nature of the foregoing remarks concerning the initiation and termination of an epileptic attack. The possible role of the corpus callosum in the etiology of epilepsy was presented earlier.

As noted earlier, the overall metabolic activity of the brain varies to a certain extent depending upon its state of functional activity. When there is a generalized acceleration of neuromuscular activity, such as occurs during convulsive states, it is not surprising that the net metabolic activity of this organ increases. Nevertheless, there is no significant alteration of the metabolic activity in specific regions of the brain that can be correlated with particular functional states.

The level of acetylcholine as well as the activity of cholinesterase have been shown to be approximately proportional to the size and density of the neurons in all regions and cortical layers of the normal brain. On the other hand, cortical foci which discharge abnormal signals resulting in epileptiform seizures in experimental animals have been shown to have an increased cholinesterase activity as well as alterations in the bound acetylcholine level during induced epileptic seizures. Such findings have been considered to be evidence that a deranged acetylcholine metabolism underlies the brain abnormalities present in epileptics.

There also is considerable experimental evidence which suggests that mechanisms other than an abnormal acetylcholine metabolism may be involved in the production of epileptic seizures. Thus an abnormal distribution of potassium has been found in the brains of experimentally convulsed animals and the onset of experimental seizures may be heralded by an increased rate of nitrogen metabolism as indicated by an elevated level of ammonia synthesis.

From an experimental and clinical standpoint, metabolic poisons, vitamin deficiencies (e.g., of pyridoxine), defects in the metabolism of certain amino acids (particularly glutamic acid), metals (e.g., aluminum), infectious agents, and even particular dietary components all have been shown capable of producing epileptiform seizures. Despite this broad spectrum of biologic models, however, the underlying mechanism(s) responsible for causing epilepsy remains unknown.

Clinical Patterns in Epileptic States. A number of systems are used in the classification of epileptic states, and these are based primarily upon etiologic factors (when known), clinical symptoms, and anatomic localization of the underlying lesion, as well as the age of the patient when the symptoms became manifest.

Several types of seizure will be discussed below in accordance with the clinical findings present in each.

Petit Mal Seizures. Epileptic seizures may occur in which the patient exhibits a transient, even momentary, loss of consciousness so brief that neither the patient nor his intimates are aware that an attack has occurred, and convulsive movements or falling of the body do not occur. Thus, the so-called triad to petit mal seizures includes myoclonic jerks, akinetic seizures, and a very transient loss of consciousness, termed "brief absences."

The *myoclonic jerks* can be manifested in either limbs or muscles and such rapid, involuntary contractions can be seen in either whole muscles, portions of muscles, or in whole groups of muscles that are either widespread or restricted to one region of the body. Such myoclonic contractions can be synchronous or asynchronous, and may occur without a loss of, or any evident change in, consciousness. Myoclonic jerks are more frequent in the morning and while falling asleep, and even normal persons may exhibit such sudden contractions while drowsy or during periods of light sleep.

An *akinetic attack*, or seizure, is characterized by an abrupt loss of postural tone such that the patient slumps over before he is able to catch himself. Alternatively, the victim may slump so that the knees or body just touch the ground before recovery is achieved.

During petit mal attacks, the EEG typically shows "doublets" that appear with a frequency of about three per second. That is, each wave consists of a spike coupled to a rounded wave.

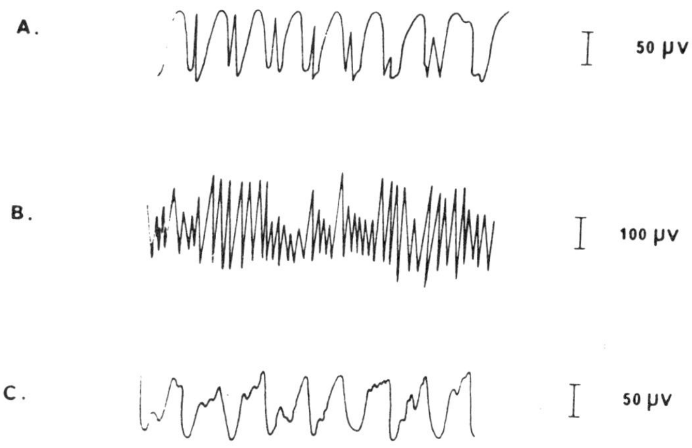

Fig. 10.2. Tracings of EEGs recorded during: A. petit mal; B. grand mal; and C. psychomotor seizures.

Grand Mal Seizures. An attack of grand mal epilepsy often is signalled by an *aura* which warns the patient that a seizure is imminent. Generally the aura is specific for each particular patient and it may consist of a somatic or visceral sensation.

Following the aura, loss of consciousness takes place and the patient drops to the ground or floor. In falling, vocalization as well as physical injury can occur. Convulsions generally ensue, the patient lying rigid for a minute or so. During this phase, the somatic muscles are in a state of sustained tonic contraction. This *tonic phase* subsequently gives way to a *clonic stage,* during which massive, rhythmic, synchronous contractions of the skeletal muscles take place throughout the body. During these convulsions, normal control over certain viscera such as the bladder and bowels often is lost so that urination and defecation occur. Rarely, fractures of the bones attend the violent convulsions; however, self-inflicted tongue injuries are common as the patient's jaw musculature contracts spasmodically.

Following the convulsive phase, a period of stuporous sleep ensues which may last for a variable interval, but generally ranges between one and four hours' duration. The patient has no clear memory for events during this postconvulsive interval, even if he is awake, and upon full recovery from the seizure the somatic musculature may be exceedingly painful.

During grand mal seizures, the EEG exhibits a fast activity pattern during the tonic phase, but at the time each clonic jerk takes place slow waves are seen, and during the recovery phases the slow waves may persist.

Interestingly, hemodialysis of the blood as part of the therapy for chronic renal failure has been demonstrated to precipitate grand mal epileptic seizures. Furthermore it has been shown that the conduction velocity of peripheral nerves in such patients is reduced. The precise mechanism whereby grand mal seizures are precipitated by dialysis is unclear, although it would seem that such episodes are related to the rapid alterations in blood biochemistry induced by dialysis and that if the dialysis procedure is prolonged the incidence of such abnormalities is reduced, as the changes in blood pH and urea concentration are induced more gradually.

Jacksonian Epilepsy. Epileptic seizures that are caused by a focal irritation of a specific region of the primary motor area of the cerebral cortex may be restricted to a specific peripheral region on the contralateral side of the body. The patient may remain conscious during the attack. The seizure also may ramify over the rest of the adjacent motor cortex rather than remaining localized in one specific focal area so that adjacent peripheral regions ultimately may become involved in the convulsive motor responses.

Jacksonian epileptic seizures generally are associated with relatively specific organic brain damage such as is associated with scar tissue following traumatic injury or following a hemorrhage. Alternatively, an epileptic focus can develop as the result of a localized neoplastic growth.

Status Epilepticus. This exceedingly dangerous situation develops when a number of major (grand mal) seizures follow each other in rapid succession so that the interval between any two seizures is relatively brief, or completely absent. The patient becomes exhausted, hyperthermia may develop, and death frequently intervenes during such attacks.

Psychomotor Seizures. Included under this heading are essentially all types of epileptic seizure that do not comply with the classic definitions of petit mal, grand mal, and focal jacksonian seizures.

Patterned, stereotyped movements, seemingly purposeful movements, incoherent speech, emotional lability, rotation of the head and eyes, lip smacking, writhing and twisting movements of the limbs, dimming of consciousness, and amnesia are common accompaniments of psychomotor seizures. EEG changes frequently associated with this form of epilepsy include slow round waves, spikes, sharp waves and/or combinations of these patterns, usually recorded from foci on the temporal lobes, and these abnormalities may become much more evident during periods of light sleep in patients who are subject to this type of seizure.

Febrile Convulsions. In very young children, fever and convulsions frequently are related. Furthermore, the first seizure manifested by an epileptic child usually is a febrile convulsion. In fact, it has been claimed that febrile convulsions are much more frequent among children whose parents have a history of epilepsy.

The relationship between fever and convulsions has been attributed to a number of possible causes. First, the fever and the convulsions both are caused by an infectious microorganism and/or its toxic metabolic byproducts. Second, the immature brain may react to high fever and/or an infectious agent by discharging random impulses that result in a convulsion. Third, excessive fluid intake (i.e., hydration) as well as any drugs employed to combat an infection may precipitate convulsions. Fourth, the fever per se develops secondarily from the liberation of excess heat energy from the muscles as they convulse. Fifth, during convulsive seizures, the hypothalamic thermoregulatory centers become "reset" at a higher level so that fever develops. Sixth, an abnormal reaction may be induced in the brain by an infection such that a local (or generalized) irritable focus develops and convulsions ensue.

Frequently children develop psychomotor seizures following one or more episodes of febrile convulsions, although the prognosis varies considerably. Nonfebrile convulsions develop subsequent to febrile convulsions in most of the patients having a history of the latter.

Coma and General Anesthesia: Dysfunctions of the Reticular Activating System

The reticular activating system (RAS) occupies a particularly exposed neuroanatomic site at the rostral end of the midbrain and in the posterior hypothalamus because it is displaced medially by other fiber systems. Consequently small lesions, such as may be induced by a tumor, hemorrhage, or other cause will produce a coma that may last for an extended period of time. Experimentally it has been shown that the trauma induced by a concussion will inhibit normal bioelectric activity in the RAS.

One major effect produced by general anesthetics such as ether, halothane, nitrous oxide, or barbituric acid derivatives is to produce a loss of consciousness. It has been demonstrated clearly that such chemical agents depress conduction in the ascending RAS as well as in the midbrain reticular formation. The excitatory influence of impulses ascending to the cortex from the RAS is inhibited markedly and consciousness is lost.

The physiologic effects of anesthetics on the RAS may reflect merely a general inhibition of synaptic conduction in all areas of the central nervous system rather than a selective (or specific) effect on the synapses of the RAS. In any event, the specific sensory pathways contain only two to four synapses, whereas the reticular pathways can involve hundreds of synapse. And at every synapse, the excitatory postsynaptic potential (EPSP) must reach a certain magnitude before that cell will fire. Since the neural pathways through the RAS contain so many synapses, on this basis alone they are far more vulnerable to inhibition by any agent, chemical or otherwise, which exerts a depressant effect on synaptic conduction.

Narcolepsy and Catalepsy

The clinical syndrome characterized by the intermittent occurrence of periods of uncontrollable and usually inappropriate sleep is termed *narcolepsy*. The hypothalamus has been implicated in some cases of this disorder.

To summarize briefly, hypothalamic lesions such as may result from influenza, encephalitis, or neoplasm can result in abnormalities of fat, carbohydrate, or water metabolism; emotional manifestations, e.g., bouts of crying or laughing; sympathetic or parasympathetic effects; derangement of normal sexual functions; and disorders of the normal sleep pattern.

Although narcolepsy can be attributed to hypothalamic lesions in many instances, frequently there is no overt damage to this region of the brain, hence the term *idiopathic narcolepsy* is applied in such cases. Nevertheless, a person suffering from attacks of idiopathic narcolepsy may exhibit such hypothalamus-related signs as obesity, polyuria, or abnormal sexual functions, which suggest a physiologic if not an evident pathologic impairment of the normal functions of the hypothalamus. The role of the RAS in the etiology of narcolepsy in obscure, but this matter would bear close experimental scrutiny as it is extremely doubtful that the narcoleptic state would develop independently of the system which normally is related so inseparably to the conscious and unconscious states.

Clinically, the duration of individual narcoleptic attacks can range from a few seconds to several hours, and a number of such episodes can occur with or without warning at generally inappropriate times throughout the day, such as while in conversation, attending a lecture, or driving an automobile. The attacks resemble normal sleep, and the diurnal nocturnal sleep pattern of a narcoleptic patient exhibits no marked peculiarities.

During a narcoleptic attack, the patient may exhibit a sudden loss of muscle tone, hence weakness, so that he sinks to the ground, particularly when the narcoleptic attack is triggered by a sudden emotional stimulus such as mirth, anger, fear, or surprise. This transient hypotonia, known as catalepsy, frequently is associated with narcolepsy; and although narcolepsy may be present without catalepsy, the reverse situation is exceedingly rare.

The simultaneous occurrence of narcolepsy and catalepsy suggests that similar pathophysiologic mechanisms may be operative in the two states. However, the hypotonus observed during a cataleptic seizure is not explicable on the basis of any presently known physiologic mechanism.

The interesting suggestion has been advanced that narcoleptic and cataleptic attacks are relics of primitive behavioral defense mechanisms which are unmasked in humans by disease. Thus certain lower organisms, such as the opossum, may enter a state similar to narcolepsy when seriously endangered.

Retrograde Amnesia

The human brain has an amazing capacity to recover functionally from irreversible damage to its structure, and it is a frequent clinical observation that a major physical or other derangement which appears immediately after traumatic or vascular injuries to the central nervous system may subsequently and spontaneously improve to such an extent that the original defects may disappear completely. Nonetheless, and despite the functional improvement, the structural damage remains. Consequently the mechanism which underlies this effect is of major importance to a better understanding of the learning and memory phenomena.

In this regard it is of interest that both experimentally as well as clinically it can be demonstrated readily that a loss of recent memory frequently occurs following a brain conclusion or electroshock therapy. That is, *retrograde amnesia* develops for those events which immediately preceded the physiologic insult. In humans, the period for which recollection is totally lost may extend backward in time for days, weeks, months, or even years, although long-term memory is completely unaffected, a fact which testifies eloquently for the stability of such memory engrams.

In experimental animals, memory for learned responses, as evidenced by behavioral studies, is lost if the subject is anesthetized or subjected to an electric shock within a few minutes after a training session. On the other hand if the physiologic insult is postponed for several hours, no such memory loss occurs. Studies such as these suggest, but do not prove conclusively, that the consolidation of recently acquired information so that stable memory engrams develop sometimes may require a fairly long interval. In humans the period for which retrograde amnesia is present may (or may not!) reflect the time required for the entire consolidation process to become complete; however this remark is largely conjectural.

Aphasia, Apraxia, and Agnosia

When the memory for learned response is lost because of damage to the cerebral cortex, this derangement of the intellectual functions, which are localized approximately in the neocortex per se, can take any of three forms; viz., aphasia, apraxia, or agnosia.

Aphasia. The term "aphasia" denotes a defect or loss of the power to express oneself in speech, writing, or gestures (i.e., by the use of symbols) or of the loss of the ability to comprehend spoken or written language due to lesions in the brain centers which are responsible for these functions. An aphasia thus is a disturbance of the sensory and/or motor areas of the brain that is caused by brain damage, regardless of the specific pathogenesis. Aphasias are not caused by defects in the sense organs themselves (i.e., in vision or audition), in the muscles which are essential to speech, or mental defects.

A number of classifications have been devised in an attempt to correlate specific brain lesions with particular functional abnormalities. As one consequence of these efforts, the terminology relating to these defects in the ability to understand and to use language is utterly confusing!

In most general terms, aphasias can be divided into two broad categories: *sensory (receptive) aphasias* and *motor (expressive) aphasias*. Each of these principal categories in turn can be subdivided further. *Word deafness* is an inability to comprehend words that are spoken. *Word blindness* is an inability to comprehend written words. *Agraphia* is the inability to express ideas by writing them down. The inability to express ideas in speech commonly is termed *motor aphasia*. The category of motor aphasia can be subdivided into *fluent aphasia*, in which normal speech occurs, and this speech even may be quite rapid although key words are missing, and *nonfluent aphasia*, in which speech is slow, labored, and the victim has difficulty in selecting any words to express himself. In fact, nonfluent aphasia in its extreme form may result in a vocabulary that contains only a few words in toto. Frequently patients with nonfluent aphasia speak only a few *automatic words*, e.g., name the months of the year, or the words being used at the time the lesion developed. A patient with nonfluent aphasia for reasons unknown may utter only obscenities in an automatic and repetitive fashion.

As discussed earlier, the cerebral hemispheres exhibit a complementary functional dominance, so that in any particular individual only one of these structures is concerned primarily with speech, the *categorical hemisphere*.

Apraxia. The term "apraxia" signifies the inability to perform a highly skilled or complex movement when requested to do so. Apraxia is not caused by muscular paralysis (or paresis), ataxia, alterations in the sensory receptors, or by a defective comprehension of the problem (i.e., confusion). Thus in the classic description of apraxia, the patient was unable to stick out his tongue when so requested, although he was able to perform normally complex semiautomatic movements of this structure such as were involved in chewing and swallowing (*motor apraxia*).

Ideational apraxia signifies that the patient is unable to formulate or to remember the concept necessary to the performance of a particular motor act. *Ideomotor apraxia* denotes a situation in which the patient is unable to carry out a specific act correctly even though older and stereotyped motor acts may be performed spontaneously as well as repetitiously.

The apraxias usually are accompanied by specific lesions of the brain. Thus ideational apraxia often is a manifestation of certain diffuse brain lesions such as cerebral arteriosclerosis, whereas motor apraxia usually is related to a lesion that is located in the precentral gyrus. Ideomotor apraxia, on the other hand, usually is related to lesions that are located within the supramarginal gyrus of the categorical hemisphere.

Agnosia. The term "agnosia" denotes an inability to recognize common objects. That is, the patient is unable to interpret sensory stimuli correctly.

Five general types of agnosia sometimes are recognized. First, in *astereognosis* (or *tactual agnosia*) objects cannot be recognized by handling them. Second, in *auditory agnosia* (or *psychic deafness*) the patient is unable to recognize objects from aural cue. This type of agnosia is similar in some respects to the aphasia called word blindness. Third, in *visual agnosia* (or *psychic blindness*), the patient neither can perceive the meaning of objects or colors that are seen, nor can he appreciate the significance of visual space. Fourth, in *autotopagnosia* (also called *body-image agnosia* or *finger agnosia*) there is a failure to recognize the different parts of the body and their relationships, to discriminate between left and right, or to perceive the relationship between the body and objects in the immediate environment. Fifth, in *anosognosia*, the patient is unaware of disease or may deny the existence of disease per se.

Like the apraxias, the agnosias generally are associated with lesions in particular areas of the brain. For example, anosognosia may be present when a lesion is evident in the supramarginal gyrus of the parietal lobe, whereas autotopagnosia may be associated with lesions that are located in the posterioinferior region of the same lobe.

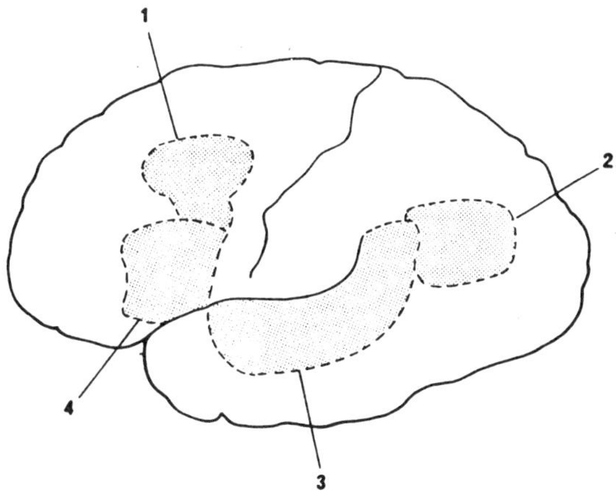

Fig. 10.3. Lateral aspect of the left cerebral hemisphere illustrating one concept of the regions of the brain responsible for language functions (shaded areas). 1. Damage affects ability to write. 2. Damage causes word blindness. 3. Damage causes word deafness. 4. Damage produces a loss of articulate speech. According to this concept, therefore, particular aphasias are related to lesions in specific areas of the brain.

Meniere's Syndrome (Paroxysmal Labyrinthine Vertigo)

Meniere's syndrome typically is manifest by intermittent bouts of severe vertigo, or dizziness, that are coupled with deafness and tinnitus. That is, an auditory nerve stimulation is present such that the patient hears "sounds" such as ringing, buzzing, or roaring, or clicking.

This syndrome frequently develops in men between the fourth and sixth decades of life for unknown reasons, although an abnormal accumulation of serous fluid in the cochlear duct is suspected. In turn this so-called endolymphatic hydrops, when maximal, could exert a mechanical pressure upon the vestibulocochlear nerve such that this structure would be excited abnormally, and this would result in the attacks of severe vertigo which is the principal symptom of this disease. A similar explanation could be offered for the tinnitus.

The vertigo may be so severe that the patient falls violently to the ground as though thrown down, and consciousness may be lost briefly during such an attack. Surrounding objects may appear to spin around the victim, and autonomic responses such as nausea, vomiting, and heavy sweating are frequent accompaniments. Any given attack may persist for a few minutes or last for up to several hours, and the frequency with which the attacks occur can vary considerably in any individual. Headache, deafness caused by defective neural conduction, and tinnitus tend to occur as well as to persist between the attacks of vertigo.

The hearing loss tends to be progressive and in the overwhelming majority of cases this loss tends to be found in one ear. Nystagmus may be seen during attacks of vertigo, and the Barany or caloric tests may reveal an abnormal labyrinthine function. The patient exhibits a hypersensitivity to loud sounds.

Meniere's syndrome can follow head injuries or infections of the middle ear; however in many instances this condition appears in the absence of any demonstrable damage to either the ear or nervous system.

Intractable Pain and Percutaneous Cervical Cordotomy

Intractable pain and percutaneous cordotomy have been selected for discussion as the concluding topics in this chapter as they not only exemplify the exceedingly complex nature of a seemingly straightforward neural phenomenon (viz, the sensation of pain) but also illustrate the pragmatic value of a knowledge of neuroanatomy and neurophysiology to the management of an exceedingly difficult clinical problem.

Neuroanatomic and Neurophysiologic Considerations. As noted earlier, pain in any form may be considered to represent the operation of an abnormal process, a biologic warning system. Viewed from a strictly physiologic standpoint, the mechanism underlying the sensation of pain consists merely of nerve impulses transmitted from the periphery, particularly in the so-called pain pathways of the nervous system. The dorsal (or anterolateral) spinothalamic system is especially significant in relaying such impulses from specific peripheral regions of the body to the thalamus and thence to the cortex where the signals are perceived as painful sensations. This view is, of course, entirely too simplistic, because pain is an exceedingly complex sensation, as the interpretation of the painful stimulus by the mind is considerably different than the mere biologic reception and transmission of information pertaining to the stimulus which is coded as nerve impulses having a certain frequency.

Although a number of hypotheses have been advanced to explain the phenomenon of pain, *the gate control theory* affords a useful and reasonable explanation of this sensation. To recapitulate briefly, this theory includes the interdependent operation of three neural systems located within the spinal cord and that are activated by signals which are transmitted centrally following stimulation of pain receptors that are located in the periphery. The three cord systems are composed of, first, neurons of the substantia gelatinosa, located in the dorsal horn of the spinal cord; second, the fibers of the dorsal column which relay signals toward the brain; and third, the first-order transmission neurons located in the dorsal column, and which convey pain signals in the dorsal horn. The substantia gelatinosa per se provides the neural matrix for the gate control system which in turn modulates the afferent impulse patterns before they excite or facilitate the transmission neurons. The afferent impulse patterns in the dorsal column in turn function as a regulatory mechanisms which can initiate selective processes in the brain that can alter the modulating characteristics of the gate control system proper. And lastly, the transmission cells are able to initiate neural mechanisms which make up the functional system that underlies the perception and response to pain. Thus pain phenomena, according to the gate control theory, are caused by the functional interplay among these three systems.

Impulses that underlie painful sensations are transmitted to the brain, once they have traversed the gate in the cord, via synapses that are located in the dorsal column. Thence neurons decussate in the ventral commissure of the cord to pass rostrally in the ascending anterolateral tracts of the cord. Most of these ascending fibers are located within the spinothalamic tract, although five discrete pathways have been implicated in the projection of pain sensations to the cerebral cortex via the thalamic projection nuclei. Thus two pathways involved in the transmission of painful sensations project to the somatosensory thalamic nuclei, thence to the related cortical regions via the dorsal column-lemniscal and dorsolateral tracts. The dorsal spinothalamic tract per se actually has been shown to contain the other three functional tracts that convey impulses related to pain. One of these tracts contains few synapses and is composed of fibers which are highly oriented in space so that this tract conveys signals related to the perception of rapidly perceived, highly localized pain. The remaining two spinothalamic subdivisions contain a greater number of synapses that does the fast-acting, tract, and these fibers terminate in the nonspecific intralaminar nuclei of the thalamus. Consequently this system transmits the signals related to slowly conducted diffuse pain. This portion of the thalamic system typically exhibits much convergence, has connections with nuclei that receive visual as well as auditory stimuli, and thus it underlies the transmission of signals that are more concerned with the perception of pain (i.e., the affective component of pain) rather than with the physiologic mechanisms that are involved in the central reception of pain signals. Consequently impulses that are related to pain inputs are not simply localized to specific neuroanatomic pathways the neurophysiologic circuits. Rather, the inputs are able to spread to neural systems that are involved with highly subjective aspects of the perception of pain in addition to the mere sensory perception of painful stimuli. Furthermore, the functional activity of the input pathways that sub-serve the phenomena related to the perception of pain can be altered by a number of descending polysynaptic influences which can operate in a reciprocal fashion, and which have their origin in the somatosensory and related cortical areas as well as in the reticular formation.